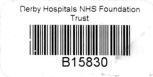
BLUEPRINTS
MEDICINE

Fifth Edition

BLUEPRINTS
MEDICINE

Fifth Edition

Vincent B. Young, MD, PhD
Assistant Professor
Departments of Internal Medicine, Microbiology, and Immunology
University of Michigan Medical School
Ann Arbor, Michigan

William A. Kormos, MD, MPH
Instructor in Medicine
Harvard Medical School
Massachusetts General Hospital
Boston, Massachusetts

Davoren A. Chick, MD, FACP
Assistant Professor
Department of Internal Medicine
University of Michigan Medical School
Ann Arbor, Michigan
Senior Faculty Advisor

Allan H. Goroll, MD
Professor of Medicine
Harvard Medical School
Physician, Medical Service
Massachusetts General Hospital
Boston, Massachusetts

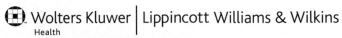
Wolters Kluwer | Lippincott Williams & Wilkins
Health

Philadelphia • Baltimore • New York • London
Buenos Aires • Hong Kong • Sydney • Tokyo

Acquisitions Editor: Charley Mitchell
Sr. Managing Editor: Stacey Sebring
Marketing Manager: Jennifer Kuklinski
Managing Editor, Production: Eve Malakoff-Klein
Art Director: Doug Smock
Composition: Maryland Composition/ASI

Fifth Edition
Copyright © 2010, 2007 Lippincott Williams & Wilkins, a Wolters Kluwer business.

351 West Camden Street   530 Walnut Street
Baltimore, MD 21201   Philadelphia, PA 19106

Printed in China

9 8 7 6 5 4 3 2 1

Library of Congress Cataloging-in-Publication Data

Young, Vincent B.
    Blueprints medicine / Vincent B. Young, William A. Kormos, Davoren A. Chick ; senior faculty advisor, Allan H. Goroll. — 5th ed.
        p. ; cm. — (Blueprints)
    Includes bibliographical references and index.
    ISBN 978-0-7817-8870-0 (alk. paper)
  1. Internal medicine—Outlines, syllabi, etc. I. Kormos, William A. II. Chick, Davoren A. III. Title. IV. Title: Medicine. V. Series.
    [DNLM: 1. Internal Medicine—Examination Questions. WB 18.2 Y78b 2010]
    RC59.Y68 2007
    616.0076--dc22

                                                        2008033567

DISCLAIMER

To purchase additional copies of this book, call our customer service department at **(800) 638-3030** or fax orders to **(301) 223-2320**. International customers should call **(301) 223-2300**.

Visit Lippincott Williams & Wilkins on the Internet: http://www.lww.com. Lippincott Williams & Wilkins customer service representatives are available from 8:30 am to 6:00 pm, EST.

Contents

Contributors

New questions and answers provided by

James T. Kwiatt, MD
Chief Resident
Department of Medicine
Medical College of Wisconsin
Milwaukee, Wisconsin

Preface

In 1997, the first five books in the *Blueprints* series were published as a board review for medical students, interns, and residents who wanted high-yield, accurate clinical content for USMLE Steps 2 & 3. Twelve years later, we are proud to report that the original books and the entire *Blueprints* brand of review materials have far exceeded our expectations.

The feedback we receive from our readers continues to be tremendously helpful and pivotal in deciding what direction each edition of the core books will take. To that end, this fifth edition includes updated material to reflect the latest developments in evidence-based medicine. This edition also includes a revised Table of Contents with separate chapters on Leukemia and Lymphoma, as well as an entirely new Neurology section. An additional 25 USMLE-style questions and answers have been added, with access to 50 more new Q&As online. We hope that this edition will continue to serve as a useful review for the USMLE, as well as a rapid reference during day-to-day activities in patient care.

What we've also learned from our readers is that *Blueprints* is more than just a board review for USMLE Steps 2 & 3. Students use the books during their clerkship rotations and subinternships. Residents studying for USMLE Step 3 often use the books for reviewing areas that were not their specialty. Students in physician assistant, nurse practitioner, and osteopath programs use *Blueprints* either as a companion or in lieu of review materials written specifically for their areas.

However you use *Blueprints*, we hope that you find the books in the series informative and useful.

Acknowledgments

We are grateful for the continued support we have received for *Blueprints Medicine*. We wish to thank all of the people at Lippincott Williams & Wilkins who helped us with preparation of this work. Finally, we wish to thank our families for all of their ongoing encouragement during this project.

Vincent B. Young, MD, PhD
William H. Kormos, MD, MPH
Davoren A. Chick, MD, FACP

Abbreviations

5-ASA	5-aminosalicylic acid	DVT	deep venous thrombosis
ABGs	arterial blood gases	EBV	Epstein-Barr virus
ACE	angiotensin-converting enzyme	ECG	electrocardiogram
ACTH	adrenocorticotropic hormone	EF	ejection fraction
ADH	antidiuretic hormone	EGD	esophagogastroduodenoscopy
AI	aortic insufficiency	EMG	electromyography
AIDS	acquired immunodeficiency syndrome	ERCP	endoscopic retrograde cholangiopancreatography
ALL	acute lymphocytic leukemia	ESR	erythrocyte sedimentation rate
ALT	alanine transaminase	FEV	forced expiratory volume
AML	acute myelogenous leukemia	FNA	fine-needle aspiration
ANA	antinuclear antibody	FTA-ABS	fluorescent treponemal antibody absorption
ARDS	adult respiratory distress syndrome		
ASD	artrial septal defect	FVC	forced vital capacity
ASO	antistreptolysin O	GFR	glomerular filtration rate
AST	aspartate transaminase	GH	growth hormone
AV	atrioventricular	GI	gastrointestinal
BE	barium enema	GU	genitourinary
BP	blood pressure	HAV	hepatitis A virus
BUN	blood urea nitrogen	HbA1C	glycosylated hemoglobin
CALLA	common acute lymphoblastic leukemia antigen	HCM	hypertrophic cardiomyopathy
		HIV	human immunodeficiency virus
CBC	complete blood count	HLA	human leukocyte antigen
CHD	coronary heart disease	HR	heart rate
CHF	congestive heart failure	IFG	impaired fasting glucose
CK	creatine kinase	Ig	immunoglobulin
CLL	chronic lymphocytic leukemia	IM	intramuscular
CML	chronic myelogenous leukemia	INH	isoniazid
CMV	cytomegalovirus	INR	international normalized ratio
CNS	central nervous system	IV	intravenous
COPD	chronic obstructive pulmonary disease	JVP	jugular venous pressure
		KUB	kidneys/ureter/bladder
CPK	creatine phosphokinase	LDH	lactate dehydrogenase
CSF	cerebrospinal fluid	LES	lower esophageal sphincter
CT	computed tomography	LFTs	liver function tests
CVA	cerebrovascular accident	LP	lumbar puncture
DHEA	dehydroepiandrosterone	LV	left ventricular
DIC	disseminated intravascular coagulation	LVH	left ventricular hypertrophy
		Lytes	electrolytes
DKA	diabetic ketoacidosis	MCHC	mean corpuscular hemoglobin concentration
DM	diabetes mellitus		
DTRs	deep tendon reflexes	MCV	mean corpuscular volume

MEN	multiple endocrine neoplasia	SGOT	serum glutamic-oxaloacetic transaminase
MHC	major histocompatibility complex		
MI	myocardial infarction	SIADH	syndrome of inappropriate secretion of ADH
MRI	magnetic resonance imaging		
NHL	non-Hodgkin lymphoma	SLE	systemic lupus erythematosus
NPO	nil per os (nothing by mouth)	s/p	status post
NSAID	nonsteroidal anti-inflammatory drug	STD	sexually transmitted disease
		STEMI	ST-elevation myocardial infarction
NSTEMI	non–ST-elevation myocardial infarction	SVT	supraventricular tachycardia
		TFTs	thyroid function tests
PA	posteroanterior	TIA	transient ischemic attack
PBS	peripheral blood smear	TIBC	total iron-binding capacity
PCI	percutaneous intervention	TIPS	transjugular intrahepatic portosystemic shunt
PCP	*Pneumocystis jiroveci* pneumonia		
		TMP-SMZ	trimethoprim-sulfamethoxazole
PE	physical exam	tPA	tissue plasminogen activator
PFTs	pulmonary function tests	TPO	thyroid peroxidase
PMI	point of maximal intensity	TSH	thyroid-stimulating hormone
PMN	polymorphonuclear leukocyte	TTP	thrombotic thrombocytopenic purpura
PT	prothrombin time		
PTH	parathyroid hormone	UA	urinalysis
PTT	partial thromboplastin time	UGI	upper GI
PUD	peptic ulcer disease	URI	upper respiratory infection
RBC	red blood cell	US	ultrasound
RPR	rapid plasma reagent (test)	VDRL	Venereal Disease Research Laboratory
RR	respiratory rate		
RS	Reed-Sternberg (cell)	VS	vital signs
RV	right ventricular	VT	ventricular tachycardia
RVH	right ventricular hypertrophy	WBC	white blood cell
SBFT	small bowel follow-through	WPW	Wolff-Parkinson-White (syndrome)

BLUEPRINTS
MEDICINE

Fifth Edition

Part 1

Cardiovascular

Chest Pain

In diagnosing the patient with chest pain, it often helps to categorize the pain by its pathophysiology. Inflammation of serous surfaces leads to **pleuritic pain**, characterized by increased pain with inspiration or cough. This pain may also be aggravated by movement or position. Pleuritic pain can be seen in pulmonary etiologies, pericarditis, and musculoskeletal disorders. **Visceral pain**, such as in myocardial ischemia and esophageal disease, often produces dull, aching, tight, or sometimes burning pain that is poorly localized.

The most important decision for the physician is to distinguish life-threatening causes, such as myocardial ischemia, pulmonary embolus, and aortic dissection, from non–life-threatening causes. The key to identifying the etiology of the pain often lies in the patient's history.

RISK FACTORS

In evaluating patients with chest pain, certain risk factors may increase the suspicion for coronary heart disease (CHD) and include the following:

- Diabetes mellitus
- Smoking
- Hypertension
- Dyslipidemia
- Family history of CHD

Abdominal (central) obesity is associated with increased CHD risk and contributes to multiple other CHD risk factors. Patients with chest pain and many cardiovascular risk factors require further workup for CHD, even if the story is atypical. CHD is uncommon (but not unheard of) before 40 years of age, and men are at greater risk than women until approximately 65 years of age. Cocaine abuse is an important consideration, especially in patients with no other cardiac risk factors.

CLINICAL MANIFESTATIONS

HISTORY

The following diseases often present with the sharp pleuritic type of pain. **Pneumothorax** has an acute onset and is pleuritic and associated with dyspnea. This occurs mostly in young patients (spontaneous) or those with underlying lung disease (secondary to blebs). **Pulmonary embolism** has symptoms similar to pneumothorax with pleurisy and dyspnea. Risk factors should be taken into account (see Chapter 16). The pain in **pericarditis** is pleuritic and positional, typically relieved by sitting forward. Substernal pain in pericarditis may radiate to the shoulder/trapezius because of diaphragmatic/phrenic nerve irritation.

In contrast, other diseases may produce a more visceral type of pain, aching, and poorly localized. Patients with **myocardial ischemia** often present with a sensation of squeezing or pressure and possibly with a burning sensation. Classic myocardial ischemic discomfort is located substernally and radiates to the ulnar aspect of the left arm, but it may also be felt in the jaw, shoulders, epigastrium, or back. Brought on by exertion or emotional stress, stable angina usually lasts only minutes. Worrisome features include prolonged pain (more than 20 minutes) with myocardial infarction and rest pain with unstable angina. **Aortic dissection** presents with abrupt pain that is most intense at onset, which distinguishes this "must-not-miss" diagnosis. Pain is often tearing and radiates to the back. In **gastrointestinal disease** (such as reflux and esophageal spasm), symptoms may be relieved with antacids, are related to food intake, and are worsened in the supine position. Esophageal spasm may be difficult to differentiate from angina.

Finally, other conditions may have a component of both types of pain. In **musculoskeletal** disorders, pain is more easily localized and worsens with movement or palpation. Pain ranges from darting, lasting seconds, to a prolonged dull ache that lasts for days. In the neuropathic pain of herpes zoster, because pain may precede rash by several days, a burning sensation in a dermatomal distribution is a key feature. With anxiety, pain is often atypical and prolonged, and workup reveals no other cause.

PHYSICAL EXAMINATION

Remember that a patient with ischemic heart disease may present (and often does) with a *completely normal* physical examination. However, some physical findings may lead to the correct diagnosis.

- **Unequal blood pressure** between arms is an important feature for aortic dissection. **Tachypnea** is seen in pulmonary cases such as pneumothorax or pulmonary embolism.
- **Reproduction of the chest pain** by palpation is a key feature of musculoskeletal causes. This is not the case in angina, pulmonary embolus, aortic dissection, or true pleuritic disease.
- **Cardiac findings** to look for include a fourth heart sound (ischemia), an apical holosystolic murmur (ischemic mitral regurgitation), a blowing diastolic murmur (aortic regurgitation as a result of aortic dissection involving the valve root), and a pericardial rub (pericarditis).
- **Pulmonary findings** of a pneumothorax include hyperresonance to percussion, decreased fremitus, and tracheal deviation to the opposite side. A pleural rub may indicate pulmonary infarction or pneumonia. Rales and basilar dullness indicate congestive heart failure, which may reflect active cardiac ischemia.

DIAGNOSTIC EVALUATION

The initial history and physical examination should guide the diagnostic workup. If the chest pain appears cardiac in nature, an **electrocardiogram** should be obtained. Furthermore, in those patients with a high probability of underlying CHD (patients over 50 years old, smokers, etc.), an electrocardiogram (ECG) should be checked even if the story is atypical. Table 1-1 lists some helpful findings. The exercise stress test may be the appropriate next step in patients with a chronic stable pattern of pain when angina is suspected (see Chapter 3).

In patients with pleuritic pain and dyspnea as predominant symptoms, a **chest radiograph** should be the initial step to rule out pneumothorax, pulmonary infiltrates, and rib fractures. A widened mediastinum on chest radiograph may be seen with aortic dissection. Chest radiograph findings seen in pulmonary embolism can be found in Chapter 16.

Other important diagnostic tests include the **chest computed tomography** (CT), by which patients with worrisome histories for aortic dissection should be further evaluated regardless of chest radiograph or ECG results. Magnetic resonance imaging (MRI) is a noninvasive diagnostic option for patients stable enough to be sent into the scanner. Transesophageal

■ **TABLE 1-1** Electrocardiogram
• Q waves in two or more leads: previous myocardial infarction
• ST depression >1 mm: ischemia
• ST elevation: acute myocardial infarction or pericarditis (the latter often has involvement of all leads and associated PR depression)
• Left bundle branch block: suggests underlying heart disease (ischemic, hypertensive)
• Right bundle branch block: may be indicative of right heart strain (as in pulmonary embolus)
• T-wave inversions and nonspecific ST changes: seen in both healthy individuals and in many diseases (therefore, not useful)

Note: A normal ECG does not rule out ischemia or serious disease, especially when recorded in the absence of pain. Right bundle branch block and early repolarization may be seen in young, healthy, normal individuals. Occlusion of the right coronary artery by an aortic dissection may present with inferior ST elevation. This is a vital distinction to make.

echocardiogram is a minimally invasive and rapid method of detecting aortic dissection at the bedside. Either helical chest CT or a **ventilation-perfusion (V/Q) scan** is used in patients with pleuritic pain and normal chest radiograph in whom pulmonary embolus is suspected. A helical chest CT is sensitive for small pulmonary emboli and may detect other chest abnormalities leading to chest pain. A normal V/Q scan rules out the diagnosis of pulmonary embolus, whereas a high-probability scan confirms the diagnosis when accompanied by a high clinical suspicion. This is further detailed in Chapter 16.

In chest pain of esophageal origin, pain induced by esophageal reflux may be confirmed by 24-hour **esophageal pH monitoring** or by an empirical **trial of antacids**. The Bernstein test (acid instillation into the esophagus, reproducing pain) is not commonly used today.

In the case of suspected musculoskeletal pain in the low-risk patient, a trial of nonsteroidal anti-inflammatory drugs is appropriate both diagnostically and therapeutically. Pericarditis also responds to this treatment.

KEY POINTS

- Patients with histories suggestive of serious causes of chest pain (e.g., ischemia, dissection, embolus) deserve further evaluation even if physical examination, chest radiograph, and ECG results are normal.

- Certain chest pain syndromes have very typical patterns, such as the acute tearing pain of aortic dissection, the dermatomal distribution of herpes zoster, or the positional pleuritic pain of pericarditis (relieved when the patient sits forward).

- Risk factors are important to determine the probability of CHD in a patient with chest pain. These include older age, male sex, diabetes mellitus, hypertension, dyslipidemia, smoking, obesity, and family history.

- The ECG is a key test in patients with a suspected cardiac origin of chest pain. The findings of Q waves, ST elevation, or ST depression all signify cardiac ischemia. A notable exception is pericarditis, which has diffuse ST elevation, often with associated PR depression.

Shock

Shock is a term used to describe decreased perfusion and oxygen delivery to the body. Shock presents with a decrease in blood pressure (BP) and may result from either a decrease in cardiac output (CO) or a decrease in systemic vascular resistance (SVR). This is best defined by the following equation:

$$BP = CO \times SVR$$

The three main syndromes leading to shock (i.e., hypovolemic, cardiogenic, and distributive) are defined by their effect on the CO or SVR. An additional clinical feature is the volume status, best assessed at the bedside by the jugular venous pressure (JVP) and in the intensive care unit by the pulmonary capillary wedge pressure (PCWP). Table 2-1 defines the syndromes and their features.

The low CO seen in cardiogenic shock may also be seen in syndromes resulting in right heart failure (such as **massive pulmonary embolism**), decreased venous filling of the heart (**tension pneumothorax**), and obstruction of outflow (**cardiac tamponade**). The low vascular resistance that occurs in distributive shock is most commonly seen in sepsis but may be mimicked by **adrenal crisis** (insufficiency) or **anaphylaxis**. CO varies in these conditions, depending on severity and volume status.

Shock can occur when systolic BP is <90 or the mean arterial pressure is <60, but a low BP alone does not indicate shock. Shock is truly defined by its **effect on other organ systems**. Organ failure is evidence of insufficient BP for organ perfusion regardless of the actual BP value. Manifestations of inadequate perfusion include the following:

- Renal dysfunction (decreased or no urine output)

- Central nervous system dysfunction (worsening mental status)
- Tissue hypoxia (lactic acidosis)

CLINICAL MANIFESTATIONS

HISTORY

History is usually not helpful because the patient often has a clouded sensorium as a result of decreased perfusion. However, these findings may be helpful:

- Recent use or discontinuation of corticosteroids (adrenal crisis)
- Ingestion of certain foods or drugs or the occurrence of bee sting (anaphylaxis)
- History of chest pain (pleuritic: pulmonary embolism or tension pneumothorax; nonpleuritic: ischemia)
- Recent urinary tract or other infection (sepsis)

PHYSICAL EXAMINATION

Vital signs are essential to evaluating the patient with shock. **Tachycardia** is almost always present; failure to increase the heart rate in the presence of hypotension suggests a primary cardiac conduction disturbance (see Chapter 7). **Pulsus paradoxus** is seen in cardiac tamponade, defined as a decrease in systolic BP of greater than 10 mm Hg with inspiration.

JVP provides a rough bedside estimate of central venous pressure. Shock from cardiopulmonary causes (see later) presents with increased JVP. Systemic causes of shock are either vasodilation or decreased

■ TABLE 2-1 Definitions of Shock Syndromes

	CO	SVR	JVP/PCWP
Hypovolemic	Decrease	Increase	Decrease
Cardiogenic	Decrease	Increase	Increase
Distributive	Increase	Decrease	Decrease

CO, cardiac output; JVP, jugular venous pressure; PCWP, pulmonary capillary wedge pressure; SVR, systemic vascular resistance.

volume; JVP is decreased or undetectable in these patients.

Absence of breath sounds on one side and **tracheal deviation** to the opposite side are findings of a tension pneumothorax. Pulmonary examination may also reveal rales in cardiogenic shock or wheezing in anaphylaxis.

DIFFERENTIAL DIAGNOSIS

CARDIOGENIC

- Pump failure from infarction, cardiomyopathy, or tamponade
- Arrhythmia
- Valve failure
- Obstructed outflow from tension pneumothorax or massive pulmonary embolism

HYPOVOLEMIC

- Hemorrhage
- Diarrhea or heat stroke
- Third spacing

DISTRIBUTIVE

- Sepsis
- Anaphylaxis
- Adrenal crisis
- Myxedema coma*

DIAGNOSTIC EVALUATION AND TREATMENT

The hypotension present in shock is easily diagnosed, and efforts are directed at discerning the

correct etiology of shock. This always begins with treating the hypotension itself. The initial approach is based on the volume status, often using the JVP as a guide. For patients with **decreased JVP**, treatment should begin with intravenous fluids (normal saline or Ringer lactate) while evaluating the cause of the hypotension. The patient should be examined for possible causes of hypovolemia, including blood loss, dehydration, and third spacing of fluid (as in pancreatitis or cirrhosis). An acute onset after ingestion of a food (especially nuts) or drug suggests an anaphylactic reaction, and 0.3 mg epinephrine subcutaneously should be given immediately.

The diagnosis of **adrenal insufficiency** is suggested by:

- Hyponatremia
- Hyperkalemia
- Hypoglycemia
- Abdominal pain
- Eosinophilia
- Mild hypercalcemia

Adrenal insufficiency is then confirmed by a suboptimal response to adrenocorticotropic hormone (ACTH). The emergent nature of an adrenal crisis requires immediate treatment with intravenous steroids (**4 mg dexamethasone IV**) while performing diagnostic studies. The **ACTH stimulation test** involves measurement of a basal cortisol level (preferably at its morning peak, 8 to 9 AM), followed by a cortisol measurement 1 hour after administration of ACTH. Basal or poststimulation values greater than 20 μg per dL rule out adrenal insufficiency. However, because stress increases cortisol levels, some authorities have recommended increasing this cutoff to 25 μg per dL in the acutely ill patient.

Patients with possible sepsis should have blood cultures drawn and urinary culture sent. Cultures of cerebrospinal fluid and sputum should be sent if suspected. **Empirical antibiotic therapy** must be started urgently, directed at the most likely pathogens.

Myxedema coma presents as a "hypo-" syndrome of severe hypothyroidism: hypothermia, hyponatremia, hypoglycemia, and hypoventilation. When suspected, blood should be drawn for TSH, T_4, and T_3 testing, and thyroid hormone should be initiated while awaiting test results. Because of the risk of coexistent adrenal crisis caused by pituitary failure, cortisol should also be tested and adrenal crisis treated while awaiting final results.

Cardiogenic shock (increased JVP) requires specific treatment aimed at the underlying pathology.

---

*Decreased cardiac contractility also responsible for syndrome.

When JVP is increased, intravenous fluids can be harmful; they may be temporizing measures in pulmonary embolism or tamponade. Along with the clinical examination and empirical treatment, the **chest radiograph** is a useful first test in hypotension with increased JVP. A chest film may show bilateral alveolar infiltrates (pulmonary edema), an enlarged cardiac silhouette (tamponade or cardiomyopathy), or a pneumothorax with mediastinal shift to the opposite side. Chest radiograph is often normal in pulmonary embolism, but certain findings may be present (see Chapter 16).

An **electrocardiogram** (ECG) may show acute myocardial ischemia, with either ST segment elevation or depression. Old Q waves may suggest past myocardial injury and a predisposition to cardiogenic shock. In pulmonary embolism, the ECG may show evidence of right heart strain, such as right bundle branch block.

Although a chest radiograph can confirm the diagnosis of tension pneumothorax, the emergent nature of the problem may demand immediate treatment. In a patient at risk for pneumothorax with typical findings (absent breath sounds, tracheal deviation, increased JVP), decompression of the affected side must be accomplished immediately. **Insertion of a chest tube** is the optimal treatment, but if one is not readily available, a large-gauge needle should be inserted in the midclavicular second intercostal space of the affected side.

In the patient with hypotension and increased JVP, an **echocardiogram** may help determine the underlying cause. For example, echocardiographic findings seen in pericardial tamponade include moderate to large pericardial effusion and diastolic collapse of the right atrium or ventricle. In addition, the echocardiogram may reveal hypokinesis (cardiogenic shock), right-sided heart failure (pulmonary embolism), or valvular or septal wall rupture.

Invasive monitoring may be necessary to evaluate and treat the patient with shock. In the patient whose etiology is unclear or in whom treatment is ineffective, a **Swan-Ganz (pulmonary artery) catheter** should be placed. This can be used to obtain a PCWP, which is a proxy for left atrial filling pressures. The PCWP is elevated only in cardiac etiologies of shock. In cardiac tamponade, equalization of pressures may occur; that is, the right atrial pressure is equal to the right ventricular diastolic pressure and the left atrial pressure.

CO may also be measured with a pulmonary artery catheter; the output is then divided by the patient's body size to yield a cardiac index. Normal values for cardiac index are 2.2 to 4 L/minute/m^2. CO is decreased in cardiopulmonary etiologies and increased in early (warm) sepsis. In late sepsis, CO may decline (cold sepsis).

In the patient who is not improved after initial treatment, **vasopressors** may be needed. The choice of drug depends on the pathophysiology and the severity of the patient's condition. **Dobutamine** is a selective β_1-receptor agonist that increases cardiac contractility. It is useful in cardiogenic shock to increase CO and decrease SVR. However, it must be used with caution when BP is below 90 because it may cause a further drop in BP when started. **Norepinephrine** has effects on both α- and β_1-receptors. It can be useful in distributive shock and cardiogenic shock. **Phenylephrine** is a pure α_1-receptor agonist and may be appropriate in early (warm) sepsis when SVR is low but CO is high. The effects of **dopamine** are dose dependent. At low doses (0.5 to 2.0 μg/kg/minute), it dilates renal and mesenteric arteries, and at intermediate doses (2.0 to 6.0 μg/kg/minute), dopamine acts similarly to dobutamine. At the highest doses, it becomes a vasoconstrictor with norepinephrinelike effects.

 KEY POINTS

- Shock, manifested by decreased BP, is the result of decreased cardiac output or decreased systemic vascular resistance.

- Shock caused by cardiopulmonary etiologies results from decreased CO and presents with increased jugular venous pressure. In hypovolemic and distributive shock, the JVP is undetectable.

- Unilateral absence of breath sounds, increased JVP, and tracheal deviation suggest tension pneumothorax. Immediate decompression is required.

- Hyponatremia and hyperkalemia in the patient with hypotension may suggest adrenal crisis. Treatment with intravenous dexamethasone is indicated. Diagnosis may be confirmed by an ACTH stimulation test.

Coronary Heart Disease

EPIDEMIOLOGY

Coronary heart disease (CHD) is the leading cause of death in people older than 45 years in the United States. An estimated 5 million people in the United States have CHD. Many more have conditions that predispose to its development. CHD is responsible for an estimated 500,000 deaths each year, but overall the death rate has been declining over the past 20 to 30 years. This is believed to be because of improvements in the management of CHD, including prevention of CHD progression, treatment of myocardial ischemia, and management of acute myocardial infarction. This chapter details the diagnosis of CHD and the management of stable angina. Chapter 4 describes the treatment of the acute coronary syndromes.

ETIOLOGY AND PATHOGENESIS

CHD results from a complex interplay of endothelial cell dysfunction, dyslipidemia, and inflammation. The formation of an **atherosclerotic plaque** within a coronary artery proceeds through a number of stages. In the first stage, endothelial dysfunction appears to predispose to formation of a "fatty streak." Smooth muscle cells migrate into the intima and proliferate, followed by accumulation of lipid. This can happen quite early in life (during the second decade). In the second stage, low-density lipoprotein (LDL) enters the endothelium in the area of the fatty streak. The LDL becomes oxidized, attracting **macrophages** that ingest the LDL. These macrophages (foam cells) release factors that recruit more macrophages, fibroblasts, and other inflammatory cells. In the final stage,

proliferating smooth muscle cells, connective tissue (produced by infiltrating fibroblasts), and lipids (cholesterol, cholesterol esters, triglycerides, and phospholipids) become incorporated into the maturing plaque. At this point, the formation of a "fibrous cap" results in narrowing of the artery lumen. In advanced lesions, areas of cell necrosis and calcification may occur within the lipid-rich core of the plaque.

Myocardial ischemia occurs in the setting of coronary artery atherosclerosis. Plaques may rupture and lead to thrombosis (see Chapter 4) or progressively grow to narrow the arterial lumen. Narrowing of the coronary artery lumen by an atherosclerotic lesion reduces blood flow to the distal myocardium. As the lesion continues to grow, oxygen supply becomes increasingly limited, and under conditions of increased demand (e.g., exercise, emotional stress), myocardial ischemia occurs. At this stage, the cross-sectional area of the coronary artery is generally <30% of normal.

Progressive luminal compromise can lead to the expansion of **collateral circulation**, alternate distal vessels that can increase blood supply to the compromised area. In some cases, complete occlusion of the diseased artery can result in little or no myocardial damage because of extensive distal collateralization.

RISK FACTORS

Chapter 1 describes standard risk factors for CHD. Diabetes mellitus and patient age are two of the strongest risk factors. Peripheral vascular disease and chronic renal failure are also strongly associated with CHD. In addition, low activity level, low intake of fruits and vegetables, lack of moderate alcohol intake, and an elevated homocysteine level or elevated inflammatory markers such as C-reactive protein all appear to confer additional risk for CHD.

CLINICAL MANIFESTATIONS

HISTORY

The typical manifestation of symptomatic CHD is **angina pectoris**, characterized as a substernal pressure, heaviness, burning, squeezing, or choking. The discomfort is rarely well localized or described as sharp pain. Radiation to the jaw, shoulder, back, or arms can occur.

In so-called **stable angina**, attacks are brought on by exertion or emotional stress. The pain increases over several minutes and is relieved by rest in several minutes. **Unstable angina** is defined as angina that occurs at rest or as a significant change in the pattern of existing chronic angina (see Chapter 4). Angina is classified by the amount of exertion needed to reproduce symptoms: class I (strenuous activity), class II (walking several blocks or up incline), class III (mild activity, such as walking short distances), and class IV (any activity or at rest).

It is important to note that not all patients describe typical anginal pain during periods of myocardial ischemia. Patients with **atypical angina** may have isolated symptoms such as jaw pain or dyspnea. This is particularly true in patients with underlying diabetes. Patients with **silent ischemia** can be completely asymptomatic. In some patients with angina who have underlying compromise of ventricular function or severe widespread ischemia, angina can be accompanied by symptoms of **heart failure** (dyspnea, orthopnea).

PHYSICAL EXAMINATION

CHD patients often have a normal physical examination, particularly if they are not symptomatic at the time of examination. They may however have findings of predisposing conditions or from atherosclerosis outside of the coronary arteries:

- Retinal vascular changes (e.g., arteriovenous nicking and/or "copper wire" changes caused by hypertension)
- Third heart sound (congestive heart failure)
- Fourth heart sound (hypertension)
- Arterial bruits (peripheral atherosclerosis)
- Absent or diminished peripheral pulses (peripheral atherosclerosis)
- Xanthomas (hyperlipidemia)

Examination during an anginal attack can reveal a fourth heart sound (because of decreased compliance of the ischemic myocardium) or signs of left ventricular failure (third heart sound, single S_2, rales, elevated jugular venous pressure). The examination should also look for findings that would prohibit safe exercise testing (e.g., critical aortic stenosis).

DIFFERENTIAL DIAGNOSIS

Chapter 1 discusses the differential diagnosis of chest pain. The probability that a patient with chest pain has significant CHD is estimated by considering the following:

- Characteristics of pain
- Patient age and gender
- Patient risk factors (especially diabetes, chronic renal failure, or the presence of known peripheral or cerebrovascular disease)
- Electrocardiogram

DIAGNOSTIC EVALUATION

Many prediction models have been tested to identify patients at high risk for CHD. Of the models, the Framingham prediction model remains the most widely accepted. This model tallies points for the major known cardiac risk factors: age, gender, diabetes, smoking, LDL, high-density lipoprotein (HDL), and blood pressure. The **resting electrocardiogram** is normal in approximately half of patients with angina pectoris. Some may have evidence of old myocardial infarction (Q waves, inverted T waves). The typical electrocardiogram (ECG) change seen during actual ischemia is **ST-segment depression**, defined as a depression of the ST segment from baseline greater than 1 mm in at least two contiguous leads.

The suspected diagnosis of CHD can be confirmed with an **exercise stress test**. During a stress test, the patient exercises on a treadmill or bicycle ergometer. The workload is increased in a standardized progressive manner, and symptoms, vital signs, and ECG are monitored. Exercise is continued to achieve 85% maximal heart rate (maximal heart rate = 220 beats per minute minus patient age). Reasons for stopping the test include moderate to

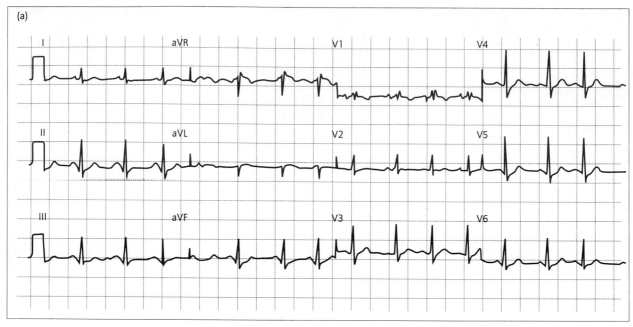

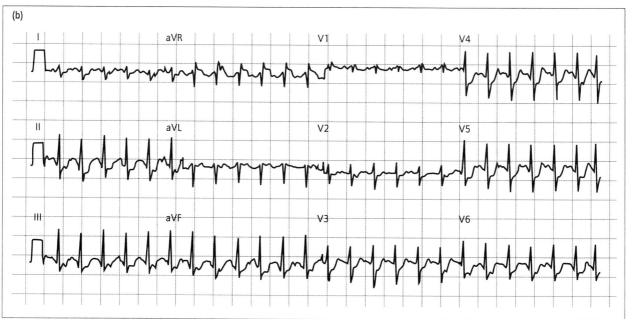

Figure 3-1 • The resting ECG **(A)** and the peak exercise ECG **(B)** of a patient with a positive exercise test. Note the ST depression in the inferior and anterior chest leads.
(This patient proved to have left main coronary artery disease.)

severe chest pain or dyspnea, dizziness, greater than 2 mm ST-segment depression, fall in systolic blood pressure (BP) of >10 mm Hg when associated with ischemia, or sustained ventricular tachycardia. Development of diagnostic **ST-segment depression** (>1 mm downsloping or horizontal) is considered to be a positive test (Fig. 3-1).

The sensitivity of exercise testing in detecting significant CHD (>70% stenosis of at least one artery) is approximately 60%. The test is more sensitive for three-vessel disease. The specificity of the test ranges from 77% to 90%. Because of this fairly low specificity, patients with low pretest probability for heart disease (estimated risk of <10%) are not

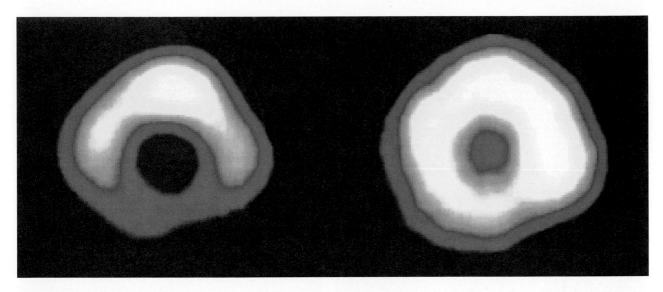

Figure 3-2 • Sestamibi-labeled myocardial perfusion scans. On the exercise scan there is a large area of very reduced uptake in the inferior wall of the left ventricle, with normal redistribution of the sestamibi on the rest scan indicating an area of ischemia. Only the left ventricular wall is demonstrated because there is too little uptake of technetium by the normal right ventricle.

generally assessed with simple exercise stress testing; a positive result would be more likely to be a false positive than a true positive. Stress testing is therefore reserved for patients with intermediate (10% to 90%) pretest probability. Left bundle branch block, left ventricular hypertrophy, preexcitation (Wolff-Parkinson-White) syndrome, and digoxin use are associated with false-positive ST depressions. Patients with these conditions or other ECG abnormalities should have **imaging studies** (see later) done along with the exercise test. The exercise test also offers prognostic information; in patients who complete an exercise study (>10 minutes) without chest pain or ST depressions, annual mortality from CHD is very low (<1% annually).

The sensitivity and specificity of exercise testing can be improved by the use of **radiolabeled tracers** (e.g., technetium, sestamibi, or tetrofosmin) to determine regional myocardial perfusion (Fig. 3-2). Images are recorded immediately after exercise, and then after a several-hour rest period, to identify ischemic areas that have decreased blood flow after exercise but normal or increased flow after rest. Infarcted areas of myocardium lack perfusion at both time points. This technique is semiquantitative, estimating the amount of ischemic or infarcted myocardium by the size of the defect seen on the images.

Patients who are unable to exercise because of orthopedic problems or severe deconditioning can have pharmacologic stress testing with the administration of **dipyridamole** or **adenosine**. These agents act as vasodilators of normal but not atherosclerotic coronary vessels and thus can cause shunting of blood flow away from diseased vessels, resulting in ischemia. They may cause bronchospasm and should be used with caution in patients with chronic obstructive pulmonary disease (COPD) or asthma. Theophylline within 72 hours and caffeine within 24 hours can both reduce the sensitivity of the vessels to these medications.

Echocardiography may be used as an alternative to radiologic imaging. **Dobutamine stress echocardiography**, which looks for wall motion abnormalities with increasing myocardial demand, has similar test characteristics to pharmacologic imaging studies. It can be safely performed in patients with asthma as well as in the presence of recent caffeine use. Exercise echocardiography is slightly less sensitive than perfusion imaging, but it is more specific. This makes it a popular option for patients with lower pretest probabilities of CHD.

The gold standard to diagnose coronary artery disease remains **coronary angiography** (Fig. 3-3). Angiography is indicated when noninvasive testing is inconclusive or when clinical parameters suggest severe (i.e., three-vessel) coronary artery disease. The parameters include severe (class III or IV) angina despite medical therapy, angina associated with congestive heart failure (CHF), ejection fraction <35%, or large perfusion defect on stress testing.

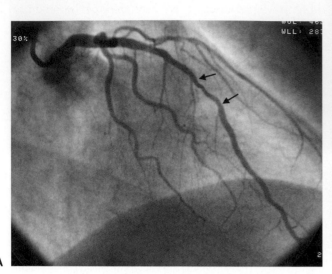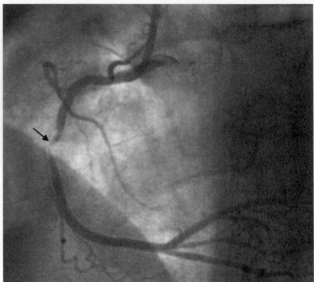

A   B

Figure 3-3 • Coronary arteriography in a patient with CHD. **(A)** Left coronary artery injection showing a moderate stenosis between the arrows in the mid left anterior descending artery. **(B)** Right coronary artery injection showing tight stenosis (*arrow*) of the mid right coronary artery.

Treatment

The initial treatment of confirmed, chronic stable angina pectoris is usually medical. The goals of treatment are to (a) prevent myocardial infarction and death from CHD and (b) decrease angina and improve quality of life. The American Heart Association suggests the following mnemonic for the important **elements in treatment of stable angina**:

A: Aspirin, angiotensin-converting enzyme inhibitors (ACEIs), and antianginals
B: β-Blocker and BP
C: Cholesterol and cigarettes
D: Diet and diabetes
E: Education and exercise

PREVENTION OF MYOCARDIAL INFARCTION AND DEATH FROM CORONARY ARTERY DISEASE

Aspirin (75 to 325 mg daily) limits platelet aggregation by inhibiting platelet thromboxane A_2. Multiple studies have demonstrated that aspirin reduces the risk of subsequent myocardial infarction (MI) as primary prevention, in patients with CHD, and for post MI. Patients who are allergic to aspirin should be placed on clopidogrel (75 mg daily),

which prevents adenosine diphosphate (ADP)-mediated platelet aggregation.

Older studies of **lipid lowering agents** suggested that every 1% reduction in cholesterol level decreased the relative risk of coronary events by 2%. Newer studies of **HMG-CoA reductase inhibitors (statins)** (see Chapter 55) demonstrate convincing benefit (25% to 35% relative risk reductions) in patients with established CHD, even when cholesterol levels are "normal." Patients with CHD should aim for an LDL level of <90 mg per dL, and there is some evidence of benefit for lowering LDL below 70 mg per dL for those with very high CHD risk.

Finally, some studies suggest higher risk patients with CHD benefit from **angiotensin-converting enzyme inhibitors** (ACEIs) or angiotensin II receptor blockers, even when BP is optimal (BP goal is less than 130/85, less than 130/80 in the presence of diabetes). ACEI are recommended for CHD patients with diabetes or left ventricular dysfunction; the role of these agents in all patients with stable angina is unclear.

ANTIANGINAL TREATMENT

β-Adrenergic blocking agents reduce myocardial workload by limiting adrenergic increases (from stress or exercise) in heart rate and contractility.

Although the data suggesting that β-blockers decrease the risk of MI or death in stable angina are limited (or nonexistent), many physicians extrapolate the benefits from post-MI patients or elderly patients with hypertension. Furthermore, β-blockers are clearly effective at reducing anginal symptoms. Contraindications to β-blockers include severe bradycardia, high-degree AV block, and decompensated CHF. Dose should be titrated to a goal heart rate of 50 to 60 beats per minute. **Side effects** include fatigue, impotence, bradycardia, and the development or worsening of heart failure.

Calcium channel blockers (CCBs) decrease myocardial contractility and increase coronary blood flow. They are equivalent antianginals compared with β-blockers and tend to cause fewer side effects. However, studies have demonstrated increased cardiac risk with short-acting dihydropyridine calcium channel blockers (nifedipine). Therefore, only long-acting dihydropyridines or nondihydropyridines (verapamil, diltiazem) are recommended. Second generation dihydropyridines (amlodipine, nicardipine) have fewer negative inotropic effects than the other options, so can be used in settings of reduced ejection fraction. Contraindications are the same as for β-blockers, and **side effects** include peripheral edema, reflex tachycardia, and constipation. When reflex tachycardia is a concern, CCBs can be combined with β-blockers.

Nitrates (nitroglycerin, isosorbide mononitrate, or dinitrate) are endothelium-independent vasodilators that reduce myocardial wall stress through venous pooling (decreased preload). They also produce coronary vasodilation, increasing myocardial blood flow. They are used in sublingual form for relief of acute ischemia and also in long-acting forms (via transdermal patches or slow-release oral formulations) for limiting frequency and severity of attacks. **Side effects** (most prominent with sublingual administration) are hypotension, lightheadedness, and headache. Constant use results in **nitrate tolerance**, which is prevented by an adequate (8-hour) nitrate-free interval.

REVASCULARIZATION

Some patients with coronary disease benefit from surgical revascularization with **coronary artery bypass grafting** (CABG). Each patient must be assessed individually, but general situations where surgical therapy is superior to medical therapy include the following:

- Left main coronary disease or left main equivalent (proximal left anterior descending [LAD] stenosis plus proximal left circumflex artery stenosis)
- Three-vessel disease, especially with decreased ejection fraction
- Severe proximal LAD stenosis with "myocardium at risk" on noninvasive testing
- Survivors of sudden cardiac death or sustained ventricular tachycardia/fibrillation

Percutaneous coronary intervention (PCI) can be used to relieve symptoms in patients who fail medical therapy but who do not have significant enough disease to require CABG. Most patients with single- or double-vessel disease will fall in this group. The routine use of drug-coated coronary stents has led to decreased risk of restenosis in the treated vessel.

 KEY POINTS

- The risk for underlying CHD is determined by patient age, gender, cardiac risk factors, and characteristics of chest pain.

- Exercise stress testing is insufficiently specific for assessment of patients with low (<10%) pretest probability of CHD. Exercise testing is best reserved for patients with intermediate pretest probability. Sensitivity and specificity can be increased with imaging studies such as radionuclide imaging or echocardiography.

- For patients with a baseline abnormal ECG, the stress test should include either radionuclide or echocardiographic imaging.

- Aspirin and HMG-CoA reductase inhibitors decrease mortality from CAD.

- β-Blockers are the first-line antianginal drugs. ACEIs, calcium channel blockers, and nitrates may be used as well.

- Severe multivessel disease, stenosis of the left main coronary artery, or equivalent lesions (proximal lesions in LAD and left circumflex artery) require CABG for survival benefit.

Myocardial Infarction

EPIDEMIOLOGY

Acute myocardial infarction (AMI) is a common manifestation of coronary artery disease (CAD). Each year, approximately a million people suffer an AMI in the United States. Many patients with AMI die suddenly before hospitalization. In patients admitted to the hospital, 30-day mortality is approximately 5% to 10%.

ETIOLOGY/PATHOGENESIS

Most myocardial infarctions (MIs) occur in the setting of underlying coronary heart disease (CHD). The formation of an **atherosclerotic plaque** within a coronary artery is a multistep process (see Chapter 3).

Spontaneous **fissuring and rupture** of a coronary atherosclerotic plaque may occur, exposing a highly thrombogenic surface. Platelet aggregation and fibrin formation follow, and the patient clinically presents with an **acute coronary syndrome**. The specific clinical manifestation depends on the extent of the thrombus. If the thrombus causes complete occlusion of the coronary artery, the result is often an **ST-elevation myocardial infarction** (STEMI). When untreated, this leads to necrosis of the myocardium previously supplied by the occluded vessel. Necrosis may occur throughout the entire thickness of the affected myocardium, resulting in **pathologic Q waves**.

Acute coronary syndromes with ischemic chest pain and elevated biochemical markers of myocardial injury, but lacking classic diagnostic ST elevation on electrocardiogram, are categorized as **non–ST-elevation myocardial infarction** (NSTEMI).

In NSTEMI, pathologic Q waves are absent. **Unstable angina** (UA) is a closely related condition, with transient thrombus and occlusion, but markers of infarction are not present (see Diagnostic Evaluation). At the time of presentation, the acute coronary syndromes of NSTEMI and UA can be difficult to differentiate.

Although rupture of an atherosclerotic plaque with thrombus formation is responsible for most AMIs, there are **other mechanisms** by which coronary blood flow or oxygen supply or both can be acutely compromised, leading to myocardial ischemia and infarction:

- "Demand ischemia" (tachycardia, hypotension, and/or severe hypoxia in setting of existing fixed CAD)
- Coronary artery dissection (often in the setting of a dissecting aortic aneurysm)
- Coronary vasospasm (idiopathic Prinzmetal angina or drug induced, e.g., cocaine)
- In situ thrombus formation (in the setting of a hypercoagulable state)
- Coronary embolism
- Vasculitis (e.g., Kawasaki disease)
- Carbon monoxide poisoning

Early death (within the first month) from AMI can be caused by a number of complications:

- Arrhythmias (ventricular fibrillation/tachycardia, complete heart block)
- Heart failure (cardiogenic shock)
- Ventricular rupture (peak incidence within 3 to 5 days of AMI)
- Other mechanical complications (ventricular septal defect, mitral papillary rupture)

Death occurring >1 month after an AMI can be caused by reinfarction, progressive heart failure, or sudden arrhythmias.

CLINICAL MANIFESTATIONS

HISTORY

Patients suffering an AMI most often complain of **retrosternal chest pain**, often starting at rest. The pain generally reaches a maximum over several minutes and then is prolonged and persistent. It may radiate to the back, neck, arms, or jaw. Administration of nitrates may provide some relief but generally not resolution of the pain. Other **associated symptoms** can include diaphoresis, dyspnea, nausea/vomiting, and anxiety.

The patient with **unstable angina** may present with rest pain, new-onset exertional pain, or increasing severity or frequency of established angina.

Some patients may not present with typical chest pain. Approximately 10% to 20% of patients with AMI present with pleuritic or sharp chest pain. The elderly (particularly patients with dementia), diabetic patients, and postoperative patients (on analgesics) may not give a history of chest pain. These patients may present with nonspecific symptoms such as fatigue, nausea, syncope, or shortness of breath.

PHYSICAL EXAMINATION

It should be noted that the physical examination can be entirely normal in the setting of an AMI. The vital signs give important prognostic and therapeutic information (see Treatment), and hypotension is indicative of **cardiogenic shock**. A fourth heart sound (because of decreased compliance of the ischemic myocardium) is common, a third heart sound may be present, and ischemia of the papillary muscle leads to a systolic murmur of acute mitral regurgitation (see Table 9-1). Signs of pulmonary edema (see Chapter 5) indicate more severe disease. The physical examination should also focus on signs of peripheral vascular disease (bruits, decreased pulses), which may increase the suspicion for coronary disease.

DIFFERENTIAL DIAGNOSIS

For a detailed discussion of the differential diagnosis of chest pain, see Chapter 1. In the patient with **chest pain and ST elevation** on the electrocardiogram (ECG), the differential diagnosis includes the following:

- AMI
- Acute pericarditis
- Prinzmetal (spontaneous vasospastic) angina

In a patient with known CHD, especially one with chronic stable angina, the distinction between worsening ischemia (unstable angina) and an AMI is often difficult to make. The pain of an AMI is often described as more severe, unrelenting, not responsive to usual doses of nitrates, and more likely to be accompanied by associated symptoms (diaphoresis, dyspnea, etc.) than typical anginal pain.

DIAGNOSTIC EVALUATION

The **ECG** should be checked early in the evaluation of possible AMI and rechecked frequently during the workup. The patient with **new left bundle branch block** is treated as having STEMI. For other patients, ECG can be helpful in differentiating between STEMI and NSTEMI/UA. The typical **evolution of the ECG** in the setting of STEMI is as follows (Fig. 4-1):

1. Increase in amplitude of the T wave (first several minutes after vessel occlusion)
2. ST-segment elevation (minutes to hours)
3. Development of Q waves (hours to days)
4. Resolution of ST-segment elevation (hours to days)

In the case of UA and NSTEMI, the ECG manifestations are more variable in the acute setting. Often there are only nonspecific ST- and T-wave changes (isolated ST depressions or elevations, inverted or flattened T waves). Hours after a NSTEMI, stable T-wave inversions in the affected region may develop. Deep inverted T waves in leads V_1 through V_4 are associated with severe disease in the left anterior descending artery (**Wellen sign**). These patients should be considered for early catheterization.

The confirmation of MI (both STEMI and NSTEMI) is generally done by **serial determinations of the cardiac enzymes**, which appear in the circulation because of damaged myocardium. The most accurate enzyme is **cardiac-specific troponin** (T or I). This marker begins to rise 6 to 9 hours after symptoms, peaks at approximately 20 hours, and remains in the circulation for 7 to 10 days. Elevated cardiac troponin T or I not only confirms the diagnosis of MI but also has prognostic significance because patients

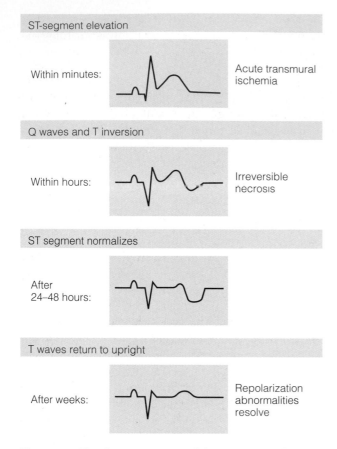

ST-segment elevation

Within minutes: Acute transmural
                   ischemia

Q waves and T inversion

Within hours: Irreversible
                   necrosis

ST segment normalizes

After
24–48 hours:

T waves return to upright

After weeks: Repolarization
                   abnormalities
                   resolve

Figure 4-1 • The changing pattern of the ECG in the affected leads during the evolution of MI.

with elevated levels have poorer outcomes than those without elevated levels. This marker should be checked on initial evaluation and then checked again 8 to 12 hours later. If troponin is elevated on the first test, it can be difficult to know whether an MI occurred in the past few days or up to 10 days ago. The more established marker of serum **creatine phosphokinase-MB** (CPK-MB) fraction is not as sensitive, but it does rise earlier (3 to 6 hours) and disappears within 48 hours. Therefore, it may help to time the cardiac event accurately. A combination of these two markers is therefore often used in patients with suspected MI.

For patients with UA or NSTEMI, further risk stratification is generally assessed using the "TIMI Risk Score," a 7 point system where more points confer higher risk. The seven prognostic factors are:

- Age >65
- At least 3 risk factors for coronary artery disease
- Known coronary artery disease with at least 50% coronary stenosis

- ST-segment changes
- At least 2 episodes of angina in the past 24 hours
- Aspirin use in the past week
- Elevated CK-MB or troponin

Cardiac **echocardiography** (both transthoracic and transesophageal) can reveal regional wall motion abnormalities indicative of ischemic or infarcted myocardium. It can also detect structural defects such as aneurysms, septal defects, pericardial effusions, valvular abnormalities, and mural thrombi. An assessment of global left ventricular function can also be made.

A **chest radiograph** can detect the presence of heart failure, cardiac enlargement, and other causes of chest pain such as pneumonia, aortic dissection, and pneumothorax.

The gold standard of diagnostic assessment for coronary artery disease is **coronary angiography**. Angiography can identify the precise location of a thrombus and detect other atherosclerotic lesions. It is usually performed early in the presentation of patients presenting with either AMI or UA with high thrombolysis in myocardial infarction (TIMI) risk score, with the goal of mechanical revascularization (see following).

TREATMENT

Acute coronary syndrome, including AMI, is a medical emergency. Prompt institution of therapy can limit the size of an infarct and preserve ventricular function postinfarction. These are the main **goals of therapy**:

- Reduction of myocardial oxygen demand (heart rate, blood pressure)
- Improvement or restoration of myocardial perfusion
- Relief of pain
- Recognition and treatment of complications

When a patient presents with a possible AMI, the following steps should be taken:

1. Perform a rapid clinical assessment with vital signs, history, physical, and 12-lead ECG within the first 10 minutes.
2. Administer oxygen and 162- to 325-mg aspirin (chewed) unless the patient has a true aspirin allergy. **Aspirin**, presumably through its antiplatelet effects, decreases mortality in AMI.
3. Sublingual **nitroglycerin** (0.4 mg every 5 minutes × 3) may be given for relief of chest pain unless

hypotension (systolic BP <90) is present. It should be given with caution in a patient with a large inferior MI (right ventricular infarction) because BP will be highly dependent on adequate preload. Intravenous nitroglycerin should be given (10 to 300 μg per minute) in patients with persistent pain or ECG changes. **Nitrates** can improve hemodynamics, reduce cardiac work, improve myocardial oxygen delivery, and limit infarct size. Intravenous **morphine** sulphate or fentanyl may be used for pain as well as to lower cardiac workload because of pain-induced sympathetic drive.

4. Intravenous **β-adrenoceptor blockers** (e.g., metoprolol, 5 mg) should be given to control heart rate and relieve myocardial demand. They also have been shown to lower mortality. Again, adequate BP must be present. Other contraindications include bradycardia (HR <50), second- or third-degree AV block, or LV dysfunction with congestive heart failure (CHF). Tachycardia in AMI may represent impending cardiogenic shock.

5. Once the above measures are initiated, patients are also treated with a statin early in the course of acute coronary syndrome.

The treatment plan will now depend on the clinical suspicion of AMI and the electrocardiogram. The possibilities include the following:

• ST elevation, with or without cardiogenic shock
• ST depression or T-wave inversion, suspicious for NSTEMI or unstable angina
• Normal ECG, consistent with low-risk unstable angina or noncardiac pain

ST-ELEVATION MYOCARDIAL INFARCTION

Patients with ST elevations are presumed to have complete occlusion of the affected artery. The earlier the infarct artery is opened, the greater the overall benefit of treatment ("time is muscle"). ST elevations that resolve with nitroglycerin may represent coronary vasospasm or subtotal occlusion with a contribution of vasospasm. In patients with persistent ST elevations (>0.1 mV) in two or more leads after nitroglycerin, reperfusion options include thrombolytic therapy or primary **percutaneous intervention** (PCI). Primary PCI is preferred when readily available because it is associated with improved outcomes and does not confer risk of serious bleeding complications. However, primary PCI needs to be performed within 90 minutes of presentation to a medical provider. Thrombolysis is therefore still performed in many settings. If thrombolysis is chosen, the onset of pain should be <12 hours before treatment. Late thrombolysis (>12 hours) has not shown benefit. PCI is also preferred over thrombolysis for patients who have had a prior coronary artery bypass graft (CABG) or who present in cardiogenic shock.

THROMBOLYTIC THERAPY

Streptokinase, **alteplase**, **tenecteplase**, and **reteplase** are thrombolytic agents that decrease mortality and preserve left ventricular function after MI. Tenecteplase has gained favor due to the ease of single bolus infusion. Successful reperfusion is heralded by relief of pain, resolution of ST elevations, and appearance of a transient reperfusion arrhythmia such as accelerated idioventricular rhythm. Rescue PCI can be performed if thrombolysis fails. The major risk of thrombolytic therapy is bleeding, including intracranial hemorrhage in 0.5% to 0.8% of patients. **Absolute contraindications to thrombolytic therapy** include:

• Previous intracranial hemorrhage
• Significant closed head injury within the past 3 months
• Stroke within 1 year
• Intracranial malignant neoplasm
• Aortic dissection (see Chapter 1)
• Active bleeding (excluding menses)

Relative contraindications, such as uncontrolled hypertension, distant history of ischemic stroke, recent trauma or surgery, pregnancy, and current use of anticoagulants, may lead to a change in therapy choice.

PRIMARY PERCUTANEOUS INTERVENTION

Patients with **cardiogenic shock** should be immediately catheterized, if possible. In other patients, evidence indicates that prompt primary PCI is more successful in producing good coronary artery blood flow and may be associated with fewer complications and shorter hospitalizations. Prompt access to the available facilities with experienced personnel is the key to PCI. Expected time to an open artery should be <90 minutes. When PCI is performed, **glycoprotein IIb/IIIa inhibitor** (abciximab) and **clopidogrel** is started prior to the procedure. The duration of clopidogrel use following successful PCI will depend on the type of procedures performed and/or stents placed. **Unfractionated heparin** should also be initiated at the time of PCI.

ANGIOTENSIN-CONVERTING ENZYME INHIBITORS

Treatment with oral **ACE inhibitors** after an AMI decreases mortality and morbidity (mainly decreased incidence of heart failure). The benefit is greatest in patients with an anterior MI or decreased ejection fraction. Hypotension is a contraindication. Angiotensin receptor blockers are used if ACE inhibitors are not tolerable.

NON–ST-ELEVATION MYOCARDIAL INFARCTION

Patients without ST elevation on initial ECG represent patients with NSTEMI, UA, and noncardiac pain. Initial cardiac markers are not reliable to distinguish these groups on presentation. All patients can receive aspirin and β-blockers. **Statins** are also provided early on presentation. Additional treatment depends on estimated risk and the presence or absence of cardiac markers.

Clopidogrel is used early in NSTEMI in combination with aspirin for patients who are not going to be treated with invasive interventions.

Unfractionated intravenous heparin (UFH) is administered in NSTEMI or UA to prevent progression of thrombus, and the dose is titrated to a goal activated partial thromboplastin time (aPTT) of 50 to 70. The **low–molecular-weight heparin enoxaparin** is superior to UFH in some studies of NSTEMI/UA, but its longer duration of action can limit its application in patients likely to require PCI. Enoxaparin is generally preferred due to its predictable effect and ease of dose (1 mg/kg subcutaneously every 12 hours). Enoxaparin is however contraindicated in severe obesity (>150 kg) due to less predictable absorption and efficacy. It is also contraindicated in thrombocytopenia or renal failure.

GP IIb/IIIa inhibitors (e.g., abciximab) block the final common pathway of platelet aggregation. These agents reduce combined endpoints of recurrent MI and death in patients with UA or NSTEMI who undergo percutaneous interventions.

Several trials have examined **early catheterization** and PCI in patients with NSTEMI/UA in the absence of recurrent ischemia. Many have shown no benefit in mortality and some increase in morbidity (often related to bleeding). Studies using newer technology have suggested that early PCI is beneficial in patients after NSTEMI. Thrombolysis is not indicated for NSTEMI.

Other **adjunctive agents** are useful in selected instances, but their **routine use is not recommended**. Calcium channel blockers do not appear to reduce mortality after AMI, and they appear to be harmful in AMI complicated by CHF. However, calcium channel blockers may be used as antianginals when β-blockers are contraindicated (e.g., with bronchospasm) or ineffective. Short-acting dihydropyridines (nifedipine) should never be used in AMI. Prophylactic antiarrhythmics are not used, and treatment of frequent PVCs or nonsustained VT (ventricular tachycardia) is not necessary. **Lidocaine** (1 mg per kg) still has a role in treating sustained VT associated with AMI. Bradycardia and high-degree AV block may occur, and treatment is indicated if symptoms (e.g., hypotension) occur.

CONTINUED CARE

Once therapy for an AMI has been initiated, including pharmacologic or mechanical revascularization, the patient requires close monitoring in an intensive care unit. Monitoring for and treating complications (arrhythmias, heart failure, mechanical complications) are the main priority. Relief of pain is also an important treatment, to decrease adrenergic tone and myocardial oxygen demand. Opiates—in particular, morphine—are useful because they provide pain relief and anxiolysis and improve hemodynamics by lowering heart rate and BP. Stool softeners limit the Valsalva maneuver, which may lead to increased ventricular loading. Bed rest with bedside commode is appropriate if the patient is hemodynamically stable. To minimize arrhythmias, potassium level should be maintained near 4.0 mEq per L. Two to 3 days after an uncomplicated AMI, patients can be transferred to a less acute-care setting.

Recurrent chest pain after AMI may be caused by pericarditis or recurrent ischemia. If ischemia is suspected, coronary angiography is indicated. Sudden hemodynamic instability or heart failure 3 to 7 days after an AMI should raise the possibility of a **mechanical complication** (ruptured free wall with pericardial tamponade, ventricular septal defect, acute mitral regurgitation from papillary muscle rupture). Patients should be carefully examined for any new systolic murmur and surgical therapy consulted immediately if detected.

Five to 7 days after an uncomplicated AMI, patients may undergo a symptom-limited submaximal exercise test (see Chapter 3). This is done to look for areas of residual ischemia that could prompt coronary angiography and mechanical intervention. Results help predict prognosis. In addition, this exercise test can provide important psychological benefit for the patient. After discharge, patients gradually increase activity over 6 weeks, avoiding maximal activity. Enrollment in a cardiac rehabilitation program and counseling can help guide activity levels. Six to 8 weeks after the AMI, the patient undergoes a maximal exercise test before resuming normal activities.

KEY POINTS

- MI is divided into ST-elevation and non–ST-elevation MI. This division drives the treatment decisions.

- The diagnosis of AMI is made by ECG changes in association with serum cardiac markers. Cardiac-specific troponins (I or T) are the most sensitive and specific test, increasing 6 to 9 hours after symptoms begin.

- Initial treatment for suspected acute coronary syndrome/MI involves oxygen, aspirin, nitrates, β-blockers, morphine, and statin.

- Patients with STEMI should be considered for primary PCI, if readily available. Unfractionated heparin or enoxaparin and clopidogrel/GP IIb IIa inhibitors should be given to patients with STEMI undergoing PCI.

- Patients with NSTEMI benefit from clopidogrel and may benefit from the addition of GP IIb/IIIa inhibitors if PCI is planned.

- Patients with anterior MI or reduced ejection fraction should benefit from ACE inhibitors.

Heart Failure

Heart failure is a clinical syndrome in which the heart has a reduced ability to fill with or eject blood. Heart failure leads to an inability to pump blood at a rate that meets metabolic demands. Heart failure can be classified according to:

- The hemodynamic state of the cardiovascular system (congestive vs. high output)
- The predominance of the ventricle affected (left vs. right)
- The predominant form of myocardial dysfunction (systolic or diastolic)
- The time course (acute or chronic)

Various combinations can exist, such as chronic congestive left-sided failure.

EPIDEMIOLOGY

Approximately a half million individuals are diagnosed with heart failure each year. The overall prevalence of heart failure in the United States is 1%, but it approaches 10% among persons older than 70 years. The prevalence has been rising, in part due to improved chronic therapy that has reduced heart failure mortality.

The overall 5-year mortality rate is 60% for men and 45% for women. When considering patients with the greatest degree of heart failure (i.e., those with symptoms at rest), the 1-year mortality rate approaches 50%.

The major **risk factors** for developing congestive heart failure (CHF) are:

- Coronary heart disease
- Hypertension
- Diabetes
- Valvular heart disease
- Cardiomyopathy (infiltrative, e.g., amyloid; toxic, e.g., drugs; idiopathic)

Obesity is also now recognized as an independent risk factor for heart failure. In the United States, 50% to 75% of individuals with CHF have developed it because of coronary heart disease. For the less common condition of diastolic heart failure, hypertension is the major risk factor.

PATHOPHYSIOLOGY

Cardiac output (CO) is determined by the heart rate (HR) and the stroke volume. **Stroke volume** (SV) is calculated as end diastolic volume minus end systolic volume and depends on the interplay among three variables: preload, contractility, and afterload. **Preload** (translated as the left ventricular end-diastolic pressure [LVEDP] or the left ventricular filling pressure) is defined as the pressure required to distend the ventricle to a given left ventricular end-diastolic volume (LVEDV). **Contractility** refers to the stroke work that the heart generates at a given preload. As such, it describes the **inotropic state** of the myocardium. Normally, as preload is increased, the stroke work, or contractility, also increases. The relationship between these two variables defines the **Frank-Starling law of the heart** and can be graphically displayed by plotting LVEDP against stroke work or cardiac output (Fig. 5-1). **Afterload** is the dynamic resistance against which the heart contracts. It is generally reflected in the systolic BP, which is the most clinically useful measure of afterload.

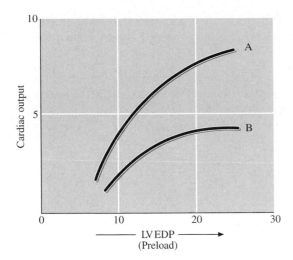

Figure 5-1 • Frank-Starling curve describing the relationship between cardiac output and preload. The position and shape of the curve depend on the level of afterload and the inotropic state of the myocardium. A, normal heart; B, decreased contractility; LVEDP, left ventricular end-diastolic volume.

The pathophysiology of most cases of heart failure begins with **decreased contractility** (systolic dysfunction). This can be caused by loss of viable myocardium by myocardial infarction or dysfunction of the individual myofibrils attributable to conditions such as myocarditis, ischemia, or toxins such as alcohol. This lowered inotropic state is quantified by a decrease in **ejection fraction** (EF), calculated as SV/LVEDV. To maintain a constant SV with a lower EF, the LVEDV must increase, which in turn results in an increase in the LVEDP (i.e., the preload). Nevertheless, the usual consequence of a decreased EF is decreased stroke volume (and cardiac output).

In the face of falling cardiac output, the **renin-angiotensin system** and the **sympathetic nervous system** are stimulated (the neurohormonal response). Systemic vasoconstriction, salt and water retention, increased afterload, and myocardial hypertrophy occur. Myocardial hypertrophy can initially decrease LV wall stress, and salt retention helps maintain a higher preload. In response to the elevated LVEDP, the cardiac ventricles produce **brain natriuretic peptide** (BNP), which attempts to decrease systemic resistance and increase natriuresis. The balance of the **neurohormonal response**, however, is detrimental and eventually leads to ventricular failure and progressive dilatation.

In **diastolic dysfunction**, the main abnormality is a **decrease in the compliance** of the ventricle, impairing the heart's ability to fill with blood. The **compliance** is defined as the relationship between the pressure and volume of the ventricle. Decreased compliance can be caused by abnormalities in the active relaxation of the myocardium during diastole or abnormalities in the elastic properties of the heart itself (or surrounding tissues). Conditions that cause these abnormalities include the following:

- Hypertension (resulting in concentric hypertrophy that can slow relaxation and increase passive chamber stiffness)
- Amyloidosis, hemochromatosis (infiltrative cardiomyopathies that increase passive chamber stiffness)
- Hypertrophic cardiomyopathy (a familial condition associated with idiopathic hypertrophy of the myocardium)
- Myocardial ischemia (acutely interferes with relaxation and over the long term can increase passive chamber stiffness)

Decreased compliance results in a higher than normal LVEDP for a given end-diastolic volume, and this higher pressure is transmitted to the pulmonary capillaries, which can lead to pulmonary congestion.

The pathophysiology of diastolic dysfunction differs from systolic dysfunction in several important ways. Contractile function is usually normal or even increased in a compensatory fashion. Avid salt and water retention and activation of the renin-angiotensin system are not prominent features in pure diastolic dysfunction. Finally, the decreased compliance results in increased sensitivity to tachycardia (by decreasing ventricular filling time) and to acute increases in intravascular volume (e.g., blood transfusion).

In unusual cases of heart failure, CO is elevated but is insufficient to meet the increased metabolic demands. Causes of such **high-output heart failure** include hyperthyroidism, arteriovenous malformation, and beriberi (thiamine deficiency). The increased CO required in these conditions eventually leads to left ventricle (LV) dilatation.

All of the preceding causes of heart failure result in increased LVEDP. The elevated LVEDP is eventually transmitted back to the left atrium and then to the pulmonary capillary bed. **Starling law** (which is different from the Frank-Starling curve discussed earlier) states that fluid filtration across a capillary is determined by a balance of the hydrostatic pressure (forcing fluid into the interstitium) and the oncotic pressure (keeping fluid in the capillary). **Pulmonary** edema occurs when the hydrostatic pressure of the pulmonary capillaries exceeds the pulmonary capillary oncotic pressure. Treatment of pulmonary edema aims to decrease the pulmonary capillary hydrostatic pressure (see "Treatment").

CLINICAL MANIFESTATIONS

HISTORY

Most symptoms caused by heart failure are pulmonary because of increased LVEDP that results in pulmonary venous and capillary congestion, including:

- Dyspnea (uncomfortable breathing that initially occurs with exertion but then also at rest)
- Orthopnea (dyspnea in the recumbent position)
- Paroxysmal nocturnal dyspnea (sudden onset of dyspnea usually occurring approximately 2 to 3 hours after falling asleep in the recumbent position)
- Cough
- Wheezing

Other symptoms can be caused by systemic fluid overload with "third space" fluid that has collected peripherally because of persistent poor forward flow (e.g., peripheral edema, weight gain), long-standing low cardiac output (e.g., fatigue), and underlying cardiac pathology (e.g., chest pain).

Symptoms (fatigue, dyspnea) in CHF are often described according to the New York Heart Association (**NYHA class**):

Class I: Asymptomatic; no limitations in ordinary activity
Class II: Slight limitation; ordinary activity causes symptoms
Class III: Marked limitation; minimal activity causes symptoms
Class IV: Symptoms at rest; all activity causes symptoms

The history should also explore possible precipitating factors for worsening CHF, including: dietary or medication noncompliance, fever/illness, new ischemic symptoms, palpitations suggesting a new arrhythmia, or recent bleeding resulting in reduced vascular volume.

PHYSICAL EXAMINATION

Physical findings generally appear once compensatory mechanisms begin to fail and significant congestion arises. They can also give clues as to whether systolic or diastolic failure is present. Cardiovascular findings include:

- Laterally displaced and/or enlarged point of maximal cardiac impulse (more in systolic dysfunction)
- Sinus tachycardia
- Accentuated second heart sound (caused by pulmonary hypertension)
- Third heart sound (systolic dysfunction)
- Fourth heart sound (hypertension and diastolic dysfunction)
- Murmurs (commonly from mitral and tricuspid regurgitation due to valvular annular dilatation, or possibly from aortic stenosis that may have been a cause of heart failure)
- Jugular venous distention and elevated jugular venous pressure

Pulmonary findings include:

- Fine-pitched inspiratory crackles (rales)
- Dullness at bases (because of the presence of pleural effusions)

Peripheral findings (because of elevated right-sided pressures) include:

- Pitting edema
- Ascites
- Hepatomegaly

Hepatojugular reflux (HJR) is elicited by application of pressure to the abdomen (traditionally in the right upper quadrant) and observation of the jugular venous pressure (JVP). Unlike the normal response (transient rise in JVP), the JVP remains elevated in HJR, indicating elevated right atrial pressures.

DIFFERENTIAL DIAGNOSIS

Chapter 12 discusses the differential diagnosis of dyspnea. In the patient with a **dilated cardiomyopathy**, the following etiologies should be considered:

- Ischemic (from old myocardial infarctions)
- Hypertension
- Valvular disease
- Toxic (alcohol, cocaine, chemotherapy such as doxorubicin)
- Viral infection (especially Coxsackievirus)
- Hemochromatosis (initially a restrictive cardiomyopathy, often dilated by time of presentation)
- Hypothyroidism

DIAGNOSTIC EVALUATION

The diagnosis of CHF should concentrate on two major issues: diagnosing the heart failure itself and identifying the precipitating factor. CHF is diagnosed clinically by the history and physical findings (see "Clinical Manifestations"). Principal diagnostic testing includes chest radiograph, electrocardiogram, blood natriuretic peptide level, and echocardiogram.

The **chest radiograph** in CHF may show the following (Fig. 5-2):

- Alveolar infiltrates (most pronounced centrally, "bat wing" pattern)
- Pulmonary venous redistribution (cephalization)
- Kerley B lines (horizontal lines located at periphery of lung)
- Peribronchial cuffing
- Pleural effusion (usually bilateral but can be right greater than left)
- Cardiomegaly (heart-to-thorax ratio >50%)

The **electrocardiogram** (ECG) is a key test in CHF because it can show the underlying etiology (e.g., Q waves in ischemic cardiomyopathy, voltage changes of ventricular hypertrophy) or a precipitating cause of CHF (e.g., ST depressions in acute ischemia, rapid atrial fibrillation). A normal ECG makes systolic dysfunction less likely.

Brain natriuretic peptide (BNP) is used as a diagnostic test for unexplained dyspnea. Elevated levels suggest CHF is the etiology of the dyspnea; a normal level (BNP <100 pg per mL) makes CHF unlikely, and a level >500 indicates likely CHF. This test is useful in diagnosis of CHF when combined with clinical diagnostic suspicion, and a low BNP is particularly helpful in ruling out CHF when it is otherwise difficult to differentiate pulmonary and cardiac causes of dyspnea. It is also helpful in monitoring CHF severity, and higher BNP levels correlate with poorer prognosis. BNP does not however distinguish between systolic and diastolic heart failure, and levels can be higher in patients with renal failure.

Other useful **blood tests** include a complete blood count (to investigate if anemia is exacerbating heart failure); electrolytes (sodium and potassium may be low); glucose (to screen for underlying diabetes); renal function (to provide baseline information about renal blood flow); and liver function tests (to assess hepatic congestion). In dilated cardiomyopathy, thyroid function tests (to screen for hypo- and hyperthyroidism) and iron studies (to screen for hemochromatosis) should be sent.

Echocardiography is useful in determining whether systolic or diastolic dysfunction predominates and to assess any valvular causes of heart failure. In systolic dysfunction, echocardiography reveals

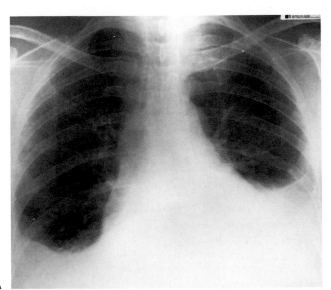
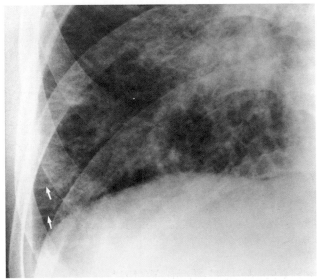

A

B

Figure 5-2 • Chest radiograph findings in heart failure. **(A)** Bilateral pleural effusions and an enlarged cardiac silhouette, the latter difficult to appreciate because the pleural fluid obscures the heart borders. **(B)** Close-up of the right costophrenic angle showing the septal lines known as Kerley B lines (*arrows*), which are horizontal, nonbranching lines that reach the pleura.

a decreased ejection fraction and cardiomegaly. In diastolic dysfunction, ejection fraction is generally normal, ventricular wall thickening without dilatation may be present, and other etiologies such as constrictive pericarditis and amyloidosis are detectable.

If the patient is an appropriate candidate for revascularization, **cardiac catheterization** is used to evaluate for possible contributing congenital heart disease (CHD). Noninvasive cardiac stress testing for viable myocardium at risk may also be indicated. In patients with a restrictive cardiomyopathy (amyloidosis, sarcoidosis), right heart catheterization to obtain an endomyocardial biopsy from the right ventricle is often indicated; however, biopsy is insensitive.

TREATMENT

The treatment of heart failure can be divided into the acute treatment of pulmonary edema focused on improving stroke volume, and the chronic treatment of CHF focused on inhibiting the neurohormonal response.

PULMONARY EDEMA

The treatment of **acute pulmonary edema** aims to decrease filling pressures because the patient is usually toward the end of the Frank-Starling curve (see Fig. 5-1). The initial treatment regimen can be summarized with the following mnemonic:

L   Lasix (furosemide) is a potent venodilator that decreases preload within minutes and a loop diuretic that decreases intravascular volume. It is given intravenously in increasing doses until a response is seen.
M   Morphine sulfate acts as a venodilator and an anxiolytic to decrease adrenergic stress (and afterload).
N   Nitroglycerin (sublingual or IV) is both an arterial and venous dilator. In addition, it is a coronary vasodilator, which can relieve ischemia when present.
O   Oxygen is used to improve systemic oxygen delivery and decrease pulmonary vasoconstriction.

Additional measures for patients with severe pulmonary edema include positive-pressure ventilation (via face mask) and inotropic agents, such as **dobutamine** (Chapter 2). In patients with severe hypertension complicating the pulmonary edema, nitroprusside and IV enalapril can be used.

SYSTOLIC DYSFUNCTION

Table 5-1 summarizes the chronic treatment of CHF **caused by systolic dysfunction**. Treatment is focused on:

- Reduction of cardiac workload by blocking the neurohormonal activation (angiotensin-converting enzyme [ACE] inhibitors, β-blockers)

■ **TABLE 5-1** Standard Medications for Congestive Heart Failure Caused by Systolic Dysfunction

Class	Examples*	Used in NYHA Class	Mortality Benefit	Other Benefits	Side Effects
ACE inhibitors	Enalapril, 10 mg bid Lisinopril, 20 mg qd	All	Yes	Fewer ischemic events; fewer hospitalizations	Hyperkalemia, cough, renal failure
Cardiac glycosides	Digoxin, 0.25 mg qd	II, III, IV	No	Fewer hospitalizations	Arrhythmias
β-Blockers	Bisoprolol, 5 mg qd Metoprolol CR, 100 mg qd	II, III	Yes		Worsening CHF
Aldosterone antagonists	Aldactone, 25 mg qd	III, IV	Yes		Hyperkalemia, gynecomastia

*Medications and dosages are representative examples, not starting doses and not applicable in all patients.
bid, twice daily; NYHA, New York Heart Association; qd, once daily.

- Control of the accumulation of salt and water (diuretics, fluid, and salt restriction)
- Augmentation of cardiac contractility (cardiac glycosides, inotrope infusions, ventricular assist device)

ACE inhibitors, which block conversion of angiotensin I to angiotensin II, reduce afterload and, attenuate sympathetic activation, and moderate ventricular remodeling. They were the first agents to demonstrate a benefit in reducing mortality in patients with heart failure. This benefit extends from asymptomatic systolic dysfunction to class IV heart failure. In patients who do not tolerate ACE inhibitors (because of cough or angioedema), **angiotensin II receptor blockers** (ARBs) (e.g., candesartan, irbesartan, losartan, valsartan) can be substituted. Although head-to-head trials show equivalence between ACE inhibitors and ARBs, ACE inhibitors remain the first-line treatment. In patients with renal insufficiency or hyperkalemia who are unable to tolerate ACE inhibitors or ARBs, the combination of isosorbide and hydralazine can be used. In comparison to placebo, this combination has been shown to reduce mortality in African American patients with NYHA class III or IV CHF.

β-Blockers were previously believed to be contraindicated in heart failure. However, several trials have shown a benefit in reducing mortality when selected β-blockers were added to stable regimens of ACE inhibitors and diuretics. The mechanism is believed to be a combination of antiarrhythmic activity and neurohormonal blockade. β-Blockers (e.g., carvedilol, metoprolol, bisoprolol) should be added in low doses and titrated up carefully. They should not be started until the patient is considered to be near euvolemia.

Spironolactone, a competitive inhibitor of aldosterone, blocks sodium–hydrogen exchange and sodium–potassium exchange in the distal tubules and collecting ducts. It is a low-potency diuretic, yet it improves mortality in advanced heart failure. This appears related to inhibition of aldosterone-promoted myocardial hypertrophy, myocardial fibrosis, and endothelial dysfunction. **Eplirinone** is an alternative aldosterone blocker that may be used if spironolactone is not tolerated due to its side effect of gynecomastia. Because both ACEI and aldosterone blockers can increase potassium, close monitoring is required.

Other diuretics are used for symptomatic treatment in CHF, but they do not improve mortality.

The most commonly used agents are the **loop diuretics** (furosemide, bumetanide, ethacrynic acid), which inhibit sodium, potassium, and chloride reabsorption in the thick ascending limb of the loop of Henle. The dosage of a loop diuretic is increased until effective diuresis occurs. IV diuretics may be needed when poor GI perfusion and absorption limit the benefit of oral medications. Thiazide diuretics (hydrochlorothiazide, metolazone), which inhibit sodium and chloride reabsorption in the distal tubule, may be added when patients are resistant to diuresis with loop diuretics. Potassium level must be closely monitored. **Sodium restriction** (2 g per day), fluid restriction, and close weight (fluid volume) monitoring are advisable in all patients.

Cardiac glycosides (e.g., digoxin) inhibit the cardiac muscle Na/K ATPase, which elevates intracellular calcium levels to augment contractility. Digoxin does not improve mortality, but it does decrease symptoms and hospitalizations. It is also useful for rate control when there is associated atrial fibrillation. The therapeutic index of digoxin is small, however, requiring monitoring of levels. The signs and symptoms of **digoxin toxicity** include:

- Anorexia
- Nausea and vomiting
- Mental status changes (generally with chronically elevated levels)
- Altered visual perception (classically a yellow tint)
- Cardiac rhythm disturbances (premature ventricular beats, AV block of varying degrees, paroxysmal, and nonparoxysmal atrial tachycardia)

Other positive inotropic agents, such as the phosphodiesterase inhibitors (e.g., milrinone, vesnarinone), have actually increased mortality when given in chronic heart failure. They may be used short term for cardiogenic shock, or they may be required as a bridge to transplantation.

DIASTOLIC DYSFUNCTION

The therapy of **diastolic dysfunction** is based on therapeutic principles because clinical trials have been inconclusive. To improve diastolic filling, treatment is aimed at control of BP and HR, with diuretics as needed. β-Blockers and calcium channel blockers are often used in these patients. Inotropic agents are not helpful. Atrial fibrillation often worsens diastolic dysfunction because of the elevated HR (decreases filling time) and loss of atrial kick. Cardioversion and antiarrhythmic medication, therefore, are sometimes necessary.

ADVANCED HEART FAILURE

In patients who do not respond to medical treatment, **dobutamine** can be initiated to improve hemodynamics. Dobutamine (via stimulation of mostly β_1- and β_2- with some α-receptor activity) increases cardiac contractility and produces peripheral vasodilatation, both of which can improve myocardial function. Side effects include tachyarrhythmias and hypotension. Once improvement is achieved, oral medications can be increased and adjusted. Invasive monitoring is sometimes used to closely measure CO and filling pressures in response to treatment (tailored therapy). It is not clear that prolonged IV infusions improve duration or quality of life.

Automatic implantable cardiac defibrillators (AICDs) are used in patients who have experienced ventricular fibrillation, symptomatic ventricular tachycardia, or cardiac arrest. AICDs also reduce mortality for patients with ischemic or nonischemic cardiomyopathy, class II to class III heart failure, and decreased ejection fractions (<35%). For patients who are not AICD candidates, **amiodarone** may be considered, despite numerous potential side effects (e.g., interstitial pneumonitis, hepatitis, cirrhosis, thyroid function abnormalities). A **biventricular pacemaker** may also be placed to provide **cardiac resynchronization therapy** in patients with low EF and left bundle branch block with prolonged QRS. In these patients, interventricular conduction delay contributes to poor coordination of ventricular contraction; resynchronization through biventricular pacing improves cardiac function.

Cardiac transplantation is a limited option because few organs are available and most patients with heart failure are older than the current age requirements. Heart transplant recipients must be maintained on immunosuppression, and accelerated atherosclerosis

in the new heart can occur. Nevertheless, survival after transplantation is much better than survival with advanced heart failure. During the waiting period for transplantation, a **ventricular assist device** (VAD) may be surgically implanted to offload blood volume from the left ventricle and return blood to the ascending aorta.

KEY POINTS

- Heart failure presents with symptoms of elevated pulmonary vascular pressures: dyspnea, orthopnea, and paroxysmal nocturnal dyspnea. Physical exam for pulmonary and peripheral edema is suggestive, and the chest radiograph confirms pulmonary congestion.

- Low cardiac output stimulates the renin-angiotensin system and sympathetic nervous systems. This neurohormonal response eventually leads to progressive ventricular failure.

- Treatment of acute pulmonary edema focuses on decreasing preload with Lasix (furosemide), morphine sulfate, nitrates, and oxygen.

- In chronic CHF with systolic dysfunction, ACE inhibitors, selected β-blockers, and aldosterone blockers decrease mortality. Digoxin, other inotropic agents, and loop or thiazide diuretics are used as required for symptoms.

- Hydralazine and nitrates in combination, when combined with standard therapy, reduce mortality for blacks with class III of IV CHF.

- Automatic implantable cardiac defibrillators improve survival when EF is <35% in class II/III CHF and nonsustained VT. Cardiac resynchronization through biventricular pacing reduces symptoms from cardiac dysfunction.

Bradyarrhythmias

The normal pacemaker of the heart is the **sinoatrial (SA) node**, located in the right atrium. Its impulse conducts through the atria to **the atrioventricular (AV) node**, where the electrical impulse is normally slowed (0.12 to 0.20 second). The impulse then travels to the **bundle of His**, which branches into three separate bundles (right, left anterior, and left posterior). The sinus node normally generates 60 to 100 impulses per minute. This rate may be increased by sympathetic stimulation or decreased by cholinergic (vagal) stimulation.

Bradyarrhythmias, or abnormally slow heart rhythms, are generally defined by a heart rate (HR) <60 beats per minute (bpm). However, a slow HR itself is not necessarily pathologic; The normal adult resting HR ranges as low as 45, and lower rates may be seen normally during sleep. Professional athletes may even have resting HRs lower than 40-bpm without any difficulty or evidence of disease. In general, pathologic bradyarrhythmias arise by delays in:

- Impulse formation
- Conduction

ETIOLOGY

Systemic causes of delayed impulse formation or conduction include:

- Hypoxia
- Increased intracranial pressure
- Hypothermia
- Hypothyroidism
- Hyperkalemia

Cardiac diseases associated with bradyarrhythmias are infiltrative heart disease (sarcoid, amyloid), degenerative disease of the cardiac conduction system, ischemic heart disease, Lyme disease, and rheumatic heart disease. Degenerative disease of the conduction system is seen most often in the elderly. It may be isolated to the conduction system (Lenègre disease) or represent generalized calcification of the cardiac skeleton that includes aortic and mitral valve involvement (Lev disease).

Commonly used cardiac **medications** slow cardiac conduction and may result in bradyarrhythmias:

- β-Blockers
- Calcium channel blockers
- Digoxin

CLINICAL MANIFESTATIONS

HISTORY

The presence of symptoms with an associated bradyarrhythmia often determines the extent of treatment. Symptoms, which may be the result of cardiac or central nervous system (CNS) hypoperfusion, include:

- Syncope
- Near-syncope or light-headedness
- Dyspnea (caused by congestive heart failure [CHF])
- Angina pectoris

Nonspecific symptoms, such as fatigue, must not be overinterpreted in the setting of bradycardia.

PHYSICAL EXAMINATION

Vital signs determine the severity of the bradyarrhythmia and assist in identifying the cause. Hypotension

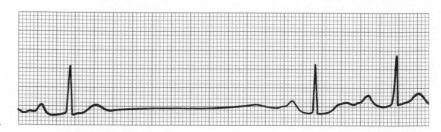

Figure 6-1 • Sick sinus syndrome.

(systolic blood pressure [BP] <90) is evidence of hemodynamic instability and requires emergency treatment when associated with symptoms.

DIFFERENTIAL DIAGNOSIS

The differential diagnosis of a bradyarrhythmia may be classified by the regularity of the HR.

Regular Rate
• Sinus bradycardia
• Complete heart block
• 2:1 AV block
• Sinus arrest with escape rhythm
• "Regularized" slow atrial fibrillation

Irregular Rate
• Sick sinus syndrome (sinus node dysfunction)
• Second-degree atrioventricular (AV) block (type I or II)
• Slow atrial fibrillation

DIAGNOSTIC EVALUATION

An **electrocardiogram** (ECG) is the first diagnostic test, and should be assessed in correlation with symptoms. One should first look for the **presence of P waves**. The absence of a P wave may indicate failure of the sinoatrial (SA) node to fire (sinus arrest) or failure of the SA node to excite the atria (sinus exit block).

These two conditions are indistinguishable by surface ECG and constitute the **sick sinus syndrome (a.k.a. sinus node dysfunction)**. The entire PQRST complex is absent (Fig. 6-1). If the syndrome is advanced, an escape rhythm (junctional or ventricular) may appear. Sinus node dysfunction is a common cause of bradycardia and contributes to approximately half of all pacemaker placements.

P waves are also completely absent in atrial fibrillation, where no organized atrial activity is present. Uncontrolled atrial fibrillation usually results in an irregular tachycardia with HRs of 80 to 140 bpm, but intrinsic AV node disease or nodal agents (β-blockers, calcium channel blockers) may slow the rate to 40 to 60 bpm. Therefore, an irregular bradycardia with no P waves is diagnostic of **slow atrial fibrillation**. In **regularized atrial fibrillation**, complete heart block is present at the AV node, and a lower escape pacemaker begins to fire (resulting in a rate of 40 to 60 bpm). This particular rhythm is seen in digoxin toxicity.

If a P wave is identified, the **PR interval** should be measured for each beat. First-degree AV block causes prolongation of the PR interval (>200 msec); this does not generally cause symptoms, nor significant bradycardia. In second-degree AV block, PR prolongation leads to a blocked beat, so a QRS complex fails to follow a P wave. In **type I (Wenckebach) second-degree block**, the PR intervals progressively lengthen each beat before a P wave fails to conduct (Fig. 6-2).

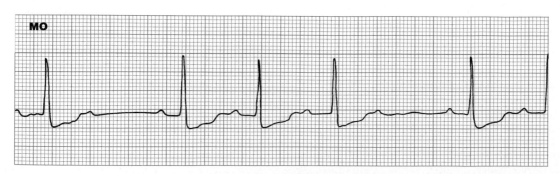

Figure 6-2 • Type I second-degree block. The PR interval progressively lengthens until the fourth P wave is not conducted.

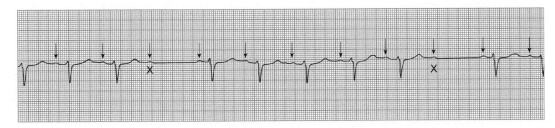

Figure 6-3 • Type II second-degree block. The "X" indicates a P wave suddenly not conducted.

This usually represents AV nodal disease. In **type II second-degree block**, the dropped beat occurs suddenly without warning, signifying infranodal disease (Fig. 6-3). Type II block has a higher risk of progression to complete heart block than type I block. If there is no relationship between the P waves and the QRS complex (variable PR interval), then **complete (third-degree) heart block** is likely to be present (Fig. 6-4). P waves, firing at a certain rate, fail to conduct to the ventricles, and a slower pacemaker begins to fire. Both atrial and ventricular rates are regular but are unrelated to each other in complete heart block.

TREATMENT

Acute treatment of bradyarrhythmia consists of treating the underlying cause (ischemia, infection, drugs, metabolic causes), if possible, and correcting the rhythm with medication or an extrinsic pacemaker. In treating the underlying cause, patients with evidence of cardiac ischemia should be treated with appropriate medications. Drugs that increase AV nodal block should be discontinued, and a digoxin level should be obtained in patients taking this medication. If hemodynamically stable (normal BP, no CHF or CNS dysfunction), patients may be observed for resolution of the bradyarrhythmia.

Emergent treatment with **atropine** is indicated in the patient with:

- Bradycardia causing hypotension
- CHF
- Syncope

Atropine, 0.5 mg, may be given intravenously or delivered through an endotracheal tube. It is most effective in bradyarrhythmias caused by increased vagal tone.

Cardiac pacemakers are used when a symptomatic bradycardia fails to resolve on its own or in response to atropine. They are also used when progression to complete heart block is likely. Pacemakers may be either temporary or permanent. If the aggravating factor is reversible (e.g., cardiac ischemia, Lyme disease), a temporary pacemaker may be inserted. Permanent pacemakers are used for patients who have degenerative conduction disease that will not improve. **Transcutaneous pacemakers** have replaced temporary IV pacemakers in many instances. Cutaneous electrodes are applied to the chest and back, and the heart is paced by applied current. The transcutaneous pacemaker may be used as a bridge to definitive therapy or as a safety net for patients who are stable but may progress to higher-degree block.

The indications for **permanent pacemaker** placement include:

- Complete heart block with symptoms
- Sinus node dysfunction with symptoms
- Bifascicular block with intermittent type II second-degree AV block

Other indications for a pacemaker are situation dependent. For example, type II second-degree AV block in the setting of a myocardial infarction (**MI**) generally requires a pacemaker because progression to complete heart block is common. Type I second-degree block (commonly seen in inferior MIs) may be observed because it often resolves. Pacemakers

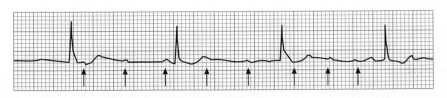

Figure 6-4 • Complete AV block. Arrows indicate regular P waves with no relation to QRS.

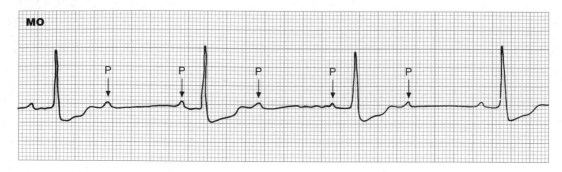

Figure 6-5 • Patients with 2:1 AV block.

are **not indicated** for asymptomatic type I second-degree AV block or asymptomatic sinus node dysfunction.

Patients with asymptomatic bradyarrhythmias should avoid drugs that may exacerbate the condition. Patients who develop symptoms should be considered for a pacemaker. Some patients may benefit from **electrophysiologic studies** to determine whether the conduction disturbance is at or below the AV node. These patients include those with 2:1 AV block (Fig. 6-5), in whom it is impossible to classify the disturbance as type I or type II. Patients with syncope and bundle branch or bifascicular block also may benefit from electrophysiologic studies.

 KEY POINTS

- A bradyarrhythmia is defined by the HR (<60 bpm) and the hemodynamic consequences (symptoms, hypotension). Asymptomatic low heart rate may not be pathologic.

- Digoxin toxicity should be considered in patients presenting with atrial fibrillation and a regular ventricular response.

- Type I second-degree block has progressively increasing PR intervals before a dropped QRS complex. This block often represents underlying AV nodal disease.

- Sick sinus syndrome (sinus node dysfunction) is a common cause of bradycardia, and placement of a permanent pacemaker is indicated for symptomatic patients.

- Pacemakers should not be inserted in patients with asymptomatic sinus node dysfunction or asymptomatic type I second-degree AV block.

- Pacemakers are indicated in type II second-degree AV block even when asymptomatic.

Tachyarrhythmias

Tachyarrhythmias are defined as heart rates exceeding 100 beats per minute (bpm). These rhythm disturbances are best divided into narrow complex tachycardias (QRS duration <0.12 second), which are almost always supraventricular in origin, and wide complex tachycardias, which may be supraventricular or ventricular. This classification helps determine the best treatment approach to a given arrhythmia.

ETIOLOGY AND PATHOGENESIS

Tachyarrhythmias occur by one of two mechanisms: abnormal impulse formation (enhanced automaticity or triggered activity) and abnormal impulse propagation (reentry). **Enhanced automaticity** refers to an increased inherent rate of depolarization; that is, certain cardiac cells simply start beating faster. **Triggered activity** relates to electrical oscillations of a cell's membrane potential during or just after repolarization. These oscillations may reach threshold potential and result in premature depolarization.

Reentry is the most common cause of tachyarrhythmias and occurs when two conduction pathways exist (Fig. 7-1). One pathway is rapidly conducting but slowly repolarizing (the fast pathway), whereas the other is slowly conducting and rapidly repolarizing (the slow pathway). As a premature impulse enters the loop, it finds the fast pathway refractory and descends down the slow pathway. When it reaches the distal end of the slow pathway, it continues distally and also enters the fast pathway, which is no longer refractory. The impulse travels retrograde up the fast pathway and

reenters the loop when it reaches the proximal aspect of the slow pathway. The tachyarrhythmia is perpetuated by recurrent reentry into the circuit. Treatments that interrupt this circuit abruptly terminate the tachycardia.

Supraventricular tachycardias may arise from the atria, ventricles, or AV node (junctional). Ventricular tachycardias occur below the AV node. The specific tachycardias are discussed here.

RISK FACTORS

Risk factors for supraventricular tachycardia (SVT) include:

- Hyperthyroidism (atrial fibrillation [AF], ectopic atrial tachycardia)
- Hypertension (AF and atrial flutter)
- Mitral valve disease (AF)
- Chronic obstructive lung disease (multifocal atrial tachycardia)
- Postcardiac surgery (nonparoxysmal junctional tachycardia)

Risk factors for ventricular tachycardia (VT) include:

- Prior MI (monomorphic VT)
- Ischemia (polymorphic VT, ventricular fibrillation)
- Long QT syndrome (polymorphic VT/torsades de pointes)
- Type IA and III antiarrhythmics (Table 7-1), phenothiazines, tricyclic antidepressants (torsades de pointes)
- Hypomagnesemia, hypo- or hyperkalemia (polymorphic VT, ventricular fibrillation)

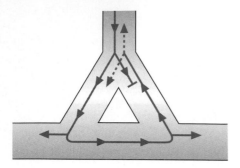

Figure 7-1 • Mechanism of reentry.

Digoxin, especially at toxic levels, can result in several characteristic arrhythmias, including:

- Paroxysmal atrial tachycardia with 2:1 AV block
- Regularized AF
- Bidirectional VT

CLINICAL MANIFESTATIONS

HISTORY

The patient with a tachyarrhythmia may be asymptomatic but frequently presents with:

- Dizziness or syncope
- Dyspnea
- Palpitations
- Diaphoresis
- Chest pain

These symptoms are not specific for a particular arrhythmia and therefore do not help in distinguishing between rhythms.

PHYSICAL EXAMINATION

Blood pressure (BP) should be measured immediately. **Hypotension** signifies a hemodynamically unstable arrhythmia that requires prompt therapy (see

Treatment). **Signs of AV dissociation**, such as cannon A waves and variability of the first heart sound, may help identify VT; AV dissociation is rarely present in SVTs.

DIFFERENTIAL DIAGNOSIS

Tachyarrhythmias should be categorized as supraventricular or ventricular in origin (on the basis of the presence or absence of P waves, and the width and morphology of the QRS on electrocardiogram [ECG]) and as regular or irregular in rhythm (this classification is used in the "Diagnostic Evaluation" section as well).

Regular SVTs include:

- Sinus tachycardia
- Ectopic atrial tachycardia
- Atrial flutter
- AV nodal reentrant tachycardia (AVNRT)
- AV reentrant tachycardias (AVRTs; e.g., Wolff-Parkinson-White [WPW] syndrome)
- Junctional tachycardia

Irregular SVTs include:

- AF
- Multifocal atrial tachycardia
- Atrial flutter with variable AV block

Ventricular tachyarrhythmias include:

- VT
- Ventricular fibrillation
- Torsades de pointes

DIAGNOSTIC EVALUATION

Figure 7-2 presents a general algorithm for the diagnosis of tachyarrhythmias.

ELECTROCARDIOGRAM

The ECG is most helpful when obtained during the tachyarrhythmia; however, the baseline ECG may also be of diagnostic use. For instance, in WPW syndrome, the baseline ECG in sinus rhythm demonstrates a short PR interval (<0.12 second) and a delta wave, a slurring of the initial deflection of the QRS complex (Fig. 7-3). The ECG during tachycardia should be carefully analyzed in regard to the regularity of the rhythm, the width and morphology of

■ **TABLE 7-1** Examples of Antiarrhythmics		
Type IA	**Type IC**	**Type III**
Procainamide	Flecainide	Sotalol
Quinidine	Encainide	Amiodarone
Disopyramide	Propafenone	

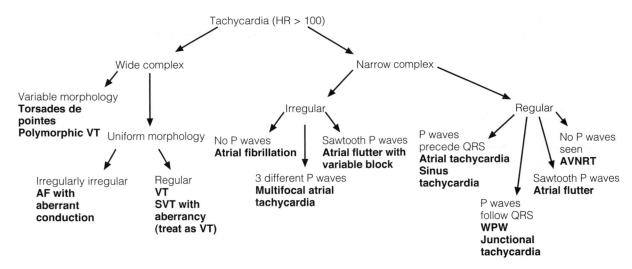

Figure 7-2 • An approach to tachycardia. The diagram shows a general algorithm for diagnosis; exceptions do occur. AF, atrial fibrillation; AVNRT, atrioventricular node reentrant tachycardia; SVT, supraventricular tachycardia; VT, ventricular tachycardia; WPW, Wolff-Parkinson-White syndrome.

the QRS complex, and the presence of P waves. Narrow QRS complex tachycardias are almost always SVT, whereas wide complex tachycardias may be VT or SVT with aberrant conduction.

REGULAR NARROW COMPLEX TACHYCARDIA

Once the tachyarrhythmia is classified as regular narrow complex, evidence of atrial activity (e.g., P waves, flutter waves) should be sought. P waves that **precede** the QRS complex are seen in sinus tachycardia and atrial tachycardia. P waves **will not be visible** or **will follow** the QRS complex in AVNRT, AVRT, and junctional tachycardia. Atrial flutter may present with a regular tachycardia, as flutter waves often conduct to the ventricles in a 2:1 pat-

tern. Waves of atrial flutter are described as "sawtooth." They are seen best in the inferior leads (II, III, aVF) and in V_1 and occur at a rate of 250 to 350 bpm (Fig. 7-4).

IRREGULAR NARROW COMPLEX TACHYCARDIA

Irregular narrow complex tachycardia also requires identifying atrial activity. Flutter waves of aproximately 300 bpm, may be conducted to the ventricles with variable (2:1, 3:1, or 4:1) AV block, thus resulting in an irregular rhythm. The presence of **P waves of three or more different morphologies** defines multifocal atrial tachycardia. The absence of P waves with an irregular ventricular response is consistent with AF.

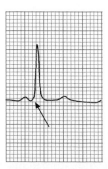

Figure 7-3 • Wolff-Parkinson-White syndrome.

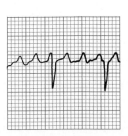

Figure 7-4 • Atrial flutter.

WIDE COMPLEX TACHYCARDIA

Wide complex tachycardias may be VT or SVT with aberrant conduction. Aberrant conduction during SVT may occur as a result of a baseline conduction abnormality (e.g., bundle branch block), a rate-related conduction abnormality, or conduction through an aberrant pathway (e.g., a bypass tract). Differentiating between VT and SVT with aberrancy can be difficult, but it is essential for the selection of appropriate therapy. ECG features that suggest VT include:

- Evidence of AV dissociation (P waves with no relation to QRS complex)
- QRS duration more than 160 msec
- Shift in QRS axis from baseline ECG
- Atypical bundle branch patterns

In the patient with known heart disease, wide complex tachycardias are most often VT (Fig. 7-5). When in doubt, it is best to err on the side of treating for VT. Torsades de pointes (French for "twisting of the points") is a form of polymorphic VT. It has a characteristic appearance on ECG (Fig. 7-6).

OTHER LABORATORY STUDIES

Underlying exacerbating conditions, such as **hypokalemia** or **hypomagnesemia**, should be excluded. A **digoxin level** should be ordered for patients taking this drug, especially when the rhythm is atrial tachycardia with 2:1 block or nonparoxysmal junctional tachycardia. **Thyroid-stimulating hormone** (TSH) level should be obtained in patients with AF to exclude hyperthyroidism. When the history is suggestive, toxin screening should be performed for **ethanol**, **cocaine**, and other cardio-irritants and stimulants.

TREATMENT: GENERAL PRINCIPLES

Synchronized countershock (cardioversion) is indicated in all patients in whom the tachyarrhythmia is associated with hemodynamic instability (hypoten-

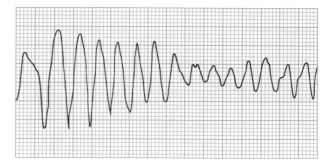

Figure 7-6 • Torsades de pointes.

sion, CHF, chest pain, decreased level of consciousness). The exceptions to use of defibrillation in the unstable patient are: torsades de pointes, in which **external pacing** to override the rhythm is the treatment of choice, and digoxin toxicity with junctional tachycardia.

In patients with hemodynamically stable SVT, maneuvers or medications that block the AV node are the treatments of choice. These include:

- Vagal maneuvers (Valsalva, carotid sinus massage)
- Adenosine
- β-Blocking agents (e.g., metoprolol, atenolol)
- Calcium channel antagonists (e.g., verapamil, diltiazem)
- Digoxin

For rhythms that are independent of the AV node (e.g., AF, atrial flutter, atrial tachycardia), these therapies will slow or block conduction through the AV node, thereby decreasing the ventricular response to the SVT and unmasking the atrial activity that may have previously been obscured by the rapid ventricular rate. For rhythms that are dependent on the AV node (AVNRT, AVRT), these therapies may terminate the arrhythmia. It is generally recommended to try vagal maneuvers before pharmacotherapy if the patient is stable. Pharmacotherapy is initially given intravenously to achieve rapid control of the HR associated with SVT. Adenosine is often used as a diagnostic (and therapeutic) agent for narrow complex tachycardias because of its marked effect on the AV node and its short duration of action ($t_{1/2} \cong 6$ seconds). Digoxin is less useful in the acute setting because of its delayed onset of action. β-Blockers may be best in situations in which adrenergic drive is contributing to the arrhythmia.

For patients with hemodynamically stable sustained VT, electrical cardioversion remains an op-

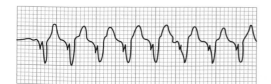

Figure 7-5 • Ventricular tachycardia.

tion. Chemical cardioversion may also be considered. Procainamide or sotalol are the drugs of choice when underlying ventricular function is normal, with lidocaine used as a second line agent. If there is underlying CHF, lidocaine or amiodarone are preferred. Lidocaine is given as a bolus (1 mg per kg), followed by an infusion of 1 to 4 mg per minute. Side effects include confusion and seizures.

TREATMENT: SPECIFIC ARRHYTHMIAS

Sinus tachycardia, multifocal atrial tachycardia, and junctional tachycardia are managed over the long term by correcting the underlying disease. Conditions that may require drug or interventional treatments are discussed in this section.

ATRIAL FIBRILLATION

The three main treatment concerns with AF are:

- Rate control
- Rhythm control
- Prevention of embolic events (i.e., cerebrovascular accident [CVA])

As noted earlier, the ventricular response to AF may be controlled with β-blockers, calcium channel antagonists, or digoxin. Amiodarone may be considered as an alternative to β-blockers and calcium channel blockers in patients with low EF.

When cardioversion to sinus rhythm is desired, electrical cardioversion is preferred. Because AF predisposes to intra-atrial thrombus formation and subsequent thromboembolism, the patient's risk for intra-atrial thrombus must be assessed prior to cardioversion. Patients at low risk for thrombus (AF duration <48 hours, no pior embolism, no valvular heart disease, preserved LVEF) may proceed directly to electrical cardioversion. All patients should first be anticoagulated for at least 3 weeks prior to cardioversion, and anticoagulation should continue for at least 4 weeks following cardioversion.

Unfortunately, AF is a recurrent problem in many patients, although continued treatment with antiarrhythmic agents increases the likelihood of maintaining sinus rhythm (amiodarone is the most effective agent in this regard). Increased left atrial size (more than 50 mm) and long duration of atrial fibrillation (more than 6 months) are predictors of relapse. More recently, outcome studies have not shown reduced embolic risk after cardioversion, and therefore simple rate control without attempted cardioversion is now a more common management choice. In the setting of AF with controlled heart rate, prevention of thromboembolism is a primary concern. Thromboembolism accounts for the 5% to 6% per year risk of CVA associated with AF, irrespective of whether it is paroxysmal or chronic AF. For this reason, anticoagulation with warfarin should be considered for almost all patients with AF (patients younger than 60 years with no other medical problems may be treated with aspirin). An international normalized ratio (INR) of 2 to 3 should be the goal of treatment.

ATRIAL FLUTTER

Atrial flutter is treated similarly to AF: rate control, rhythm control, and anticoagulation.

SUPRAVENTRICULAR REENTRANT TACHYCARDIAS

Patients with AVNRT or AVRT may be treated with AV nodal blocking agents, both acutely during the arrhythmia and to prevent recurrences. Catheter-based radiofrequency ablation of one arm of the reentrant loop offers definitive treatment, with a success rate of approximately 90%. This option may be best for young patients with recurrent symptoms and avoids lifelong drug therapy. Complications, such as procedure-related AV block or thromboembolism, may occur in rare instances.

Specific note should be made of AVRT. This arrhythmia is a reentrant rhythm that uses the AV node as one limb of the reentrant loop and an accessory pathway between the atria and ventricle as the other. The most common form of AVRT is WPW preexcitation syndrome. In sinus rhythm, atrial activity may reach the ventricles either through the AV node or via the accessory pathway. This may be evident on ECG by the presence of a delta wave (Fig. 7-3), representing ventricular preexcitation. Patients with WPW are prone to developing both AVRT and AF. The acute treatment of AVRT involves AV nodal blockade; however, the acute treatment of AF in patients with WPW should not include AV blockade because this will preferentially shunt the atrial activity down the accessory pathway at very rapid rates. The appropriate treatment of AF in the setting of WPW is procainamide or electrical cardioversion.

VENTRICULAR TACHYCARDIA

Ischemic heart disease often is the underlying cause of VT and should be appropriately evaluated and treated. Asymptomatic nonsustained VT (NSVT) in patients with preserved LV systolic function is usually treated with β-blocking agents. Patients with more malignant ventricular arrhythmias (symptomatic NSVT, sustained VT, VF) have a high risk of subsequent sudden cardiac death and require more aggressive therapy. In general, antiarrhythmic therapy is inadequate in this setting, and placement of an implantable cardioverter defibrillator (ICD) is required. Even with ICD placement, β-blocking agents or the class III agent sotalol may still be used to control symptoms and reduce the incidence of ICD firing. In patients who are believed to be at intermediate risk, electrophysiological studies may help guide therapy.

TORSADES DE POINTES

As noted earlier, torsades de pointes is a polymorphic VT and is almost always associated with a prolonged QT interval. **Causes of prolonged QT interval** are:

- Medications (type IA and III antiarrhythmics [see Table 7-1], phenothiazines, tricyclic antidepressants)
- Electrolyte disorders (hypokalemia, hypomagnesemia, hypocalcemia)
- Congenital long QT syndrome
- Ischemia

This rhythm tends to be self-limited but may be associated with hemodynamic instability if prolonged, and it may progress to ventricular fibrillation. Torsades de pointes is unique among the VTs in that acute treatment is with IV magnesium and overdrive pacing. Removal of the inciting agent is essential.

KEY POINTS

- Digitalis toxicity can lead to paroxysmal atrial tachycardia with 2:1 block or nonparoxysmal junctional tachycardia.

- The WPW syndrome is characterized by a short PR interval, delta wave, and AVRT. AV nodal blocking agents should be avoided when AF is present with WPW.

- AVNRT and AVRT should be treated initially with AV nodal blocking agents. Radiofrequency ablation should be considered for long-term management.

- Torsades de pointes is a multifocal VT, associated with a long QT interval. Treatment is overdrive pacing and magnesium.

- Adenosine is the drug of choice to treat regular narrow complex tachycardias after vagal maneuvers have been unsuccessful.

- Treatment of AF and atrial flutter involves rate control, rhythm control, and prevention of thromboembolism.

Hypertension

Hypertension is a major risk factor for the development of cardiovascular disease and affects up to 30% of people in developed countries. Uncontrolled hypertension may lead to multiorgan dysfunction, including stroke, heart disease, kidney failure, retinopathy, and peripheral vascular disease.

No biologic threshold separates normal from abnormally elevated blood pressure (BP); the cardiovascular risk of blood pressure increases linearly starting at a BP of 115/75. Hypertension has been somewhat arbitrarily defined as a persistent systolic BP >140 mm Hg or diastolic pressure >90 mm Hg, on two or more occasions (and at least three occasions prior to starting medication treatment). Isolated systolic hypertension has been traditionally defined as a systolic pressure >160 mm Hg with a diastolic pressure <90 mm Hg, but a systolic BP goal of <140 is now considered standard for all patients. Prehypertension is a newer category, which describes the levels between hypertension and optimal blood pressure. Hypertension can be further classified based on the absolute magnitude of the pressure elevation (Table 8-1).

EPIDEMIOLOGY AND RISK FACTORS

An estimated 20% to 30% of the American population has hypertension, with 2 million new cases diagnosed each year. However, the actual prevalence of hypertension depends on the definition used and the population studied. For example, in the Framingham study of a predominantly white suburban population, nearly half of the cohort had at least stage 1 hypertension. Among patients with hypertension, 75% have stage 1 disease, and only 25% to 30% are optimally controlled on their present medications. Furthermore, 30% of patients are unaware they have hypertension.

Various risk factors for the development of hypertension have been identified and include:

- Increasing age
- Smoking
- Male sex
- Race (African Americans more than whites)
- Obesity
- Family history of hypertension
- High sodium intake (applies more to populations than individuals)
- Ethanol intake
- Psychological stress

ETIOLOGY AND PATHOPHYSIOLOGY

More than 95% of hypertensive individuals have **essential hypertension**; that is, they do not have an identifiable etiology for their elevated pressure. Current research has suggested that most hypertension results from the interplay of a large number of physiologic and environmental factors (see the list of risk factors given earlier); thus, essential hypertension is a bit of a misnomer. However, the concept is still useful to distinguish essential hypertension from hypertension in which there is a well-defined etiology (i.e., secondary hypertension).

Major **causes of secondary hypertension** include:

- Renovascular disease (atherosclerosis, fibromuscular dysplasia)
- Intrinsic kidney disease (e.g., glomerulonephritis, polycystic kidney disease)

■ TABLE 8-1 Staging of Hypertension

	Systolic BP (mm Hg)		Diastolic BP (mm Hg)
Normal	<120	*and*	<80
Prehypertension	120 to 139	*or*	80 to 89
Stage 1 hypertension	140 to 159	*or*	90 to 99
Stage 2 hypertension	≥160	*or*	≥100

- Primary aldosteronism
- Pheochromocytoma
- Cushing syndrome
- Hyper- or hypothyroidism
- Obstructive sleep apnea
- Coarctation of the aorta
- Drugs (e.g., oral contraceptives, alcohol)

Suspicion of secondary hypertension should be increased in patients with the following characteristics:

- Age of onset <20 years or >50 years
- No family history of hypertension
- Severe, rapid acceleration of hypertension
- Hypertension refractory to maximal therapy with three or more medications

Poorly controlled hypertension may result in **complications** in a number of organ systems, including:

- Cardiac (myocardial infarction, congestive heart failure, ventricular hypertrophy)
- Cerebrovascular (stroke, intracerebral hemorrhage)
- Vascular (peripheral vascular disease including limb ischemia, aortic dissection)
- Renal (acute/chronic renal failure)
- Ophthalmologic (retinopathy, blindness)

CLINICAL MANIFESTATIONS

HISTORY

Most newly diagnosed hypertensive patients are **asymptomatic** but may report a family history of hypertension. History should assess for secondary causes in appropriate patients, including symptoms of thyroid disease (changes of skin, hair, and heat/cold tolerance); obstructive sleep apnea (morning headache, daytime sleepiness); and kidney disease (flank pain of polycystic kidney disease or urinary pattern changes). About two-thirds of patients with pheochromocytoma will have the classic **spells**, which can be remembered by the seven "P's": pounding (headache), perspiration,

palpitations, pallor, pyrexia, (blood) pressure elevations, and postural symptoms. These spells often last 10 to 60 minutes.

A complete history should also assess the patient's sodium intake and activity level, alcohol intake, over-the-counter or illicit drug use, and cardiovascular risk factors.

In the symptomatic patient, symptoms reflect **target-organ damage**:

- Cardiac (chest pain, dyspnea)
- Neurologic (headache, confusion, numbness, and weakness)
- Aortic and peripheral vascular (chest pain, claudication)
- Ocular (visual changes)
- Peripheral edema (may reflect nephrosis or heart failure)

PHYSICAL EXAMINATION

The most important aspect of the physical examination is the accurate measurement of **blood pressure**. The patient should be resting in the seated position for at least five minutes, and the arm should be supported at the level of the heart. Systolic blood pressure is defined as the pressure where the first sound is heard; diastolic blood pressure is the pressure when sound disappears. The remainder of the physical examination should focus on recognition of target-organ damage and clues of secondary causes. The major manifestations of **target-organ damage** include:

- Cardiac (e.g., left ventricular heave, S_4, pulmonary or peripheral edema)
- Cerebrovascular (e.g., carotid bruits, neurologic deficits)
- Peripheral vascular (e.g., diminished pulses, aneurysms)
- Ocular (e.g., arteriovenous nicking, hemorrhages, exudates, papilledema) (see Color Plate 1)
- Renal (e.g., peripheral edema, renal bruits)

Clues to the presence of a secondary cause of hypertension relate to the underlying condition. Examples are violaceous striae in Cushing disease, thyroid abnormalities in hypo- or hyperthyroidism, renal masses in polycystic kidney disease, and the presence of renal bruits in renovascular disease.

DIAGNOSTIC EVALUATION

Laboratory studies focus on defining the presence and extent of target-organ damage and identifying secondary causes. A generally accepted panel of **initial laboratory studies** to be used when evaluating a newly diagnosed hypertensive patient includes:

- Serum creatinine, potassium and glucose
- Fasting lipid profile
- Urinalysis (including assessment of proteinuria and microalbuminuria)
- Electrocardiogram

This relatively simple and inexpensive panel defines end-organ damage (renal failure, heart disease), assesses overall cardiac risk and suggests possible secondary etiologies (e.g., hypokalemia in primary aldosteronism). Assessment of thyroid function (e.g., TSH) should also be considered. Limited echocardiography to assess for left ventricular hypertrophy should be ordered only when clinical decision making is affected.

The patient with hypertension and hypokalemia, as well as the patient with difficult to control blood pressure, should be evaluated for primary aldosteronism. The key feature is a suppressed renin level (from excess aldosterone production). A **ratio of aldosterone to plasma renin activity** (PRA) of greater than 20 is suggestive of primary aldosteronism. Attempts are then made to suppress the excess aldosterone level with a high-sodium diet. Continued high aldosterone levels (on urine collection) confirm the diagnosis. If primary hyperaldosteronism is confirmed, an abdominal CT is obtained to look for an adrenal adenoma (seen in about 30% of cases).

Testing for pheochromocytoma should be pursued if the patient has difficult to control blood pressure, "spells" of palpitations, headache, and marked elevation in blood pressure, or a suggestive family history (e.g., multiple endocrine neoplasia syndrome). No single test is usually adequate, but the high sensitivity of **plasma metanephrines** (measured while patient is resting comfortably) makes this a useful initial test. If normal, pheochromocytoma is very unlikely. If elevated, urinary catecholamines and metanephrines may be measured. Careful attention must be paid to the numerous medications (including antihypertensives such as labetalol) that interfere with these urinary tests.

More specialized tests for other secondary causes should be undertaken as suggested by the history and physical. Patients with renal insufficiency and/or vascular disease may have atherosclerotic renal stenosis. Magnetic resonance angiography (MRA) or Doppler ultrasound of the renal arteries can diagnose this condition. In younger women (age less than 40) with new onset hypertension, fibromuscular dysplasia may be suggested by Doppler ultrasound, although angiography is often required for definitive diagnosis.

TREATMENT

The treatment of patients with secondary causes of hypertension is directed at correction of the underlying disorder. Endocrine dysfunction should be treated, pheochromocytomas and adrenal adenomas resected, and aggravating drugs and medications discontinued. Revascularization should be considered for patients with renal artery stenosis, although this rarely results in complete resolution of hypertension.

For patients with essential hypertension or uncorrected secondary hypertension, antihypertensive therapy is initiated with the aim of reducing the patient's risk of target-organ damage by lowering BP to established goal levels. Generally, accepted goals include:

- BP <140/90 mm Hg in patients with uncomplicated hypertension
- BP <130/80 mm Hg in patients with renal failure, heart failure, or diabetes

For patients with isolated systolic hypertension (baseline diastolic BP <90), treatment should avoid lowering the diastolic BP below 65 because low diastolic pressures in such patients are associated with increased stroke risk.

Goal BPs should be achieved through graduated, stepwise interventions, taking into consideration a variety of specific factors (see later). The exception to this gradual approach is in the setting of **hypertensive emergencies**, including:

- Hypertensive encephalopathy
- Intracranial hemorrhage
- Acute myocardial infarction
- Acute pulmonary edema
- Aortic dissection

In these cases, rapid lowering of BP is necessary and usually requires parenteral therapy and monitoring in the intensive care setting. Intravenous medications for hypertensive emergencies include labetalol (combined α/β-blocker), nicardipine (calcium channel blocker), or fenoldopam (dopamine-1 agonist). The initial goal reduction in mean arterial pressure is approximately 25%. β-Blockers are a necessary therapy for patients with aortic dissection to decrease wall stress.

In the absence of symptoms or evidence of acute target-organ injury, most other hypertensive patients can be managed in the outpatient setting. As a first intervention for gradual BP reduction, **nonpharmacologic modalities** may be effective. Their use is encouraged in all hypertensive patients and, in some patients with prehypertension or stage 1 hypertension, they may be effective as isolated therapy. These modalities mostly consist of lifestyle changes and include:

- Weight reduction
- Smoking cessation
- Sodium restriction (2 to 3 grams per day)
- Regular physical exercise
- Stress reduction
- Lowering or discontinuing alcohol intake

The Joint National Committee on the Prevention, Detection, Evaluation, and Treatment of High Blood Pressure has established guidelines regarding the institution of therapy for hypertensive patients. All hypertensive patients should be treated with lifestyle modification as part of their therapeutic regimen. Antihypertensive medications should be started in patients who do not attain goal BP levels after 6 to 12 months of nonpharmacologic therapy. Antihypertensive agents should also be started in all patients with stage 2 hypertension (BP more than 160/more than 100) and in all patients with target-organ damage, CAD, or diabetes who have a BP >130/80 mm Hg.

Antihypertensive **medications** fall into several major classes (Table 8-2):

- Diuretics
- Angiotensin-converting enzyme (ACE) inhibitors and angiotensin II receptor blockers (ARBs)
- Adrenergic blocking agents (alpha-1 and β-blockers)
- Calcium channel blockers
- Vasodilators (e.g., hydralazine)
- Centrally acting agents (e.g., clonidine, methyl-dopa)

There are many things to consider when choosing a specific antihypertensive agent. Low-dose thiazide diuretics are preferred initial agents because they have a proven beneficial effect on mortality and morbidity, and they are well tolerated as well as cost effective. ACE inhibitors or ARBs are first-line therapy for patients with diabetes, proteinuric kidney disease, and cardiovascular diseases. ACE inhibitors or ARBs also work synergistically with thiazide diuretics for BP

■ **TABLE 8-2** Antihypertensive Medications			
Medication Class	**Mechanism**	**Examples (starting dosages)**	**Side Effects**
Diuretics	Increased urinary sodium excretion	Hydrochlorothiazide 12.5 to 25 mg daily	Urinary frequency Muscle cramps
ACE inhibitors	Decreased angiotensin II production	Lisinopril 5 to 10 mg daily Captopril 12.5 to 25 mg t.i.d.	Cough Angioedema (0.05%)
Angiotensin II receptor blockers	Blockade of angiotensin II receptor	Losartan 25 mg daily Valsartan 80 mg daily	Dizziness
β-Blockers	Blockade of beta-1 receptors	Atenolol 25 to 50 mg daily Metoprolol 25 to 50 mg b.i.d.	Bradycardia Sexual dysfunction
Calcium channel blockers	Direct vasodilation	Nifedipine XL 30 to 60 mg daily Amlodipine 5 mg daily	Edema
Alpha-1 antagonists	Blockade of peripheral alpha-1 receptors	Doxazosin 2 mg daily Terazosin 2 mg daily	Orthostatic hypotension
Direct vasodilators	Direct vasodilation	Hydralazine 25 mg four times daily	Hypotension, headache
Alpha-2 agonists	Decreased sympathetic output	Clonidine 0.1 mg daily	Orthostatic hypotension, dry mouth

control, so they are often used together as initial therapy. Aldosterone antagonists (e.g., spironolactone) are used to treat primary aldosteronism. β-Blockers are added for patients with coexisting CAD, a history of MI, or compensated heart failure because of their mortality benefit in these settings. However, the overall effectiveness of β-blockers as monotherapy for hypertension has recently been questioned.

Several recommended strategies should be considered once the decision has been made to start antihypertensive medication:

- Maintain lifestyle modifications irrespective of the effect of pharmacologic therapy.
- Start medications at lower doses and titrate every 1 to 2 weeks as needed.
- If there is an inadequate response to therapy, (a) increase drug dosage *or* (b) substitute another drug if the first agent is ineffective at high doses *or* (c) add a second agent from a different class if the first agent is effective but the patient is not yet at the goal BP.
- If there is still not an adequate response, add a second or third agent (include a diuretic if one is not already prescribed).

Using this aggressive approach, ideal BP control is achievable in 75% to 80% of patients. However, on average it takes three to four medications to attain the goal BP.

In the patient with refractory hypertension (poor control to 3 or more medications), the following possibilities are considered:

- Nonadherence to low sodium diet or medications
- Medication interaction (nonsteroidal anti-inflammatory drugs, oral contraceptives, corticosteroids)
- Secondary hypertension

FOLLOW UP

Patients on antihypertensive therapy should have regular assessment of electrolytes and renal function. An electrocardiogram and urinalysis can be periodically monitored to assess for end-organ damage. Additional cardiovascular risk factors (smoking, high cholesterol, diabetes) should also be treated.

KEY POINTS

- Optimal blood pressure is 120/80 or less. Hypertension is defined as blood pressure over 140/90.
- Uncontrolled hypertension results in injury to the heart (MI, heart failure); vasculature (peripheral vascular disease, aortic dissection); brain (encephalopathy, stroke); kidneys (renal failure); and eyes (retinopathy).
- In most (more than 95%) hypertensive patients, no single etiology for hypertension can be found. Secondary causes include primary hyperaldosteronism, pheochromocytoma, sleep apnea, renal artery stenosis, and medications.
- Initial treatment of stage 1 hypertension includes nonpharmacologic measures (low sodium diet, exercise, and weight reduction). Initial pharmacologic therapy should begin with a thiazide diuretic. ACE inhibitors are appropriate first line agents for patients with diabetes, heart disease, or proteinuria.

Valvular Heart Disease

Valvular heart disease in the **adult** population is usually the result of **acquired valvular defects**. This is in contrast to the situation in the **pediatric** population, in which **congenital defects** predominate. Valvular abnormalities result in either valvular thickening with limitation of forward blood flow (stenotic lesions) or valvular incompetence with resultant reversal of blood flow (regurgitation). The most commonly affected valves are the aortic and mitral valves. This chapter focuses on the major clinical entities of aortic stenosis (AS), aortic regurgitation (AR), mitral stenosis (MS), and mitral regurgitation (MR).

EPIDEMIOLOGY

Acquired AS is three times more common in men than in women. AR is likewise more common in men, whereas MS is more common in women. Rheumatic MR is more common in men; nonrheumatic MR is more common in women. Patients with congenital valve disease frequently develop symptoms in infancy or childhood, but they may be asymptomatic until their third or fourth decade of life. Rheumatic valve diseases tend to cause symptoms by the fourth to fifth decades of life, whereas degenerative valve diseases tend to present one to two decades later.

ETIOLOGY

Historically, the most common cause of valvular heart disease was **rheumatic fever**. Although the inci-

dence of acute rheumatic fever has declined in the United States, rheumatic fever remains a worldwide problem and therefore remains the major cause of acquired valvular disease in the world. Acute rheumatic fever produces a chronic inflammatory valvulitis resulting in **thickening of the valve apparatus and retraction of the valve leaflets**. These changes predispose to malcoaptation of the leaflets during valve closure and development of regurgitation. Furthermore, progressive valvular scarring and **fusion of the valve leaflets** lead to progressive impairment of valve opening with resultant stenosis. The mitral valve is most commonly affected, followed in decreasing order by combined mitral and aortic valve involvement, isolated aortic valve involvement, and then tricuspid (almost always with associated mitral) valve involvement. The pulmonic valve is rarely affected. Rheumatic valves are prone to infection (**infective endocarditis**), which in turn can result in further valvular degeneration.

Other common disorders associated with specific valvular lesions include the following:

Aortic Stenosis
- Congenitally bicuspid valve
- Rheumatic fever
- Calcific (senile) degeneration

Aortic Regurgitation
- Congenitally bicuspid valve
- Infective endocarditis
- Rheumatic fever
- Aneurysm of the aortic root (e.g., Marfan syndrome, syphilitic aortitis, spondyloarthropathies)
- Connective tissue disease (e.g., systemic lupus erythematosus)

Mitral Stenosis
- Rheumatic fever
- Mitral annular calcification
- Iatrogenic (following mitral valve repair or replacement)

Mitral Regurgitation
- Mitral valve prolapse (the most common cause of MR requiring surgery)
- Myocardial infarction or ischemia (papillary muscle dysfunction)
- Infective endocarditis
- Rheumatic fever
- Left ventricular (LV) dilatation

PATHOGENESIS

In general, **stenotic** valvular lesions lead to a state of **pressure overload**, whereas **regurgitant** lesions cause **volume overload**. The following pathophysiologic changes occur in **response** to various valvular diseases:

Aortic Stenosis
- Elevated LV systolic and diastolic pressure
- Concentric hypertrophy (initial response to elevated pressures)
- Left atrial enlargement (secondary to increased LV diastolic pressure)
- Decreased LV systolic function (late)

Aortic Regurgitaton
- LV dilatation (primary response to volume overload)
- LV hypertrophy (secondary response)
- Decreased LV systolic function (late)

Mitral Stenosis
- LA enlargement (early; frequently associated with subsequent atrial fibrillation [AF])
- Pulmonary venous congestion (early)
- Pulmonary hypertension (late)
- Right ventricular (RV) hypertrophy and failure (late; secondary to pulmonary hypertension)

Mitral Regurgitaton
- Left atrial (LA) enlargement (early; also frequently associated with AF)
- Pulmonary congestion (late in chronic MR; early in acute MR)
- Pulmonary hypertension (late)
- LV failure (late because LV is no longer able to compensate for regurgitant flow by increased systolic emptying)

- RV failure (late; secondary to pulmonary hypertension)

Note that most of the changes just listed occur only if the valvular abnormality develops slowly over time, as is the case in rheumatic heart disease. Initially, these responses are compensatory but only at the eventual cost of chamber failure. Stenotic lesions develop slowly, whereas regurgitant lesions may be acute or chronic. If valvular dysfunction occurs rapidly (as in acute AR or MR from infective endocarditis or acute MR in the setting of MI), there is no time for compensatory responses to develop. In this setting, an acute elevation in pulmonary pressure occurs, resulting in acute pulmonary edema.

CLINICAL MANIFESTATIONS

HISTORY

In a patient with valvular disease, a thorough history may give etiologic clues. Murmurs present since childhood often reflect congenital valvular disease. A history of rheumatic fever is an important finding. A history of recent dental work or invasive procedures should prompt consideration of endocarditis. Patients with associated chest pain should be carefully questioned because this symptom may be related to the valve disorder or to concomitant coronary artery disease (CAD). Patients should be questioned in regard to their exercise capacity because symptoms may be masked by inactivity. Dyspnea is common to all left-sided valvular disorders due to the elevated pulmonary pressures these lesions eventually cause.

The **symptoms** common in each valvular lesion are as follows:

Aortic Stenosis
- Exertional angina related to increased LV pressure or concomitant CAD (associated with life expectancy of approximately 5 years without surgical therapy)
- Effort-related syncope (associated with life expectancy of approximately 3 years without surgical therapy)
- Dyspnea resulting from LV systolic and/or diastolic dysfunction (associated with life expectancy of approximately 1 to 2 years without surgical therapy)

Aortic Regurgitation
- Forceful heartbeat/palpitations (because of increased LV stroke volume)

- Exertional dyspnea (resulting from LV systolic and/or diastolic dysfunction)
- Angina

Mitral Stenosis
- Exertional dyspnea (because of elevated pulmonary pressure)
- Palpitations (because of atrial ectopy or fibrillation)
- Hemoptysis

Mitral Regurgitation
- Dyspnea (with chronic MR)
- Pulmonary edema (with acute MR)
- Palpitations (because of AF)
- Fatigue, chest pain, palpitations, presyncope (the mitral valve prolapse syndrome)

Patients with valvular disease may present with symptoms or syndromes that are indirectly related to valve dysfunction. Embolic phenomena (e.g., transient ischemic attack [TIA], CVA, peripheral emboli) may result from associated AF but can also occur without atrial arrhythmias in patients with rheumatic disease or severe LV dysfunction.

PHYSICAL EXAMINATION

Table 9-1 outlines the classic physical findings in valvular heart disease. In addition, several specific features are important to note, according to the clinical entity.

Aortic Stenosis
- The more severe the stenosis, the longer it takes for the systolic murmur to reach peak intensity.
- Severe AS is associated with a late-peaking murmur, diminished and delayed carotid pulses (*pulsus parvus et tardus*), and a single S_2.

■ TABLE 9-1 Clinical and Diagnostic Features of Valvular Lesions

	Aortic Stenosis	Aortic Regurgitation	Mitral Stenosis	Mitral Regurgitation
Etiologic factors	RF, bicuspid valve, degeneration	RF, aortic root dilation, endocarditis	RF	RF, myocardial infarction, dilated cardiomyopathy
Age at presentation (years)	30 to 40 (rheumatic), 40 to 50 (bicuspid), >60 (degenerative)	Variable depending on etiology	20 to 50	Variable depending on etiology
Gender preference	4:1 male-female (rheumatic)	None	2:1 female-male	None
Symptoms	Angina, dyspnea, syncope	Dyspnea on exertion, CHF	Dyspnea on exertion, CHF, palpitations	CHF
Murmur	Systolic, crescendo-decrescendo, at upper sternal border	Decrescendo diastolic "blow," parasternal	Diastolic rumble at LV apex	Holosystolic at LV apex, radiates to axilla
Associated physical findings	Sustained apical impulse, single S_2, pulses parvus et tardus	Peripheral signs of increased pulse pressure (see text)	Opening snap, presystolic accentuation of diastolic rumble	Midsystolic click (with MVP)
ECG	LVH, LAE, LAD	LVH	L + RAE, RVH, AF	LAE, AF
Chest radiograph	Dilated aortic root, calcified aortic valve	Dilated LV	LAE, pulmonary hypertension	LAE, dilated LV

AF, atrial fibrillation; CHF, congestive heart failure; LAD, left axis deviation; LAE, left atrial enlargement; LV, left ventricle; LVH, left ventricular hypertrophy; MVP, mitral valve prolapse; RAE, right atrial enlargement; RF, rheumatic fever; RVH, right ventricular hypertrophy.

- Bicuspid AS may be associated with an early systolic click.

Aortic Regurgitation
- AR may be associated with a diastolic rumble at the apex due to functional mitral stenosis from the regurgitant jet (Austin Flint murmur).
- Peripheral manifestations reflect increased pulse pressure:
  - Pulsatile flow in nail beds (Quincke pulses)
  - Head bobbing (de Musset sign)
  - Rapidly rising and falling carotid pulse (Corrigan pulse)
  - To-and-fro bruit over the femoral artery (Duroziez sign)
  - Bobbing uvula (Müller sign)

Mitral Stenosis
- As the severity of MS increases, the interval between S_2 and the opening snap decreases (due to higher left atrial pressure).
- There is presystolic accentuation of the diastolic rumble in patients in sinus rhythm.

Mitral Regurgitation
- Mitral valve prolapse is associated with a mid-systolic click followed by a mid to late systolic murmur.

DIFFERENTIAL DIAGNOSIS

Many of the symptoms of valvular disease are nonspecific. Chest pain from AS or MS may mimic angina. The dyspnea associated with valvular disease is indistinguishable from that caused by other cardiac disorders (e.g., hypertension, cardiomyopathy). High-output states (e.g., anemia, pregnancy) can result in dyspnea and chest pain and may be associated with a systolic flow murmur, thereby mimicking AS. However, a thorough history and physical examination usually limits the differential diagnosis.

Valvular AS needs to be differentiated from supravalvular AS (rare in adults) and subvalvular AS (most commonly caused by a subvalvular membrane or obstructive hypertrophic cardiomyopathy). The murmur of obstructive **hypertrophic cardiomyopathy** (HCM) begins later (after S_1) than does the murmur of valvular AS because early systolic flow in HCM is fairly unimpeded. Also, with HCM, the obstruction is dynamic, not fixed, and any interventions that increase myocardial contractility (such as exercise) or decrease LV volume (such as Valsalva maneuver) will increase the obstructive gradient and therefore the murmur.

DIAGNOSTIC EVALUATION

The principal initial studies are the **electrocardiogram**, **chest radiograph**, and **echocardiogram**. The latter is indicated when the history, physical examination, ECG, and/or chest film is highly suggestive of valvular disease. The detection of a diastolic murmur or holosystolic murmur warrants echocardiography. A mid-systolic murmur is often an ejection murmur in the young or aortic sclerosis in the elderly. Evaluation is needed only if the patient has symptoms, or if there are other findings of cardiac disease (such as left ventricular hypertrophy).

Echocardiography is useful not only in determining the presence of valvular disease but also in **assessing the severity of the lesion**, quantifying LV function, estimating valvular calcification, assessing valve mobility, and identifying associated abnormalities. Serial echocardiograms (every 6 to 12 months) are used to follow disease progression. Regurgitant lesions are graded on a scale of 1 (mild) to 4 (severe). Stenotic lesions are graded based on the associated valve area. The normal aortic valve (AV) is approximately 3.5 cm². An AV area of 1.0 to 1.5 cm² reflects mild AS, 0.8 to 1.0 cm² reflects moderate AS, and <0.8 cm² reflects severe AS. The AS is often termed *critical* if its area is 0.6 cm² or less. The normal mitral valve area is 3.5 to 4.5 cm². Mild MS is defined as a valve area of 1.5 to 2.0 cm², moderate MS as 1.0 to 1.5 cm², and severe MS as <1.0 cm².

Once valve replacement surgery becomes necessary (see later), **cardiac catheterization** is performed. This allows for direct measurement of transvalvular pressure gradients, calculation of stenotic valve area, assessment of intraventricular and pulmonary pressures, and identification of concomitant coronary artery disease (Fig. 9-1).

TREATMENT

The treatment of mild to moderate valvular disease is usually conservative, especially in the absence of symptoms. **Mitral stenosis** impairs diastolic LV filling. Initial medical therapy involves heart rate control, especially in patients with AF (bradycardia prolongs diastole and improves LV filling). This can be achieved with β-blockers or calcium channel blockers. Diuretics are frequently added to control symptoms of pulmonary congestion. Patients with acutely symptomatic **mitral regurgitation** can be treated with afterload reduction using nitroprusside or hydralazine, and they frequently

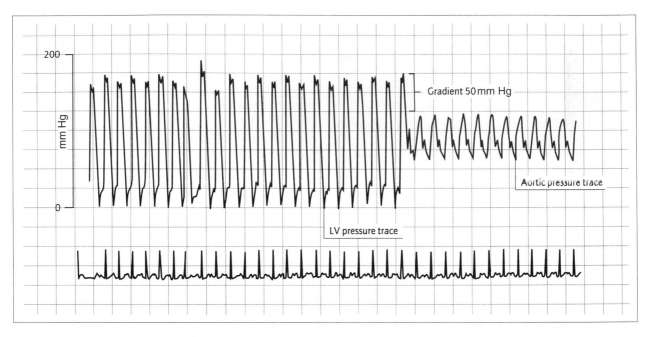

Figure 9-1 • The pressure trace on catheter withdrawal across a stenosed aortic valve at cardiac catheterization.

require diuretic therapy. Medical management for symptomatic MR is less effective than surgical therapy, however, and symptomatic control with chronic medications should be considered only for patients who are not surgical candidates. Afterload reducing vasodilators for chronic symptomatic MR include angiotensin-converting enzyme (ACE) inhibitors, angiotensin II receptor blockers, or the combination of hydralazine/nitrates. Medical therapy for **aortic regurgitation** includes afterload reduction with ACE inhibitors or vasodilating calcium channel blockers. These agents may decrease the regurgitant volume and delay the need for surgery, but the studies are conflicting. Patients with AR who are not surgical candidates otherwise need standard treatment for heart failure (see Chapter 5). No effective medical therapy for **aortic stenosis** is available, and several medications (nitrates, β-blockers, calcium channel blockers, ACE inhibitors) may precipitate hemodynamic instability in patients with severe or critical disease.

If medical management is pursued, patients should be monitored closely for signs and symptoms of clinical decompensation. If this occurs, the valve in question should be reassessed by echocardiogram, and if progressive disease is present, surgery should be considered.

Antibiotic prophylaxis against infective endocarditis is no longer recommend for patients with native valve disease, but is still required in patients who have undergone valve replacement (see Chapter 33).

Aggressive therapy of concomitant cardiac disease is essential. The treatment of chronic valvular-associated congestive heart failure (CHF) is the same as in other causes of CHF and includes ACE inhibitors, β-blockers, and diuretics, although care must be taken when using these agents in patients with AS. AF frequently complicates valvular heart disease and must be treated with rate control and anticoagulation (risk of thromboembolism is approximately 12% per year in patients with AF associated with rheumatic heart disease).

Acute AR or MR is poorly tolerated, frequently results in acute pulmonary edema, and requires urgent surgical treatment. **Indications for surgery** in patients with chronic valvular heart disease include the following:

Aortic Stenosis
- Symptomatic AS
- Asymptomatic critical AS or asymptomatic severe AS with associated LV dysfunction

Aortic Regurgitation
- Symptomatic moderate to severe AR
- Asymptomatic AR associated with progressive LV dilatation (LV end-systolic diameter >55 mm) or progressive LV dysfunction (LV ejection fraction <50%)

Mitral Stenosis
- Symptomatic moderate or severe MS
- Progressive pulmonary hypertension

Mitral Regurgitation
- Symptomatic severe MR
- Asymptomatic severe MR associated with LV dysfunction (LV ejection fraction <60%) or progressive LV dilatation (LV end-systolic diameter >45 mm)

Valve replacement is the most common surgical approach, although valve repair should be considered in patients with MR from mitral valve prolapse or endocarditis. If valve replacement is to be done, a choice needs to be made regarding use of a bioprosthesis (tissue valve) or mechanical prosthesis. The decision usually hinges on the age of the patient and the estimated risks of anticoagulation. Mechanical valves are extremely durable but require lifelong anticoagulation (INR 2.0 to 3.0 for most aortic valves, 2.5 to 3.5 for mitral valves). Available tissue valves (e.g., porcine valves) have a life expectancy of 10 to 15 years, but they do not require anticoagulation. Generally, mechanical valves are preferred. However, tissue valves are frequently placed in patients older than 75 years of age, women of child-bearing age, and patients with medical (e.g., bleeding) or psychosocial (e.g., noncompliance, patient preference) contraindications to anticoagulation. Following valve replacement, patients should be monitored for signs of prosthetic valve dysfunction. Aspirin (75 to 100 mg) should be given to patients with bioprosthetic valves and to patients with mechanical valves (in addition to warfarin) who also have risk factors for thromboembolism (atrial fibrillation, previous thromboembolism, LV dysfunction).

Percutaneous balloon valvuloplasty is a minimally invasive technique for management of stenotic valvular lesions. Although it is associated with relatively good results in certain cases of MS, balloon valvuloplasty for AS is associated with a high rate of early recurrence of AS as well as serious complications (stroke, aortic regurgitation, MI). Nonetheless, it may provide temporary relief of symptoms in patients with severe AS who are not surgical candidates, and it can provide urgent hemodynamic improvement for patients awaiting surgical intervention.

 KEY POINTS

- Degenerative valve disease has superseded rheumatic disease as the most common cause of valvular heart disease.
- Valvular lesions can be stenotic, leading to pressure overload; or regurgitant, resulting in volume overload.
- Systolic murmurs are heard in aortic stenosis and mitral regurgitation. Diastolic murmurs are heard in aortic regurgitation and mitral stenosis.
- Symptomatic valvular lesions require surgical intervention. Asymptomatic lesions can be followed closely and monitored with cardiac ultrasound.
- No effective medical therapy is available for symptomatic aortic stenosis. Vasodilators can be dangerous by lowering systemic pressure in the face of a fixed pressure gradient.

Vascular Disease

Cardiovascular disease comprises a very broad spectrum of diseases including coronary heart disease (CHD), peripheral vascular disease, and cerebrovascular disease. Cardiovascular disease is the most common cause of death in the United States and most other industrialized nations. This is in large part the result of CHD and cerebrovascular disease; however, diseases of the aorta and the peripheral vasculature contribute significantly to overall cardiovascular morbidity and mortality. Accordingly, this chapter reviews the diseases affecting the aorta and the peripheral vasculature. Cerebrovascular and carotid disease are discussed in Chapter 75.

EPIDEMIOLOGY

Cardiovascular disease accounts for approximately 900,000 deaths in the United States each year. The majority of these deaths are due to coronary artery disease (CAD) and cerebrovascular disease. However, aortic disease is responsible for 15,000 deaths per year, mostly due to ruptured aneurysms. In addition, peripheral arterial disease (PAD) is a strong predictor of underlying coronary disease. Angiography identifies coronary disease in about 90% of patients with PAD, and stress testing demonstrates reversible ischemia in about two-thirds. The highest incidence of peripheral arterial disease occurs in the sixth and seventh decades.

ETIOLOGY

The spectrum of vascular diseases arises from a variety of pathogenic mechanisms, the most common of which is atherosclerosis. Atherosclerotic plaque

formation (see Chapter 3) results in progressive vascular obstruction. The resultant reduction in distal blood flow predisposes to ischemia of the organs subserved by the diseased vessels. The atherosclerotic process may also produce vascular dilatation, resulting in the formation of **arterial aneurysms**. Aneurysms may be focal (saccular) or diffuse (fusiform). They may develop anywhere within the vascular tree; however, they are most common in the infrarenal aorta because of the absence of vasa vasorum in this region. As an aneurysm expands, it becomes more susceptible to rupture. Furthermore, the vascular intima in the region of the aneurysm is prone to tear, resulting in an **aortic dissection**. Propagation of the dissection flap along the course of the aorta may lead to occlusion of branch vessels, with resultant acute limb or organ ischemia. A similar process may occur following spontaneous rupture of the vasa vasorum within the aortic wall with subsequent hemorrhage into the aortic media (**intramural hematoma**).

Acute arterial occlusion can occur via **embolization**, in situ thrombosis, dissection, or trauma. Arterial emboli may be thrombotic or atherosclerotic and originate from cardiac or proximal vascular sources. Cardiac emboli are most common and arise from the left atrium (usually in the setting of atrial fibrillation); the aortic or mitral valves (in the setting of rheumatic or degenerative valvular disease, endocarditis, or from prosthetic valves); or the left ventricle (most often in the setting of ventricular dysfunction resulting from CAD). Rarely, thromboemboli may originate in the venous system and reach the systemic vasculature via an atrial or ventricular septal defect (paradoxical embolism). In situ thrombosis most often occurs at sites of preexisting atherosclerotic disease but can occur in relatively normal arteries in patients with coexisting hypercoagulable states (e.g., malignancy).

Arterial disease may also result from a variety of nonatherosclerotic disorders, including the following:

- Marfan syndrome, Ehlers-Danlos disease, bicuspid aortic valve, hypertension—result in cystic medial necrosis and predispose to aortic aneurysms and dissection
- Takayasu arteritis and giant cell arteritis—result in vasculitis of the aorta and its major branches
- Thromboangiitis obliterans—results in vasculitis of small and medium-size arteries of the extremities
- Infectious diseases (e.g., syphilis)—may cause ascending aortic aneurysms

RISK FACTORS

The same factors that predispose to the development of PAD are risk factors for the development of atherosclerotic vascular disease in general, and they include:

- Smoking
- Diabetes mellitus
- Hypertension
- Dyslipidemia
- Male gender
- Family history of vascular disease

CLINICAL MANIFESTATIONS

The clinical manifestations of vascular disease vary depending on the severity of the disease, the rapidity of its development, and the anatomic location of the vessel affected. Nonetheless, all of the manifestations reflect tissue ischemia.

HISTORY

Acute peripheral arterial occlusion results in acute limb ischemia, is a medical emergency, and is characterized clinically by the "six Ps":

- Pulselessness
- Pallor
- Poikilothermia (temperature of affected extremity varies with the ambient temperature)
- Pain
- Paralysis
- Paresthesia

In **acute mesenteric arterial occlusion**, the major clinical feature is severe diffuse abdominal pain, frequently out of proportion to findings on physical examination. **Chronic occlusive disease involving the mesenteric circulation** can manifest as **abdominal angina**, a syndrome of abdominal pain that occurs most often after a meal. Weight loss is common. Nausea, vomiting, and early satiety may also occur.

In **chronic peripheral arterial disease**, the most common symptom is **intermittent claudication**. Claudication is usually described as a muscular pain, aching, or numbness that occurs during exercise and is relieved by rest. It is to be distinguished from pseudo-claudication caused by lumbar spinal stenosis, which may result in similar discomfort but requires a change in position (e.g., sitting down) for resolution. Claudication is most common in the lower extremities because of the higher incidence of obstructive lesions in the distal aortic, iliac, and femoral systems. Aortoiliac disease may cause claudication in the buttocks and thighs and may be associated with impotence (Leriche syndrome), whereas femoral-popliteal disease results in calf claudication. As the degree of vascular obstruction increases, the symptoms progress, occurring with progressively less exertion until they occur at rest. Once pain occurs at rest, ischemic ulcers and frank gangrene can be the most prominent complaints.

Aortic aneurysms are usually asymptomatic until a complication develops. Patients occasionally complain of a dull ache or prominent pulsation in their abdomen, or they may develop symptoms related to compression of surrounding structures by the enlarging aneurysm. **Aneurysmal rupture** is usually heralded by acute chest or abdominal pain and frequently results in hemodynamic collapse. The pain of **aortic dissection** is often described as sudden, severe, chest pain that is tearing in quality and often associated with diaphoresis (see Chapter 1 for discussion of dissecting aortic aneurysm). It may be associated with evidence of limb or organ ischemia related to occlusion of branch vessels, aortic valve insufficiency, myocardial ischemia, or spinal cord ischemia (paraplegia).

PHYSICAL EXAMINATION

Physical examination findings depend on the anatomic distribution and nature of the vascular disease. A careful examination of the peripheral pulses and auscultation for bruits are the key elements.

- PAD: Often associated with diminished distal pulses and vascular bruits. As the degree of obstruction increases, a bruit may diminish and eventually disappear, making bruit intensity a poor indicator of the severity of disease. Smooth, shiny, hairless skin may be seen in the affected extremity, and ischemic ulceration may develop. Gangrene is a late finding.
- Acute peripheral arterial occlusion: Findings are the "6 Ps" as listed earlier.
- Aortic aneurysm: May be associated with a pulsatile abdominal mass (abdominal aortic aneurysm), prominent pulsation in the sternal notch, and findings of aortic valve insufficiency (thoracic aortic aneurysm).
- Aortic dissection: May be associated with asymmetric pulses and blood pressure, evidence of limb or organ ischemia, and/or findings of aortic insufficiency.

DIAGNOSTIC EVALUATION

Diagnostic testing is done to confirm the presence of vascular disease and to evaluate its severity. A variety of invasive and noninvasive tests are available to diagnose peripheral arterial disease, including segmental BP measurement (**ankle-brachial index**, or **ABI**), ultrasound (US), magnetic resonance angiography (MRA), and contrast angiography. ABIs are frequently the first test used to assess the severity of chronic peripheral vascular disease and may be performed sequentially to follow disease progression. The BP on the legs is usually slightly greater than that in the arms (measured with Doppler at the ankle and the brachial vessels); the normal ABI is thus >1.0. An ABI <0.95 suggests PAD, and an ABI <0.5 is consistent with severe disease. Generally, claudication can be present when ABI is below 0.95, rest pain begins when ABI is <0.5, and gangrene may occur at ABI <0.4. Angiography for chronic PAD is generally reserved until the patient requires surgical therapy. In the setting of arterial occlusion (both acute and chronic), the diagnosis is usually confirmed by **MRA or contrast angiography**. If an occlusion is documented and an embolic event is suspected, **cardiac ultrasound** is generally performed to exclude potential cardioembolic sources.

Abdominal aortic aneurysms (AAA) can be assessed with US, computed tomography (CT) scan, or MRA, although US is the most frequent method used for the serial assessment of aneurysmal size. Thoracic aneurysms are best assessed with CT scan or MRA. Based on well-designed randomized trials, screening for AAA with US is now recommended for all men age 65 to 75 who have ever smoked.

Aortic dissections can be diagnosed with **transesophageal echocardiography** (TEE), **contrast CT**, or **MRA**. Contrast angiography, once the gold standard, is now rarely required. All three studies appear to have similar sensitivity and specificity to diagnose dissection. MRA is not frequently utilized since the patient is rarely sufficiently stable for the exam; TEE is the test of choice for diagnosing acute aortic dissections at the bedside because it can be performed quickly for unstable patients.

TREATMENT

ACUTE ARTERIAL OCCLUSION

An acute arterial occlusion is a medical/surgical emergency, generally requiring immediate referral to a vascular surgeon. Heparin is usually started immediately, but definitive restoration of blood flow is essential to avoid tissue necrosis. This can occasionally be achieved with thrombolytic agents; however, percutaneous or surgical thrombectomy is usually required. Following revascularization, chronic anticoagulation with warfarin is required if occlusion was embolic in nature.

AORTIC DISSECTION

The treatment of an acute aortic dissection depends on its location (Fig. 10-1). Dissections involving the ascending aorta and/or arch (Stanford type A) require emergent surgical repair irrespective of whether they extend to the descending aorta (DeBakey type I) or are confined more proximally (DeBakey type II). The mortality of type A aortic dissection approaches 1% per hour for the first 24 hours; therefore, rapid recognition and early surgical intervention are essential. Dissections limited to the descending thoracic and/or abdominal aorta (Stanford type B, DeBakey type III) are generally managed medically with aggressive BP control (β-blockers, vasodilators) unless there is compromise of branch vessels, development of a pseudoaneurysm, or progressive expansion of the aneurysm.

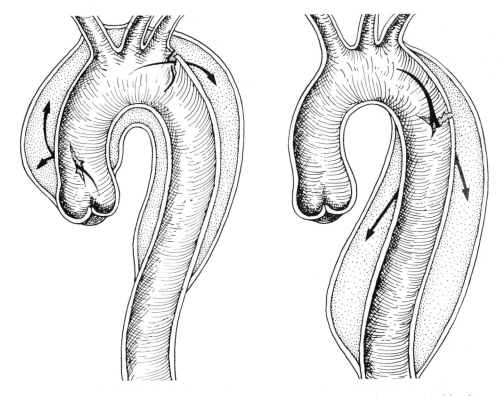

Figure 10-1 • Acute aortic dissection. In acute aortic dissection, an intimal tear permits blood to dissect the media, separating the intima from the adventitia. Type A is located in the ascending aorta and is more common. Type B is located in the descending aorta.
LifeART image © 2009 Lippincott Williams & Wilkins. All rights reserved.

AORTIC ANEURYSMS

Symptomatic (leaking) aortic aneurysms require urgent surgical treatment. Small, stable aortic aneurysms may be managed conservatively and followed with annual ultrasound; β-blockers may decrease the rate of aneurysm expansion and reduce the risk of rupture. The risk of rupture and death from an abdominal aortic aneurysm varies with its size and location. The 2-year risk of rupture is approximately 80% for aneurysms with a diameter >6 cm and 10% to 30% for aneurysms between 4 and 6 cm in size. **Indications for elective aneurysm repair** include:

- Rate of aneurysm expansion >0.5 cm per year
- Thoracic aortic aneurysm >6 cm (>5.5 cm in patients with Marfan syndrome)
- Abdominal aortic aneurysms >5.5 cm
- Abdominal aortic aneurysms in the presence of iliac or femoral aneurysms that require treatment

In patients who are high risk for surgical repair due to comorbid diseases, endovascular repair through a catheter-based approach can be attempted.

PERIPHERAL ARTERIAL DISEASE

The initial treatment of chronic arterial occlusive disease is generally conservative and includes:

- **Pharmacologic therapy**. Antiplatelet agents (e.g., aspirin, clopidogrel) may improve symptoms and decrease the need for surgical revascularization. Rheologic agents, specifically cilostazol, appear to be the most effective agents at reducing time to claudication and improving exercise capacity. Vasodilators *do not* improve outcome.
- Regular **exercise** (to the point of discomfort but not beyond; will improve exercise tolerance).
- Aggressive **risk factor modification** (control of hypertension, diabetes, dyslipidemia). Lipid lowering with HMG CoA reductase inhibitors (statins)

should be started to target a low density lipoprotein level (LDL) less than 100 mg/dL.

• **Smoking cessation**.
• **Meticulous foot care** (wearing protective, properly fitted shoes; keeping feet clean and dry; using moisturizing creams).

In patients with symptoms at rest or with progressive symptoms despite medical therapy, surgical or percutaneous revascularization is usually required. Percutaneous revascularization with balloon angioplasty combined with intravascular stenting may be effective for iliac and femoral arterial disease, but it is relatively ineffective for more distal disease. Surgical approaches depend on the anatomic location and extent of disease. Diseases of the distal aorta and iliofemoral system are frequently treated with aortofemoral bypass grafting using a segment of the patient's saphenous vein or synthetic graft material. Patency rates for vein grafts are superior compared to synthetic grafts. More distal disease may be treated with femoral-popliteal or popliteal-distal bypass, depending on the level of the vascular disease. Occasionally, extra-anatomic bypass using a distant arterial source (e.g., axillary-femoral or femoral-femoral bypass) is necessary because of diffuse proximal vascular disease. When considering surgery for peripheral vascular disease, it must be kept in mind that peripheral vascular disease is a marker for CAD. Therefore, a thorough assessment of the cardiac risk of surgery must be performed preoperatively.

KEY POINTS

- Peripheral arterial disease is a coronary artery disease equivalent. Patients should be treated with aspirin, statins, and tight blood pressure control.

- Intermittent claudication can be managed medically, but ischemic rest pain requires immediate evaluation by a vascular specialist.

- Acute arterial occlusion is manifested by the six "Ps": pulselessness, pallor, poikilothermia, pain, paralysis, paresthesia

- Connective tissue disease (e.g., Marfan, Ehlers-Danos) or bicuspid aortic valve should be considered in a young person with a thoracic aneurysm.

- Aortic dissection is best diagnosed by transesophageal echocardiogram at the bedside. Surgical repair is required for dissections involving the ascending aorta.

Syncope*

Syncope is a sudden, transient loss of consciousness and postural tone followed by spontaneous recovery. Presyncope is the sensation of impending syncope without loss of consciousness.

EPIDEMIOLOGY

Syncope is a common clinical entity, accounting for approximately 3% of emergency department visits and 6% of all hospital admissions. The incidence of syncope increases with advancing age, and approximately a third of the population will suffer an episode of syncope at some point in their lifetime.

PATHOPHYSIOLOGY

The common physiologic link among all causes of syncope is a transient decrease in cerebral blood flow. This is usually related to a primary cardiovascular problem or to an inability to maintain blood pressure (due to hypovolemia or neurally mediated vasodilation and bradycardia). Infrequently, cerebrovascular disease can lead to bilateral cortical or brainstem hypoperfusion. Unilateral carotid artery disease is unlikely to cause syncope.

Metabolic abnormalities (such as hypoglycemia or hypoxia) and seizures produce loss of consciousness by inducing diffuse brain dysfunction via electrical or metabolic derangement. However, there is no loss of postural tone, so these are not causes of true syncope.

*Adapted from Gururaj A. In: Awtry EH, Ware M, Jeon C. *Blueprints in Cardiology*. Malden, MA: Blackwell Publishing, 2003.

DIFFERENTIAL DIAGNOSIS

The main causes of syncope can be separated into neurally mediated (reflex) syncope, orthostatic hypotension, and primary cardiac problems (Table 11-1). The most common type of neurally mediated syncope is **vasovagal syncope** (also known as **neurocardiogenic syncope**) in which various stimuli trigger the sudden development of vasodilation ("vaso") and bradycardia ("vagal"), resulting in hypotension. Vasovagal syncope precipitated by a specific trigger (such as coughing or micturition) is referred to as situational syncope. A similar reflex can be provoked in some people by applying gentle pressure over the carotid artery (carotid sinus hypersensitivity). This may result in vasodilation (vasodepressor response), bradycardia, or both.

Orthostatic hypotension is another frequent cause of syncope, often provoked by hypovolemia or medications. This can also be secondary to an underlying disease, such as diabetes, amyloidosis, or Parkinson disease. Another provoked cause of orthostatic hypotension is postprandial hypotension. This is more common in the elderly and is a result of splanchnic venous pooling 30 to 60 minutes after a meal.

Structural cardiac disease and arrhythmias account for approximately 15% to 20% of all episodes of syncope. Common mechanical causes include aortic stenosis and hypertrophic obstructive cardiomyopathy (HCM). Mitral stenosis, atrial myxoma, and cardiac tamponade are less common causes. Both bradyarrhythmias (sick sinus syndrome, atrioventricular [AV] node blockade, etc.) and tachyarrhythmias (ventricular tachycardia [VT] or supraventricular

■ TABLE 11-1 Common Causes of Syncope

Neurally Mediated (Reflex)

Vasovagal (neurocardiogenic)

Situational

   Micturition

   Tussive

   Valsalva

   Carotid sinus hypersensitivity

Orthostatic Hypotension

   Volume depletion

   Medications

   Postprandial

Systemic disease (diabetes, amyloidosis, Parkinson disease)

Primary Cardiac Causes

Structural

   Aortic stenosis

   Mitral stenosis

   Hypertrophic cardiomyopathy

   Atrial myxoma

Arrhythmic

   Supraventricular tachycardia

   Ventricular tachycardia

   Sinus node dysfunction

   AV nodal block

Decreased cardiac output

   Myocardial infarction

   Pericardial tamponade

   Pulmonary embolism

   Aortic dissection

lation as well. However, an unusual shunting of blood can occur with subclavian stenosis. With activity of the upper extremity, blood from the ipsilateral vertebral artery provides flow to the subclavian artery in a retrograde fashion. This shunts blood from the contralateral vertebral and basilar arteries, resulting in cerebral hypoperfusion and syncope (**subclavian steal syndrome**). The most common cause of subclavian stenosis is atherosclerotic disease, although vasculitis and congenital malformations occur as well.

CLINICAL MANIFESTATIONS

HISTORY

The history is the most important aspect in evaluating a patient with syncope. It is important to obtain the history not only from the patient but also from any witnesses, and to ask the following questions:

1. What was the patient doing at the time of the syncopal episode?
2. Were there any symptoms (e.g., chest pain, palpitations, light-headedness, nausea) that preceded the event?
3. Is the patient on any medications?
4. Does the patient have a history of heart disease?
5. Was there any sign of seizure activity? Any incontinence or tongue biting?
6. How long did the patient remain unconscious?
7. When the person awoke, was he or she confused?

A typical vasovagal prodrome is a reassuring finding. The patient will describe a feeling of weakness, light-headedness, diaphoresis, and nausea before the event. Syncope is often triggered when the symptoms cause the patient to stand up and try to leave the area.

It is important to identify patients who have a primary cardiac cause of their syncope because their prognosis is much worse than if they have an alternative etiology. Cardiac syncope is always sudden in onset, may be preceded by chest pain or palpitations, and resolves spontaneously (usually in <5 minutes). The following findings on history suggest true cardiac syncope:

- Syncope following chest pain (suggests myocardial ischemia or infarction)
- Syncope preceded by palpitations (suggests an arrhythmic cause)

tachycardia [SVT]) can result in a fall in cardiac output, thereby precipitating syncope. It is noteworthy that SVT rarely causes syncope in the absence of underlying structural heart disease or an atrioventricular bypass tract. Pulmonary embolism and aortic dissection can present with syncope, but rarely is syncope the predominant symptom.

Infrequently, severe cerebrovascular disease can result in syncope. Due to collateral circulation of the circle of Willis, this requires bilateral carotid stenoses and some disturbance of the posterior circu-

TABLE 11-2 Alternate Causes that May Mimic Syncope

Central Nervous System

Cerebrovascular accident

Seizure

Metabolic Abnormalities

Hypoglycemia

Hypoxia

Psychiatric

Anxiety

Pseudo-syncope and pseudo-seizure

Falls

- Exertional syncope (suggests ischemia, aortic stenosis, or hypertrophic cardiomyopathy [HCM])
- Syncope without prodrome or aura (consider arrhythmia)
- Syncope in the setting of known heart disease

Table 11-2 lists alternate causes of loss of consciousness, and Table 11-3 outlines important historic features of syncope and associated diagnoses.

PHYSICAL EXAMINATION

The physical examination should ensure that no significant trauma was suffered because of the syncopal fall. Then the exam should be directed at identifying potential causes of syncope. It is important to evaluate the patient for orthostatic blood pressure changes or unequal blood pressures. Cardiac exam should focus on the murmurs of aortic stenosis, mitral stenosis, or obstructive hypertrophic cardiomyopathy (see Chapter 9). Carotid and subclavian arteries are auscultated for bruits. Carotid sinus massage should be performed if the history is suggestive, but should not be performed if the patient has a carotid bruit or history of recent stroke. Neurologic examination should look for focal deficits or underlying peripheral neuropathy.

TABLE 11-3 Historical Features of Syncope and Suggested Etiologies

Historical Feature	Suggested Cause(s)
Exertional	Aortic or mitral stenosis, HCM, pulmonary hypertension
Associated with chest pain	Myocardial ischemia, pulmonary embolism, aortic dissection
Associated with palpitations	Tachyarrhythmias or bradyarrhythmias
Family history of syncope or sudden death	Hereditary long QT syndrome, HCM
Associated with emotional stress, pain, unpleasant auditory or visual stimuli	Vasovagal episode
Following cough, micturition, or defecation	Situational syncope
After arising from lying or sitting position	Orthostatic hypotension, hypovolemia
After turning head; during shaving	Carotid sinus sensitivity
Associated with certain body position	Atrial myxoma or "ball valve" thrombus
Diuretic medication use	Hypovolemia
Antiarrhythmic or antipsychotic medication use	Ventricular tachyarrhythmias
Parkinson disease, diabetic neuropathy	Orthostatic hypotension (especially postprandial)
Premonitory aura, tonic-clonic movements, incontinence, or tongue-biting	Seizure
History of stroke or head trauma	Seizure
Syncope precipitated by arm movement	Subclavian steal syndrome

HCM, hypertrophic cardiomyopathy.

DIAGNOSTIC EVALUATION

Many procedures are available to aid in determining the etiology of syncope (Table 11-4); however, the use of these ancillary tests should be guided by results of the history and physical examination. In at least a third of cases of syncope, a specific diagnosis cannot be determined; however, in approximately half of cases in which a diagnosis is made, it is suggested by the history or physical examination, with the assistance of an **electrocardiogram** (ECG).

A 12-lead **ECG** should be obtained in all patients with syncope. The exception may be the young patient where the history clearly suggests vasovagal syncope. The ECG may reveal the actual cause (e.g., heart block, tachyarrhythmias) or suggest potential causes (e.g., evidence of ischemic heart disease, atrioventricular bypass tracts, etc.).

In the patient with a high suspicion for cardiac etiology, further testing is indicated. These patients may have a worrisome history (see above) or multiple risk factors for cardiac disease. An **echocardiogram** can indicate structural abnormalities (valvular disease, cardiomyopathy), or demonstrate a wall motion abnormality (raising concern for myocardial ischemia and arrhythmia). An **exercise test** is often useful to rule out underlying myocardial ischemia as a concern.

In patients in whom an arrhythmia is suspected but not documented on ECG, prolonged monitoring with an **event recorder** may be helpful. If the episodes are very infrequent but severe, an implantable recorder that can monitor the patient for up to 2 years can be placed. If the history, physical examination, or initial diagnostic tests suggest an arrhythmic cause for syncope, an **electrophysiologic study** (EPS) may be indicated, especially if the patient is also suspected of having CAD. During EPS, the arrhythmia that caused the syncope can frequently be reproduced. This may also be necessary in the patient with a cardiomyopathy, regardless of prior testing. In patients without underlying heart disease, EPS rarely identifies the cause of syncope.

Most patients without structural heart disease or clinical evidence of arrhythmias have a reflex cause of syncope (usually vasovagal), and further invasive diagnostic studies are usually not indicated. In such patients who have recurrent syncope, the diagnosis of neurocardiogenic syncope is sometimes evaluated with **tilt-table testing**. In this test, the patient is strapped supine to a table and is then elevated to 60 to 90 degrees. This stimulates venous pooling, and can precipitate vasovagal syncope. Medications, such as isoproterenol (a beta-adrenergic receptor agonist) or nitroglycerin, can be used to further provoke syncope during the test. The sensitivity of this test is reported to be between 70% and 80%, but the reproducibility and specificity are poor. In addition, the tilt-table is not useful to guide therapy. The AHA/ACCF guidelines recommend against routine use of this test.

PROGNOSIS

Young patients (<60 years) with syncope but without underlying heart disease have an excellent prognosis. Syncope patients with a normal ECG have a low probability of an arrhythmic cause and a low risk of sudden cardiac death. Patients who have a cardiac

---

■ TABLE 11-4 Diagnostic Modalities in the Evaluation of Syncope

Diagnostic Procedure	Syncope Types in Which it May be Helpful
ECG	Arrhythmias, heart block, conduction disease
Tilt-table testing	Neurocardiogenic syncope (vasovagal)
Electrophysiologic testing	VT, some SVT, some bradycardias
24-hr Holter monitor	Arrhythmias that occur frequently
Event monitor	Infrequent arrhythmias (can monitor for ~1 week)
Implantable loop monitor	Very infrequent arrhythmias (can monitor up to 18 mo)
EEG, Head CT scan	Seizure disorder
Carotid sinus massage	Carotid sinus hypersensitivity

CT, computed tomography; ECG, electrocardiogram; EEG, electroencephalography; SVT, supraventricular tachycardia; VT, ventricular tachycardia.

cause of syncope have an annual mortality rate as high as 30%. The risk of recurrent syncope in patients with vasovagal (neurocardiogenic) syncope is about 30% at 5 years.

TREATMENT

The treatment of syncope depends entirely on its cause. Most types of situational or vasovagal syncope require no specific therapy. Therapies aimed at preventing neurally mediated syncope have yielded inconsistent results. Although small randomized trials suggested a benefit to pacemaker placement, a larger blinded study showed no benefit. In an attempt to block the sympathetic signal that triggers the reflex, β-blockers have been utilized. Again, a larger randomized trial showed no difference in recurrent events.

Arrhythmias require specific therapy based on the type of arrhythmia present. In general, SVTs can be treated with rate-lowering medications (e.g., β-blockers, calcium channel blockers, digoxin), antiarrhythmic drugs, or occasionally radiofrequency ablation, whereas VT almost always requires treatment with antiarrhythmic drugs and/or implantation of a defibrillator. Syncope resulting from brady-arrhythmias requires placement of a pacemaker unless a reversible cause is identified (e.g., medications, metabolic abnormalities).

Syncope resulting from underlying heart disease requires correction of the structural abnormality. For example, aortic and mitral stenoses require valve replacement, and ischemic heart disease (ischemia or infarction) requires coronary revascularization with percutaneous coronary intervention or coronary artery bypass surgery. Outflow obstruction from hypertrophic cardiomyopathy may be improved with calcium channel blockers, β-blockers, right ventricular apex pacing, or myectomy. However, given the concern for associated ventricular arrhythmias in this population, an implantable defibrillator is often required.

Syncope caused by orthostatic hypotension that results from autonomic dysfunction may benefit from nonmedical therapies such as crossing/tensing the legs when standing, using compression stockings, and taking care to stand up slowly. Fludrocortisone and a high-salt diet expand the vascular volume but can lead to edema and hypertension.

KEY POINTS

- Syncope refers to the sudden, transient loss of consciousness and postural tone. The most common etiologies are neurally mediated (reflex), orthostatic hypotension, and cardiac (structural or arrhythmic).

- History is the most important aspect of the workup. Cardiac syncope is always sudden in onset, with little prodrome. Exertional syncope is very worrisome for a cardiac disorder. Patients with underlying heart disease have presumed cardiac syncope until proven otherwise.

- Vasovagal (neurocardiogenic) is the most common cause of syncope. A prodrome of weakness, lightheadedness, diaphoresis, and nausea is usually present.

- Workup should focus on history, physical examination, and electrocardiogram. Additional cardiac testing may be needed if the etiology is unclear or suspicion for cardiac disease is high.

- There is no effective treatment for vasovagal syncope, but prognosis is excellent.

Part 2

Respiratory

12 Dyspnea

Dyspnea is an **uncomfortable awareness of breathing**. The awareness and control of respiration by the central nervous system (CNS) are influenced by the input of a number of peripheral receptors:

- Central and peripheral chemoreceptors (which measure blood oxygen content, carbon dioxide content, and pH)
- Mechanical receptors in pulmonary parenchyma, airways, and respiratory muscles

These receptors provide information to the CNS concerning the efficiency of respiration (i.e., gas exchange) as well as the work of breathing. It is important to note that there is a **large subjective component** as the same quantitative respiratory defects in different patients can elicit different degrees of dyspnea.

DIFFERENTIAL DIAGNOSIS

Disorders affecting the cardiopulmonary system and the blood's oxygen-carrying capacity are generally the most common causes of dyspnea. It is useful to divide dyspnea into acute and chronic etiologies.

ACUTE DYSPNEA

Pulmonary causes include:

- Asthma
- Bronchitis
- Pneumonia
- Pneumothorax
- Pulmonary embolism
- Large airway obstruction (aspiration of foreign body, epiglottitis)
- Airway irritants (smoke, aerosols)

Cardiac causes include:

- Heart failure (including failure related to an acute myocardial infarction)
- Tamponade

Other causes include:

- Hemorrhage
- Hemolysis
- Carbon monoxide poisoning
- Psychogenic (hyperventilation syndrome, panic attack)
- High altitude
- Exercise

CHRONIC DYSPNEA

Pulmonary causes include:

- Chronic obstructive pulmonary disease (COPD)
- Pleural effusions
- Interstitial lung disease
- Pulmonary hypertension
- Neuromuscular disease
- Severe kyphoscoliosis

Cardiac causes include:

- Heart failure (e.g., related to decreased cardiac output or valvular disease)
- Restrictive pericarditis

Other causes include:

- Chronic anemia
- Severe obesity

Among outpatients, the most commonly encountered causes of dyspnea are COPD, asthma, heart failure, and anxiety. Among inpatients, in particular those who are severely ill with another process, the onset of dyspnea may signal an urgent process such as pulmonary embolus or hospital-acquired pneumonia.

CLINICAL MANIFESTATIONS

HISTORY

When a patient presents with a complaint of dyspnea, the clinician must establish whether the onset of dyspnea was acute or if the condition is chronic. If the onset was acute, life-threatening conditions such as pulmonary embolus, spontaneous pneumothorax, and pneumonia need to be sought. The decision regarding hospitalization and empirical treatment often will need to be made quickly in cases of acute-onset dyspnea.

Historical features in acute dyspnea that can provide a clue as to the underlying etiology are:

- Cough (bronchitis, asthma, pneumonia, airway irritation)
- Sputum production (bronchitis, pneumonia)
- Pleuritic chest pain (spontaneous pneumothorax, pulmonary embolus, pneumonia)
- Visceral chest pain, angina (heart failure)
- Hemoptysis (pulmonary embolus, bronchitis, pneumonia)

The **evaluation of chronic dyspnea** can be more problematic, requiring a stepped diagnostic workup (see "Diagnostic Evaluation"). Historical features that should be sought in the evaluation of chronic dyspnea include:

- Smoking (COPD; bronchitis)
- Cardiac history (heart failure)
- Occupational/environmental exposures (e.g., asbestos, metal dust, allergens leading to interstitial lung disease)

In addition, because chronic dyspnea usually manifests initially as exertional dyspnea, a determination of the **baseline fitness** of an individual is important. Any significant change from baseline indicates possible severe pathology and necessitates further evaluation.

PHYSICAL EXAMINATION

A directed physical examination in the setting of **acute dyspnea** should evaluate the patient for:

- Wheezing (asthma, heart failure)
- Stridor (upper airway obstruction)

- Consolidation (pneumonia)
- Rales, S_3, jugular venous distention (heart failure)
- Cardiac murmurs (valvular disease)
- Tracheal shift from midline, absent unilateral breath sounds (pneumothorax, tension pneumothorax)
- Leg swelling or pain, especially if unilateral (deep vein thrombosis [DVT] leading to pulmonary embolism)

In **chronic dyspnea**, physical finding of note include:

- Hyperexpansion (COPD)
- Rales (fine rales in interstitial lung disease, more coarse in heart failure)
- Evidence of congestive heart failure (CHF)/valvular disease (S_3, jugular venous distention, murmurs)
- Pulmonary hypertension (fixed split of S_2, loud pulmonic component of second heart sound, right ventricular heave, jugular venous distention)

DIAGNOSTIC EVALUATION

In the setting of **acute dyspnea**, a **chest radiograph** should be obtained and examined for:

- Pneumothorax (loss of lung markings, pleural reflection)
- Pneumonia (consolidation)
- Heart failure (Kerley B lines, effusions)

Measurement of **ABGs** (see Chapter 20) usually does not suggest a specific etiology but can help quantitate the degree of respiratory compromise. Peak expiratory flow measurements are useful in the evaluation of possible asthma (see Chapter 15). Measurement of brain natriuretic peptide (BNP) can be useful in diagnosing heart failure (see Chapter 5).

The diagnosis of **pulmonary embolus** is a critical one to make in the setting of acute dyspnea. Ventilation-perfusion (V/P) scanning, lower extremity venous ultrasound (US), helical computed tomography (CT) with contrast, measurement of D-dimers, and pulmonary angiography can all be used in the evaluation (see Chapter 16).

Evaluation of **chronic dyspnea** should also start with a chest radiograph. Conditions such as COPD, interstitial lung disease, and heart failure can have specific radiographic findings (see individual chapters for details). Further imaging with CT can be useful.

A complete blood count (CBC) to screen for underlying anemia should be performed. If after a

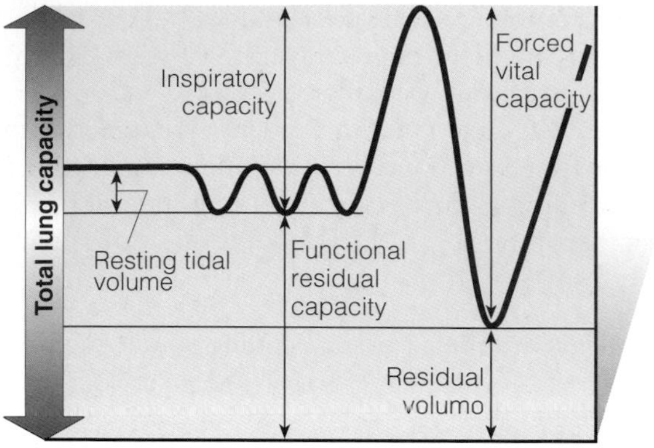

Figure 12-1 • Spirogram tracing showing static lung volumes.

routine history, physical examination, and these initial tests, a cause for chronic dyspnea is not apparent, then more specialized testing, often in consultation with a pulmonary specialist, needs to be done.

Chest radiographs, ABG measurements, screens for pulmonary embolus, and peak flow measurements generally yield a diagnosis in **acute dyspnea**. In rare instances, more invasive diagnostic tests such as right-heart catheterization or bronchoscopy are required.

As mentioned, **chronic dyspnea** can be difficult to diagnose. A common scenario is a patient who presents with chronic, progressive exertional dyspnea and who has evidence of both chronic pulmonary disease and coronary artery disease. An ordered evaluation is required to make the diagnosis without unnecessary expensive and invasive tests.

Pulmonary function testing (PFT), commonly used in the evaluation of chronic dyspnea, can range from simple **spirometry** that measures expiratory flow rates and volumes (see Chapter 14) to more sophisticated measurement of lung volumes and diffusion capacity. The following parameters can be measured and calculated (Fig. 12-1):

- Forced vital capacity (FVC): The volume of air that can be exhaled going from maximal inhalation to maximal exhalation
- Forced expiratory volume in 1 second (FEV_1): The volume of air exhaled in 1 second starting at maximal inhalation
- FEV_1/FVC (FEV_1%): Calculated ratio of FEV_1 to FVC
- Total lung capacity (TLC): The volume of gas contained within the lung after maximal inspiration
- Residual volume (RV): The volume of gas remaining in the lungs after maximal expiration
- Diffusion capacity of lung for carbon monoxide (DLCO): The ability of gas to diffuse across the alveolar-capillary membrane

Specific patterns of PFT abnormalities are associated with particular pulmonary diseases (Table 12-1).

Evaluation of the cardiovascular system (see Chapter 5) can reveal a cardiac cause for dyspnea. Generally, an assessment of valvular and ventricular function via an echocardiogram is sufficient. Radionuclide ventriculography can also assess ventricular function and is used during cardiopulmonary exercise testing (see later).

In a patient with chronic exertional dyspnea, if the preceding pulmonary and cardiac evaluations fail to reveal significant abnormalities or if the individual abnormalities do not appear to explain the

Disease	FVC	FEV_1	FEV_1%	TLC	RV	DLCO
Emphysema	↓	↓	↓	↑	↑	↓
Chronic bronchitis	↓	↓	↓	↔	↑	↔
Asthma (active flare of disease)	↓	↓	↓	↔	↑	↔↑
Interstitial lung disease	↓	↔	↔↑	↓	↓	↓
Extrapulmonary restriction (e.g., kyphoscoliosis)	↓	↓	↔	↓	↔↓	↔
Heart failure (early, increased blood flow)	—	—	—	—	—	↑
Heart failure (late, with pulmonary edema)	—	—	—	—	—	↓
Pulmonary embolus	—	—	—	—	—	↓

TABLE 12-1 Patterns of Pulmonary Function Testing Abnormalities

DLCO, diffusion capacity of lung for carbon monoxide; FEV_1, forced expiratory volume in 1 second; RV, residual volume; TLC, total lung capacity.

degree of impairment, **cardiopulmonary exercise testing** (CPEx) may be necessary. CPEx involves graded exercise (much as with a cardiac stress test) with cardiopulmonary monitoring, and it is generally performed in consultation with a pulmonary specialist.

CPEx will be able to determine if the limitation to exercise is because of a cardiac or pulmonary limit. In normal individuals, pulmonary capacity is greater than cardiac. By determining the function of both the cardiac and pulmonary systems, the relative degree of impairment can be used to guide therapy.

 KEY POINTS

- Dyspnea is an abnormally uncomfortable awareness of breathing.
- Dyspnea can arise from abnormalities in the pulmonary, cardiac, hematologic, and musculoskeletal systems.
- Acute dyspnea can be the result of life-threatening conditions such as pulmonary embolism, pneumothorax, and pneumonia.

- Chronic dyspnea is most commonly caused by COPD or heart failure.
- Evaluation of chronic exertional dyspnea requires a careful and orderly assessment of the function of the cardiac and pulmonary systems. CPEx can determine the physiologic limitations to exercise.

Cough is an important defense mechanism that allows the clearance of secretions and foreign particles. There are **three phases to a cough**:

1. Deep inspiration
2. Glottic closure and buildup of intrathoracic pressure
3. Opening of the glottis with rapid release of pressure

Cough is triggered by receptors located throughout the upper and lower respiratory tract; therefore, a wide variety of **stimuli** can trigger the cough reflex, including:

- Upper respiratory infection
- Lower respiratory infection
- Environmental pollutants
- Mechanical irritation
- Chemical irritation
- Chronic inflammatory states
- Drugs

The final common pathway of most of these causes of cough is mechanical or chemical irritation. These nervous inputs are transmitted to the integrative cough centers in the brain that coordinates the cough reflex just outlined. It is important that **cigarette smoking** is a very common cause of chronic cough. Cough associated with smoking is often dry and worse on awakening in the morning. Many of the irritants that cause cough can also produce bronchospasm in some patients, which may present as wheezing.

DIFFERENTIAL DIAGNOSIS

Causes of cough can be grouped according to the pathogenic stimuli listed in the previous section.

Upper Respiratory Infection (generally viral)
- Pharyngitis
- Sinusitis (via persistent nasal secretions into the pharynx—"postnasal drip")
- Tracheitis

Lower Respiratory Infection
- Bronchitis
- Pneumonia
- Tuberculosis

Environmental Pollutants
- Dust
- Pollen, animal dander, and other allergens
- Cigarette smoke

Mechanical Irritation (of upper or lower respiratory tract)
- Tumor
- Aortic aneurysm
- Cerumen
- Pulmonary edema

Chronic Inflammatory States
- Asthma
- Chronic aspiration
- Gastroesophageal reflux disease
- Sarcoidosis

Drugs
- Angiotensin-converting enzyme (ACE) inhibitors
- Psychogenic

Acute cough is most commonly due to acute upper respiratory tract pathology (general viral infection) while chronic cough is most commonly secondary to chronic upper airway conditions (allergies, sinusitis), asthma, and gastroesophageal reflux disease.

CLINICAL MANIFESTATIONS

HISTORY

When a patient presents with the complaint of a cough, a number of important historical features should be elicited:

- Is the cough acute (less than 2 to 3 weeks in duration) or chronic?
- Does the patient smoke, and, if so, is there any history of obstructive airway disease?
- Is there sputum production? (If so, what color is it? Is there any blood?)
- Are there any environmental exposures (e.g., dust, fumes, animal dander)?
- Are there any associated constitutional symptoms (e.g., fever, weight loss)?

These historical points can begin to aid in sorting through the differential diagnosis.

PHYSICAL EXAMINATION

Several elements of the physical examination may provide etiologic clues:

- Sinus tenderness (sinusitis)
- Conjunctival injection, rhinitis (URI)
- Tympanic membrane erythema (otitis)
- Oropharyngeal "cobblestoning" (chronic sinusitis)
- Loose rhonchi (infection; i.e., bronchitis or pneumonia)
- Consolidation (pneumonia)
- Fine crackles (pulmonary edema)
- Focal wheezing (local obstructing lesion; i.e., tumor or foreign body)
- End-expiratory wheezing (obstructive airways disease; i.e., asthma/chronic obstructive pulmonary disease [COPD])

The nature of the cough itself can give clues to the etiology: for example, the dry, irritant, nonproductive cough secondary to ACE inhibitors or the productive early morning cough encountered in chronic bronchitis.

DIAGNOSTIC EVALUATION

Many times the etiology of a cough is suggested by the history and physical. In other cases, if no diagnosis becomes readily apparent, a **chest radiograph** may be useful. It can reveal an infiltrate, mass, or pulmonary edema. A clear chest radiograph can steer the diagnosis toward tracheobronchitis, asthma, or environmental exposure as the etiology of the cough.

Examination of a Gram stain of **sputum** may also aid in diagnosis. Purulent sputum with many white blood cells (WBCs) suggests bronchitis or pneumonia (see Chapter 28). Eosinophils and mucus casts (so-called Curschmann spirals) suggest asthma. The presence of red blood cells (RBCs; with or without frank hemoptysis) may indicate chronic bronchitis, bronchiectasis, or tumor.

A therapeutic trial, such as a course of antibiotics based on the findings of a sputum Gram stain, or the institution of inhaled β-agonists for a suspected asthmatic, may help establish a diagnosis.

In some instances, usually with chronic cough, the etiology may not be readily apparent, even after trials of therapy. **Pulmonary function testing** (with or without provocative challenge such as methylcholine; see Chapter 12) may reveal chronic obstruction or reactive airways disease. Computed tomography (**CT**) of the chest may reveal anatomic lesions such as extrinsic compression, bronchiectasis, or parenchymal masses. **Bronchoscopy** may be of use, particularly in cases where findings on radiography require biopsy. **Purified protein derivative (PPD) testing** is indicated if tuberculosis (see Chapter 31) is suspected. Additionally, **pertussis** has been increasingly encountered as a cause of chronic cough, even among previously immunized individuals.

TREATMENT

Treatment should be directed at the underlying cause. Because mechanical or chemical irritation is the common etiology for most coughs, elimination or avoidance of these irritants is vital. Smoking cessation and avoidance of polluted environments are major components of management. Allergic rhinitis can be managed with antihistamines, nasal corticosteroids and decongestants. Empirical antibiotic therapy is generally initiated when a bacterial etiology is suspected (keeping in mind the caveat that most URIs are generally viral in etiology) in particular when sinusitis is considered.

The use of **antitussives** is often considered. Absolute suppression of the cough reflex is seldom medically necessary or even desired because the purpose of coughing is to clear foreign particles and secretions. For example, in chronic bronchitis, adequate clearance of secretions is a major component of management. **Reduction** of cough to prevent interference with sleep and improve comfort, rather than full cough suppression, should be the goal of antitussive therapy.

Antitussives suppress the cough reflex either by anesthetizing the peripheral irritant receptors or increasing the threshold of the central cough center. **Peripheral anesthetics** include:

- Benzonatate
- Phenol preparations
- Menthol preparations

Of these agents, benzonatate probably is the most effective. It is chemically related to other local anesthetics such as tetracaine.

Central antitussive agents include narcotics such as codeine, which are generally the most effective agents. **Dextromethorphan**, a nonnarcotic agent, can be useful in some patients, but studies have revealed variable efficacy.

KEY POINTS

- Cough is usually caused by mechanical or chemical irritation of the upper or lower respiratory tract or both.

- A wide variety of agents and conditions can lead to this irritation.

- History and physical examination alone can often suggest an etiology for a cough.

- Chest radiograph is a useful initial test in cases in which diagnosis is not readily apparent after history and physical examination.

- Further diagnostic testing is usually reserved to rule in or rule out specific diagnoses suggested by history, physical examination, and chest radiograph.

- Treatment should be directed at the underlying etiology of the cough, with cough suppression used only to deal with side effects of cough (sleep disturbance, etc.).

Chronic Obstructive Pulmonary Disease

Chronic obstructive pulmonary disease (COPD) refers to conditions that chronically impair expiratory airflow. Two major entities encompass COPD: emphysema and chronic bronchitis. Although their pathophysiologies differ, both result in airflow obstruction that is not fully reversible. **Chronic bronchitis** is defined as excess tracheobronchial mucus production resulting in a productive cough that occurs for at least 3 months a year for 2 or more consecutive years. **Emphysema** is defined as abnormal dilatation of terminal airspaces with destruction of the alveolar septa. Thus, chronic bronchitis is defined **clinically**, whereas the diagnosis of emphysema is made **pathologically**.

Asthma (see Chapter 15) is another obstructive disease that results in airway obstruction. It differs from COPD in that the obstruction is generally reversible and there is no association with smoking. Note that a subset of asthmatics can develop a component of irreversible obstruction, but these patients are not discussed here.

EPIDEMIOLOGY

Chronic bronchitis and emphysema are associated with cigarette smoking and affect approximately 16 million Americans. COPD is responsible for 80,000 deaths a year, making COPD the most preventable cause of morbidity and mortality. Although cigarette smoking is by far and away the most important etiologic factor (accounting for at least three-fourths of all cases), occupational and environmental exposures (e.g., air pollution, asbestos, heavy metals) can also have an additive (and independent) effect on risk. In addition, hereditary deficiencies in the protease inhibitor α_1-antitrypsin predispose to a distinct histologic form of emphysema (see "Pathology and Pathophysiology").

In the past, men had a much higher incidence of COPD. With the increase in the rate of cigarette use by women, there has been a corresponding rise in the incidence of COPD in women, and COPD deaths in women now exceed the number of deaths in men.

PATHOLOGY AND PATHOPHYSIOLOGY

In **chronic bronchitis**, there is distinctive hypertrophy and hyperplasia of the mucus-producing glands that line the airways. In addition, there is chronic mucosal and submucosal inflammation, intraluminal mucus plugging, and smooth muscle hypertrophy. These latter changes are more pronounced in the most distal, smaller caliber airways. The loss of ventilation in regions distal to the airway obstruction results in ventilation/perfusion (V/Q) mismatches and hypoxia.

In **emphysema**, two patterns occur: **centrilobular emphysema**, in which the areas most affected are the respiratory bronchioles and the central alveolar ducts, and **panacinar emphysema**, in which there is destruction throughout the acinus. Generally, cigarette smoking is associated with centrilobular emphysema, and α_1-antitrypsin deficiency with the panacinar form. In severe cases, however, it may be difficult to make a definite pathologic distinction as to which pattern is predominant. The destruction of lung parenchyma reduces elastic recoil, resulting in increased airway collapsibility and outflow obstruction. The destruction of airspace and blood vessels is equal; therefore, marked V/Q mismatch does not occur. Most patients with COPD have elements of both chronic bronchitis and emphysema, but usually one or the other predominates clinically.

The pathophysiologic changes seen in COPD contribute to expiratory obstruction and resultant decrease in forced expiratory volume (FEV_1). The FEV_1 depends on a number of variables:

- Airway diameter
- Collapsibility of the airways
- Elastic recoil of the lung parenchyma

Other physiologic changes that result from COPD are as follows:

- V/Q mismatches (generally shunt, i.e., blood flow to nonventilated areas, resulting in hypoxia)
- Pulmonary hypertension (in part because of loss of blood vessels from alveolar destruction, but more important is vessel constriction caused by hypoxia)
- Abnormal ventilatory responses (blunted response to hypercapnia and a reliance on hypoxic respiratory drive, generally seen in patients with chronic bronchitis)
- Right heart failure (caused by long-standing pulmonary hypertension, so-called *cor pulmonale*)

The natural history of COPD is generally one of inexorable decline in pulmonary function. Patients with chronic bronchitis have a course that is usually punctuated with multiple exacerbations with episodic increases in sputum production and worsened obstruction. In emphysema, the decline in pulmonary function is generally more continuous and steady.

CLINICAL MANIFESTATIONS

Many patients with COPD manifest elements of both chronic bronchitis and emphysema. To contrast the clinical presentations, it is useful to consider the presentation of patients who present primarily with one disease or the other.

HISTORY

The hallmark of **chronic bronchitis** is **cough** with **sputum** production. Early in the disease, symptoms are much worse during the winter months, but as the disease progresses, they become continuous and increase in frequency and severity. Dyspnea is not a predominant symptom initially, but the onset of **exertional dyspnea** often triggers medical attention. **Weight gain**, **lethargy**, and **cyanosis** are late findings.

In contrast, patients who present primarily with **emphysema** have minimal cough that may be productive of scant amounts of thin sputum. The major symptom is that of **dyspnea**, initially with exertion, but then quite significant at rest. **Weight loss** is common, but cyanosis is rare.

PHYSICAL EXAMINATION

On examination, patients with **chronic bronchitis** are generally comfortable at rest. Because of the common **obesity** and **cyanosis** associated with this disease, they are often referred to as "blue bloaters." If right-sided heart failure has developed, **peripheral edema** contributes to this picture. Lung examination is usually **resonant**, often with coarse **rhonchi** and wheezes. Cardiac examination may reveal signs of **right ventricular overload** (sternal heave, tricuspid regurgitation with neck vein distention, and large V waves). Despite cyanosis, marked clubbing of the digits is rare and, if present, is suggestive of an additional condition, most ominously a lung cancer.

The patient with **emphysema** reports **dyspnea at rest** and appears **thin** without cyanosis. This leads to the description of emphysematous patients as "pink puffers." They have a markedly **prolonged expiratory phase**, often through pursed lips. **Hypertrophy of the accessory muscles of respiration** in the neck is common, as is retraction of the intercostal muscles with inspiration. The lung examination is **hyperresonant**, with **decrease in breath sounds**, an **increased anteroposterior chest diameter**, and **lowered diaphragms**. The heart sounds are often distant, and signs of right heart overload are absent.

DIAGNOSTIC EVALUATION

Spirometry, the measurement of flow rates and volumes generated during forced expiration (see Fig. 12-1), is the primary means of quantifying airway outflow obstruction. The main measurements obtained are:

- **Forced vital capacity** (FVC): The volume of air that can be exhaled going from maximal inhalation to maximal exhalation
- **Forced expiratory volume in 1** second (FEV_1): The volume of air exhaled in 1 second, starting at maximal inhalation
- **FEV_1/FVC (FEV_1%):** The calculated ratio of FEV1 to FVC

The calculated FEV_1% (normally 0.75 to 0.8) is usually considered the most accurate, sensitive, and reproducible measure of airway outflow obstruction. With early obstructive disease, the FEV_1% may be normal, and the only measurable defect would be a slight decrease in midexpiratory flow rates, but for most patients with symptomatic COPD, the FEV_1% is a very useful assessment of the severity/stage of disease (Table 14-1) and can help predict mortality.

Other measurements of pulmonary function can be determined, including measurement of the **residual volume** (the amount of air that remains in the lungs at the end of maximal expiration), **total lung capacity**, and **diffusing capacity**. These require more sophisticated instrumentation than simple spirometry and are generally used for more extensive evaluation, usually in consultation with a pulmonary specialist.

■ **TABLE 14-1** Spirometric Classification of COPD Severity Based on Post-Bronchodilator FEV_1

Stage I: Mild	FEV_1/FVC <0.70 FEV_1 ≥80% predicted
Stage II: Moderate	FEV_1/FVC <0.70 50% ≤ FEV_1 <80% predicted
Stage III: Severe	FEV_1/FVC <0.70 30% ≤ FEV_1 <50% predicted
Stage IV: Very Severe	FEV_1/FVC <0.70 FEV_1 <30% predicted *or* FEV_1 <50% predicted plus chronic respiratory failure

FEV_1, forced expiratory volume in one second; FVC, forced vital capacity; respiratory failure, arterial partial pressure of oxygen (PaO_2) less than 8.0 kPa (60 mm Hg) with or without arterial partial pressure of CO_2 ($PaCO_2$) greater than 6.7 kPa (50 mm Hg) while breathing air at sea level. From GOLD Science Committee. Global Initiative for Chronic Obstructive Lung Disease. Global strategy for the diagnosis, management, and prevention of chronic obstructive pulmonary disease. Executive summary, 2007. Available online at http://www.goldcopd.com/.

Determination of ABGs at rest is often useful. Patients with emphysema generally have normal $PaCO_2$ and only slightly lowered PaO_2, whereas patients with chronic bronchitis often have elevated $PaCO_2$ (50 to 60 mm Hg) and depressed PaO_2 (45 to 60 mm Hg). In addition, patients with chronic bronchitis may have an elevated hematocrit (in the range of 50% to 55%) in response to the hypoxia.

TREATMENT

A key intervention in the management of COPD is **cessation of smoking**. Unfortunately, this does not usually reverse the damage that already exists, but it will usually slow the progression of disease and also limit exacerbations. Other environmental airway irritants should be avoided, including hairsprays, dust, insecticides, and spray deodorants. All patients with COPD should receive yearly **influenza vaccines**. In addition, they should receive **pneumococcal vaccine**.

Patients with significant airway obstruction (i.e., FEV_1 <1.0 L) require an understanding that a reduced life span is likely. Prospective discussions with such patients concerning endotracheal intubation when there is reduced likelihood of recovery are important. It is much less stressful for the patient and his or her family if these discussions can take place when the patient is clinically stable, rather than during an acute and potentially life-threatening exacerbation.

As stated earlier, patients with chronic bronchitis often experience acute increase in symptoms (so-called **acute exacerbations of chronic bronchitis**, or **AECB**). Patients with AECB generally present with increased dyspnea and an increase in purulence and/or volume of sputum. Some experts advocate administration of empirical antibiotics for AECB, although this is not a universally accepted intervention. Approximately half of episodes of AECB are felt to be related to viral or noninfectious causes. If administered, antibiotic coverage should encompass pathogens such as *Streptococcus pneumoniae*, *Moraxella catarrhalis*, and *Haemophilus influenzae*.

Bronchodilator therapy can alleviate symptoms significantly in some patients. Agents fall into three classes:

- Anticholinergics (e.g., ipratropium, tiotropium)
- β-Adrenergic agonists (e.g., albuterol, salmeterol)
- Methylxanthines (e.g., theophylline)

Inhaled **anticholinergic agents** cause bronchodilation through inhibition of vagal stimulation of the airways. Ipratropium bromide was traditionally used as the first-choice bronchodilator for use in COPD because tolerance does not develop and systemic side effects are minimal. The availability of the long-acting anticholinergic agent tiotropium bromide has led to a shift toward using this agent as first-line therapy. Evidence indicates that tiotropium can reduce the incidence of exacerbations and hospitalizations and improves health-related quality of life. Inhaled **β-agonists** can be added to provide additional bronchodilation, but dependence on these agents alone can lead to decreased effectiveness as well as systemic side effects such as tremulousness and cardiac rhythm disturbances. Oral **theophylline** is infrequently used for patients who are not controlled on standard bronchodilators. In some cases, it is useful for the prevention of nocturnal symptoms. Serum levels need to be monitored because nausea, palpitations, and seizures can result from toxic levels. In addition, multiple drug interactions can alter the levels of theophylline.

Systemic corticosteroids can be useful in the setting of acute exacerbations. Some patients benefit from long-term inhaled steroids for prevention of frequent exacerbations. Generally, empirical treatment is the only real way to determine which patients will have a beneficial response from long-term inhaled steroid use.

In patients with documented persistent hypoxemia (i.e., PaO_2 <60 mm Hg or SpO_2 <90%), **continuous supplemental oxygen** is indicated. Patients with signs of cor pulmonale and right heart failure should also receive supplemental oxygen even with less severe hypoxemia. Note that **oxygen therapy is the only pharmacologic therapy that has been proven to improve survival and quality of life.** Some patients do not require oxygen supplementation during the day but have significant desaturation during sleep and thus benefit from nocturnal oxygen therapy. Patients who do not normally require supplemental oxygen may need supplementation during air travel.

A comprehensive **pulmonary rehabilitation** program provides significant benefit to many patients. This program involves nonpharmacologic interventions such as nutritional support (as up to a third of patients with COPD may have protein-calorie malnutrition), exercise therapy, and psychological support, generally combined with smoking cessation interventions. Exercise training is a key component, resulting in improved exercise tolerance and quality of life.

Some patients remain severely incapacitated despite maximal therapy. In selected patients, lung transplantation can restore pulmonary function and relieve symptoms. Organs are in very limited supply, however, and the selection criteria are generally quite strict, making this a viable option for only a small minority of patients. Additionally, it is not clear if there is a significant decrease in long-term morbidity. For patients with documented α_1-antitrypsin deficiency, IV replacement therapy is indicated.

In some patients with emphysema who have a small number of large bullae, surgical resection of these bullae can relieve symptoms as well as improve respiratory function, although information conflicts concerning the absolute benefit of this intervention. Again, this is only an option for selected patients. Consultation with a pulmonologist and a thoracic surgeon is necessary.

KEY POINTS

- COPD is generally a smoking-related disease that results in a long-term decrease in maximal expiratory airflow.

- COPD can be divided into chronic bronchitis, which is characterized by cough and excess sputum production, and emphysema, in which destruction of the terminal airspaces is predominant.

- Spirometry, the measurement of expiratory volumes and flow rates, is the primary means for quantitating the degree of airflow obstruction and can be used to follow the progression of disease.

- The natural history of COPD is generally one of progressive increase in airflow obstruction. In chronic bronchitis, there are often periodic exacerbations, whereas in emphysema, the decline is steadier.

- Smoking cessation is critical to management and improvement in mortality in patients with COPD.

Asthma

Asthma is a disease of the airways characterized by chronic inflammation and abnormally heightened responsiveness of the tracheobronchial tree, leading to reversible expiratory airflow obstruction. A key feature of asthma is its episodic nature: acute exacerbations separated by symptom-free periods.

EPIDEMIOLOGY

Asthma affects an estimated 4% to 5% of the U.S. population. Onset is generally among younger patients; about half of cases manifest prior to 10 years of age, and another third before 40 years of age. In childhood, there is a 2:1 male-to-female preponderance, but by 30 years of age, the sexes are equally affected until a female predominance emerges after age 40. A documented increase in the prevalence of asthma has occurred in the United States over the past several decades. Numerous theories have been proposed for this increase, but the exact reasons are still unclear. It does not appear that increased awareness of the disease is the reason for the increased prevalence. One theory holds that decreased exposure to childhood infections results in skewing of the immune system toward Th2 responses (see following section).

Death related to asthma is infrequent (approximately 1 for 100,000 population), but there are indications that the mortality rate has been rising over the past 10 to 15 years. The precise reason for this rise in asthma-related mortality is not known, but it has been suggested it is a reflection of improper management of asthma, in particular an overreliance on beta-agonist bronchodilators.

ETIOLOGY AND PATHOGENESIS

Asthmatics have greater degrees of **airway reactivity** (i.e., bronchoconstriction) to inhaled stimuli such as histamine, methylcholine, and cold air when compared with nonasthmatics. Similarly, asthmatics exhibit heightened response to bronchodilators.

The pathophysiology of this airway hypersensitivity is not entirely clear. However, **chronic airway inflammation** appears to have an important role. A number of **stimuli can lead to chronic airway inflammation**:

- Inhaled allergens (e.g., animal dander, molds, dust mites)
- Viral and *Mycoplasma* infections
- Low-molecular-weight chemicals (including industrial dusts and gases)

Inhaled allergens are the most commonly encountered and important causes of chronic airway inflammation. Patients with so-called **allergic asthma** have increased serum IgE levels and positive skin-test results to airborne antigens. In some patients, chronic inflammatory stimuli cannot be identified, yet they still have severe airway inflammation. These patients are referred to as having **intrinsic asthma**.

An **acute asthma attack** is triggered by **stimuli that cause bronchoconstriction**:

- Cold air
- Exercise
- Inhaled irritants (cigarette smoke, dust, aerosols such as hairspray or perfume)
- β-adrenergic blockers
- Emotional upset
- Nonsteroidal anti-inflammatory drugs

- Food additives (e.g., sulfites)
- Inhaled allergens

Given the key role that inflammation appears to play in the pathogenesis of asthma, significant attention has been directed at studying the precise nature of the inflammatory response in the disease. Studies of biopsies of patients with asthma have documented that lymphocytes in the airways of asthmatics are predominantly of the Th2 phenotype along with mast cells and eosinophils. These lymphocytes secrete IL-4, IL 5, IL 9, and IL-13 and thus promote synthesis of IgE, an important mediator of allergic responses. The underlying defect responsible for this Th2 predominance in asthma is not known, but the "hygiene hypothesis" speculates that this is caused in part to decreased childhood exposure to infectious agents. By an as yet undetermined mechanism, this decreased exposure to infectious agents and thus decreased immune stimulation has led to an increased prevalence of dysregulated immune responses, which can be of a Th2 (as in the case of asthma) or a Th1 (as in the case of Crohn's disease) phenotype.

CLINICAL MANIFESTATIONS

HISTORY

An acute asthma attack is heralded by **symptoms** of:

- Dyspnea
- Wheezing
- Cough
- Sputum production (mucorrhea)
- Sleep disturbance
- Increased use of bronchodilators

In many patients, these **symptoms develop over days to weeks** following an inciting event. In some patients, however, the onset of an attack can occur acutely, over **hours or even minutes**. This is particularly true if attacks are triggered by nonsteroidal anti-inflammatory agents, beta-adrenergic blockers, or food additives.

PHYSICAL EXAMINATION

During an acute attack, an asthmatic will be in **respiratory distress** with **tachypnea**, **wheezing**, and possibly a **cough**. On lung examination, patients usually have audible **wheezes**, scattered **rhonchi**, and a **prolonged expiratory phase**. The chest is often **hyperinflated**, with an increased anteroposterior diameter.

Vital signs reveal sinus tachycardia in addition to tachypnea. A **pulsus paradoxus** (an increase in the normal fall in systolic blood pressure [BP] of ≤10 mm Hg or less observed during inspiration) can be seen. Severe paradox (≥25 mm Hg) is indicative of a severe attack. Note that as respiratory muscle fatigue develops and the patient can no longer generate increased intrapleural pressure, the paradox can disappear.

Further signs of **respiratory muscle fatigue** are **accessory muscle use** and **paradoxic breathing pattern** (inward movement of the abdominal wall and lower thorax during inspiration). Note that with a severe attack, wheezing may disappear as fatigue and obstruction increase.

DIFFERENTIAL DIAGNOSIS

In a patient with known asthma, the diagnosis of an acute attack is relatively straightforward; however, the respiratory signs and symptoms can resemble those seen in:

- Heart failure (pulmonary edema)
- Pulmonary embolism
- Pneumonia/bronchitis
- Upper airway obstruction

DIAGNOSTIC EVALUATION

The primary test used to determine severity of an acute asthma attack and monitor primary response to therapy is measurement of **peak expiratory flow (PEF) rates** (in L per minute). Simple handheld devices for measuring PEF are available that can be used in the physician's office and by patients at home. Accurate measurements require appropriate patient effort and technique. The results are most useful when they can be expressed as a **percentage of normal**, or, better still, as the percentage of the patient's best obtainable value during an asymptomatic period while on optimal treatment. Most patients present during an **acute attack** with a PEF in the range of 20% to 30% of predicted. **Symptoms generally resolve** when PEF returns to approximately 50% of normal and **signs** of an attack (e.g., wheezing) disappear at approximately 60% to 70% of normal. Therefore, signs and symptoms may be absent when the patient still has severe residual airflow limitation, making measurement of PEF important.

ABG values are normal early in an attack. Because dyspnea and anxiety result in hyperventilation, respiratory alkalosis, and hypocapnia result. If respiratory failure develops secondary to respiratory muscle fatigue, an initial **pseudonormalization** of the P_{CO_2} and eventual hypercapnia with respiratory acidosis develop. Hypoxemia is generally not seen until respiratory acidosis develops. Routine measurement of ABGs during an acute attack is not generally recommended. If improvement in the PEF and symptoms occur with initial treatment, ABG measurement is unnecessary.

Chest radiographs are generally unnecessary but typically reveal hyperinflation and possibly atelectasis secondary to mucous plugging. Chest radiographs can reveal pneumonia as well as complications of a severe attack such as pneumothorax and pneumomediastinum and should be obtained if such conditions are suspected.

TREATMENT

Given the pathophysiology of asthma, prevention of acute attacks depends on **limiting the degree of chronic inflammation**, whereas treatment of an acute attack involves the **relief of bronchoconstriction**. The use of **anti-inflammatory agents** limits acute attacks, and the use of **bronchodilators** provides **symptomatic relief** during exacerbations. Patient education is a key aspect of effective management. Patients need to know the basic pathophysiology of asthma and to understand the difference between preventive treatment and symptomatic treatment. Patients need to be taught how to recognize exacerbations early and to institute prompt treatment.

Control of the patient's environment is another important aspect of asthma management. It is crucial to avoid sensitizing agents such as inhaled allergens and bronchospastic triggers such as nonsteroidal anti-inflammatory agents.

Corticosteroids are the **most potent anti-inflammatory agents** available. They are generally administered via the inhaled route using a metered-dose inhaler (MDI). For stable patients, inhaled steroids can provide benefits equivalent to ingested steroids with fewer systemic effects. Oral steroids are generally reserved for the treatment of acute attacks or for maintenance in the rare patient who is not controlled with inhaled steroids alone.

A newer class of anti-inflammatory agents includes drugs that modify the inflammatory mediators known as leukotrienes. **Montelukast** and **zafirlukast** are leukotriene receptor antagonists, whereas **zileuton** inhibits the synthesis of leukotrienes. These drugs are possible alternatives to inhaled corticosteroids in patients with mild asthma or combined with inhaled steroids for patients with more severe disease.

Sodium cromoglycate and **nedocromil** are two related noncorticosteroid agents that are able to blunt the effect of inflammatory inducers and certain bronchospastic triggers (especially cold air and exercise). They are particularly effective in patients who have a significant **allergic component** to their asthma. The precise mechanism of action of the agents is not yet clear.

β-agonists are the most potent and widely used **bronchodilators**. Generally administered via MDI to limit systemic side effects (e.g., tachycardia, tremors), they provide prompt symptomatic relief, but because they do not have intrinsic anti-inflammatory action, they do not alter the underlying pathophysiology. Inhaled, medium-acting β_2-selective agonists (e.g., albuterol, terbutaline, pirbuterol, metaproterenol) are generally used for immediate relief. Long-acting agents (salmeterol) can be used in combination with anti-inflammatory agents for long-term control but generally never on their own.

Theophylline and related **methylxanthines** have moderate bronchodilatory action but may also improve respiratory muscle function and increase respiratory drive. Administered via the oral route (although sometimes used intravenously during an acute attack), they can be useful for the prevention of nocturnal symptoms. Serum levels need to be monitored because nausea, palpitations, and seizures can result from toxic levels. The advent of more potent topical agents as well as multiple drug interactions has resulted in decreased use of these agents.

Inhaled anticholinergic agents such as **ipratropium bromide** cause bronchodilation through inhibition of vagal stimulation of the airways. It has a slower onset and usually a lower peak effect in most asthmatics when compared with the β-agonists. Although ipratropium bromide is the first-choice bronchodilator for use in patients with chronic obstructive pulmonary disease (COPD), only certain asthmatics, particularly older patients with intrinsic asthma, benefit from its routine symptomatic use.

During an acute attack, most asthmatics benefit from supplemental oxygen to maintain oxygen saturation at 90% or higher. Hypoventilation caused by loss of hypoxic drive is extremely rare in asthma, as opposed to the case in chronic bronchitis.

The National Heart, Lung, and Blood Institute has published guidelines for the classification of asthma, along with recommendations for long-term and symptomatic therapy (Table 15-1). The emphasis is on proper maintenance therapy (with anti-inflammatory medication) with minimal reliance on short-acting β-agonist agents.

Key reasons for **failure in asthma control** are:

- Patient noncompliance
- An overreliance on β-agonists
- Improper use of MDIs (requires significant patient education and effort to use properly)
- Failure to recognize acute exacerbations early and institute proper therapy

It is important to note that failure related to these reasons can be avoided by aggressive patient education.

TABLE 15-1 National Heart, Lung, and Blood Institute's Asthma Guidelines

Classification	Symptoms	Nighttime Symptoms	Lung Function	Long-Term Control	Quick Relief
Mild Intermittent	Symptoms ≤2 times a week Asymptomatic and normal PEF between exacerbations Exacerbations brief (from a few hours to a few days); intensity may vary	≤2 month	FEV_1 or PEF ≥80% predicted PEF variability <20%	No daily medication required	Short acting β_2-agonist as needed for symptoms Use of short-acting β_2-agonist <2 times a week may indicate long-term control therapy
Mild persistent	Symptoms >2 times a week but <1 time a day Exacerbations may affect activity	>2 times a month	FEV_1 or PEF ≥80% predicted PEF variability 20% to 30%	One daily medication: Inhaled corticosteroid (low dose) *or* cromolyn *or* nedocromil Leukotriene modifier may be considered (exact position in therapy not fully established)	Short acting β_2-agonist as needed for symptoms Use of short-acting β_2-agonist on a daily basis may indicate need for additional long-term control therapy
Moderate persistent	Daily symptoms Daily use of inhaled short acting β_2-agonist	>1 time a week	FEV_1 or PEF >60% to <80% predicted PEF variability >30%	Daily medication: *Either* inhaled corticosteroid (medium dose) *or* inhaled corticosteroid (low-medium dose) and long-acting bronchodilator, esp. for nighttime symptoms (either long-acting β_2-agonist, sustained-release theophylline, or leukotriene modifiers)	Short acting β_2-agonist as needed for symptoms Use of short-acting β_2-agonist on a daily basis indicates need for additional long-term control therapy

■ TABLE 15-1 National Heart, Lung, and Blood Institute's Asthma Guidelines *(continued)*

Classification	Symptoms	Nighttime Symptoms	Lung Function	Long-Term Control	Quick Relief
	Exacerbations affect activity			*If needed*: High-dose inhaled cortico-steroid *and* long-acting bronchodilator *Consider* referral to asthma specialist	
	Exacerbations ≥2 times a week; may last days				
Severe persistent	Continual symptoms Limited physical activity Frequent exacerbations	Frequent	FEV$_1$ or PEF ≥60% predicted PEF variability >30%	Daily medication: Inhaled cortico-steroid (high dose) *and* long-acting bronchodilator, esp. for nighttime symptoms (either long-acting β$_2$-agonist, sustained-release theophylline, or leukotriene modi-fiers) *and* cortico-steroid tablets/syrup long term (make repeated attempt to reduce systemic steroids) and maintain control with high-dose inhaled steroids *Recommend* referral to asthma specialist	Short acting β$_2$-agonist as needed for symptoms Use of short-acting β$_2$-agonist on a daily basis indicates need for additional long-term control therapy

FEV$_1$, forced expiratory volume in 1 second; PEF, peak expiratory flow.

 KEY POINTS

- Asthma is an episodic disease characterized by abnormally heightened responsiveness of the tracheobronchial tree, leading to expiratory airflow obstruction.
- Chronic airway inflammation appears to be a key pathophysiologic feature of asthma.
- Acute attacks of asthma are often triggered by stimuli that produce bronchoconstriction in the setting of chronic airway inflammation.

- Management of asthma involves avoiding environmental stimuli that produce inflammation and/or bronchoconstriction, control of chronic inflammation by the use of anti-inflammatory drugs (e.g., inhaled steroids), and the limited symptomatic use of bronchodilators (e.g., β-agonists).

Pulmonary Embolism

EPIDEMIOLOGY

Pulmonary embolism (PE) is a common, but often unrecognized, medical disease with approximately 500,000 cases and an estimated 150,000 deaths annually in the United States. Without treatment, approximately 30% of all pulmonary emboli are fatal, although this statistic decreases to <10% with effective anticoagulant therapy, making rapid, accurate diagnosis essential.

ETIOLOGY

The great majority of pulmonary emboli (95%) arise from deep vein thrombosis (DVT) in the lower extremity. The development of thrombosis is increased by three major factors (Virchow's triad): **stasis, alteration in blood vessels** (injury), and **hypercoagulability**. **High-risk conditions** may be classified by these factors:

Stasis
- Surgery
- Heart failure
- Chronic venous stasis
- Immobility

Alteration in Blood Vessels (injury)
- Fractures or surgery of lower extremity
- Major trauma

Hypercoagulability
- Postpartum period
- Malignancy
- Oral contraceptives
- Deficiencies of protein S, protein C, and antithrombin III

- Lupus anticoagulant
- Activated protein C resistance (e.g., factor V Leiden)
- Prothrombin gene mutations
- Hyperhomocysteinemia

CLINICAL MANIFESTATIONS

HISTORY

The most prominent symptom in pulmonary embolism is a **sudden onset of unexplained dyspnea**. **Pleuritic chest pain** (increased with respiration) occurs in almost as many patients. **Cough** can be present in roughly a third of patients. **Hemoptysis**, although considered a classic finding, is relatively uncommon and usually indicates pulmonary infarction.

Other presentations include syncope, supraventricular tachycardias (SVTs), and worsening of underlying heart failure or lung disease. Hospitalized patients, particularly those who are severely ill or on pain medications, may present primarily with anxiety or agitation.

Overall the signs and symptoms are generally not helpful diagnostically as they can be seen in a wide variety of conditions, making it important to have a high level of suspicion when attempting to diagnosis a possible PE.

PHYSICAL EXAMINATION

Vital sign abnormalities are common in PE. **Tachycardia** is often found, and **tachypnea** is almost universal. Low-grade fever (<101°F [38.3°C]) may be encountered, but high fevers (>103°F) are rare.

The pulmonary examination in PE is often completely normal with less than half of all patients presenting with scattered rales as the sole finding. Cardiac examination may reveal signs of **right-sided heart strain** if the embolus is extensive. These include:

- Loud pulmonic component of second heart sound (P2), best heard in left second intercostal space
- Right-sided S3 (increased with inspiration)
- Right ventricular heave (palpable lift over left sternal border)

Physical findings related to underlying lower extremity thrombosis is seen in only approximately a third of all patients. In summary, there is a distinct lack of sensitive or specific clinical findings in patients with PE, making laboratory diagnosis essential (see later).

DIFFERENTIAL DIAGNOSIS

In the patient who presents with **shortness of breath and chest pain**, the differential diagnosis includes:

- Pneumothorax
- Myocardial ischemia
- Pericarditis
- Asthma
- Pneumonia

In the patient with a massive PE who presents with **hypotension** and hemodynamic instability, also consider:

- MI with shock
- Cardiac tamponade
- Tension pneumothorax
- Aortic dissection

DIAGNOSTIC EVALUATION

ABG classically shows hypoxia, hypocapnia, and a respiratory alkalosis. However, a normal ABG does not conclusively rule out pulmonary embolus, and patients with massive PE may have hypercapnia and a metabolic/respiratory acidosis, making ABG measurement of limited diagnostic utility

Chest radiograph most often shows atelectasis, seen in 60% to 70% of patients. Some classic, but less common, **radiograph findings** include:

- Increased lung lucency in the area of embolus (Westermark sign)
- Abrupt cutoff of vessel

- Wedge-shaped pleural-based infiltrate ("Hampton hump")
- Pleural effusion, which if sampled by thoracentesis, is often hemorrhagic

The last two signs occur 12 to 36 hours after symptoms begin and usually indicate pulmonary infarction.

The classic pattern on an **electrocardiogram** (ECG) for PE in the context of **right heart strain** is an S wave in lead I with a Q-wave and T-wave inversion in lead III ("S1-Q3-T3 pattern"). Other signs of right heart strain are new right bundle branch block and ST-segment changes in V_1 and V_2. However, the most common ECG finding is simply **tachycardia and nonspecific ST-segment and T-wave changes**.

Ventilation/perfusion (V/Q) scan identifies a "mismatch" between areas that are ventilated but not perfused and is the best initial test for PE in patients with a clear chest film. Prospective studies in large numbers of patients evaluated for PE have shown the following:

- A **normal** scan basically rules out the diagnosis of PE.
- A **high-probability** scan is diagnostic if the clinical suspicion is also high (i.e., a "classic" story for PE in a patient with risk factors).
- A **low-probability** scan rules out the diagnosis only in a patient with a low pretest clinical probability because PE can be found in roughly 15% of patients with "low-probability" scans.
- An **indeterminate** scan is just that—indeterminate. Chance of PE in these patients ranges from 16% to 66%, depending on the physician's pretest probability.

Unfortunately, the clinical and V/Q scan combination in the majority of patients is unable to confirm or exclude the diagnosis of PI, thus leading to the development of additional tests as listed below.

A newer modality for the noninvasive diagnosis of PE is the use of **helical computed tomography (CT) with intravenous contrast**. Several studies initially indicated that the use of contrast helical CT may eventually replace V/Q scanning as the initial screening test of choice. However, subsequent studies have revealed varying sensitivities. Variation in reader expertise appears to greatly influence the sensitivity of the test. The consensus among experts is that helical CT is a useful adjunctive diagnostic modality, but additional prospective studies are required to arrive at more firm recommendations regarding the routine use of the technique. It is likely that determination of clinical pretest probability (as with V/Q scanning) may improve the diagnostic utility of helical CT. One advantage of CT is that it may reveal an alternative diagnosis for the patient's symptoms (e.g., tumor or lymphadenopathy).

Color-flow Doppler ultrasound (US) with compression is a noninvasive test of the lower extremities that accurately detects **proximal** DVT (70% to 80% of all patients with PE have a concomitant proximal DVT). It is **not** useful in asymptomatic post–hip replacement patients (sensitivity <50%). Some clinicians advocate using this test before going to invasive procedures because a positive result establishes a need for anticoagulation.

The detection of D-dimers (a biochemical marker for thrombosis) in a patient's blood has been evaluated in ruling out DVT/PE in patients with a low clinical probability of DVT/PE. In patients with no risk factors coupled with a poor history and physical examination for DVT/PE, the negative predictive value of a negative D-dimer test is >99% and thus obviates the need for additional testing.

Several schemes for the diagnosis of PE using a panel of noninvasive tests have been proposed and validated. A combination of clinical assessment, V/Q scanning, D-dimer testing, and venous US can confirm or exclude the diagnosis of acute PE in many patients. In one study, a list of criteria, the "modified Wells' criteria" (Table 16-1), was used to assign clinical likelihood of PE. Using a specific D-dimer assay, a negative D-dimer coupled with a low clinical probability effectively ruled out PE. Other studies have the used the Wells' criteria in multimodal testing schemes (see Key Points).

Performance of a **pulmonary angiogram** remains the gold standard for diagnosis. This invasive procedure is generally safe (approximately 1% mortality) and is indicated if the diagnosis remains uncertain after noninvasive testing, which can be the case in up to 20% of cases in recent studies.

TREATMENT

In the high-risk patient with PE, **heparin** should be started while awaiting the diagnostic workup. Delay in therapy will likely increase morbidity, whereas the risk of a brief period of anticoagulation is small. **Contraindications** for anticoagulation include:

- Active GI bleeding
- Intracranial neoplasm
- Recent major surgery (relative contraindication)
- Known bleeding diathesis (relative contraindication)

Patients with DVT should also be treated with heparin. The treatment of **below-the-knee DVT** is more controversial. These clots have a low risk of embolizing, although 15% to 20% progress to above the knee. Recommendations vary from conservative treatment with elevation of the extremity and nonsteroidal anti-inflammatory drugs to treatment with standard anticoagulation therapy. Others advise follow-up with noninvasive tests every 3 to 4 days over the next 10 to 14 days to detect progression.

In the hypotensive patient with massive pulmonary embolus, **thrombolytic therapy** may be indicated. More stable patients are believed not to benefit from this high-risk therapy.

Adequate anticoagulation should be achieved within the first 24 hours; if not, the risk of postphlebitic complications and DVT recurrence is increased. Heparin dosage can be calculated by a weight-based nomogram (e.g., an initial IV bolus, equal to 80 U per kg, followed by a continuous drip of 18 U/kg/hour), although other nomograms have been found to be effective in achieving adequate anticoagulation within 24 hours. The partial thromboplastin time (PTT) should be checked every 4 hours, with appropriate dose adjustments (as per protocol) to reach the goal of 1.5 to 2.0 times the control value of PTT.

During heparin therapy, platelet counts should be monitored. **Heparin-induced thrombocytopenia** manifests as a dramatic drop in platelets 1 to 20 days after initiation of therapy and is believed to be an autoimmune destruction mediated through IgG.

TABLE 16-1 Modified Wells' Criteria for the Clinical Assessment of Pulmonary Embolus (PE)

Criteria	Score
Clinical symptoms of DVT	3.0
Other diagnoses less likely than PE	3.0
Heart rate >100	1.5
Immobilization or surgery in past 4 wk	1.5
Previous DVT/PE	1.5
Hemoptysis	1.0
Malignancy	1.0
Probability of PE	**Score**
High	>6.0
Moderate	2.0 to 6.0
Low	<2.0

Changing from bovine to porcine heparin or vice versa has not proven to be effective (nor is a change to low-molecular-weight heparin). Discontinuation of heparin is recommended if the platelet count is below 75,000.

Once the heparin dose is therapeutic, **warfarin** therapy should be instituted (although some studies have found comparable efficacy and safety to initiation of oral anticoagulation at the same time as heparin therapy). The goal for warfarin therapy is an international normalized ratio (INR) of the PT of 2 to 3. Heparin is normally continued for at least 5 days and overlapped with a therapeutic warfarin dose for 2 to 3 days. Warfarin is then continued for 3 to 6 months in patients who have no complications.

Recently, low-molecular-weight heparin (LMWH) has begun to replace standard heparin as initial therapy for DVT. This is generally recommended only for hemodynamically stable patients, otherwise IV unfractionated heparin remains the treatment of choice. **Advantages of LMWH** include:

- Fixed dosages administered subcutaneously (possibly at home)
- No need for laboratory monitoring
- Decreased risk of DVT recurrence in some studies

Some patients are candidates for placement of an **inferior vena cava filter**. Indications include:

- Contraindication to anticoagulation (see earlier)
- Formation of thrombosis despite adequate anticoagulation
- Large burden of thrombosis in lower extremities that could be fatal if embolized

The use of thrombolysis in patients with PE has been studied, with the theory that certain patients, in particular those with massive thrombus loads, may benefit. However, well-controlled prospective randomized clinical trials need to be completed before preliminary recommendations can be made regarding this mode of treatment.

CONTINUED CARE

Morbidity from pulmonary emboli is best avoided by preventing the development of DVTs. For patients at risk of DVT, low-dose subcutaneous heparin (5,000 U twice a day) or intermittent lower extremity compression is effective. **Indications for prophylaxis** include:

- Major surgery
- Acute myocardial infarction
- Stroke
- Prolonged immobility

Special consideration is given to patients at extremely high risk, such as those with hip fractures or hip/knee replacements. Warfarin to achieve an INR of 2 to 3 is indicated in these situations. LMWH appears to be effective in these instances as well.

Although cancer is associated with thromboembolism, most cancers are known or obvious at the time of PE diagnosis. However, approximately 10% of patients with idiopathic PE (no known risk factors) develop cancer within a few years of diagnosis. Routine cancer screening (stool guaiac, mammograms, etc.) is recommended, but extensive testing is not.

 KEY POINTS

- Patients at risk for DVT/PE are those with an abnormality of blood vessels, stasis, or hypercoagulability. The most common predisposing causes are orthopedic injuries, surgery, and malignancy.

- Sudden onset of dyspnea and pleuritic pain is the classic presentation, but physical findings are neither sensitive nor specific for the diagnosis of PE. A normal chest radiograph and normal ABG level do not rule out the diagnosis but are useful to exclude other causes.

- V/Q scanning (or potentially helical CT with contrast) should be performed on all patients suspected of PE. In the high-risk patient, heparin therapy should be initiated if testing is delayed.

- The diagnosis of PE and the need for anticoagulation can be documented by any of the following: angiogram positive for PE, DVT confirmed by US or venogram, or a high-probability V/Q scan in a patient with a high suspicion of PE.

- Anticoagulation can safely be withheld in patients with a normal V/Q scan or negative D-dimer test.

- Anticoagulation can also be withheld in patients with low pretest clinical probability (based on Wells' criteria) with non–high probability lung scan and either negative venous Doppler studies or negative D-dimer test.

- Adequate anticoagulation with heparin, followed by oral anticoagulation, is the mainstay of treatment of PE.

Interstitial Lung Disease

Interstitial lung disease (ILD) refers to a heterogeneous group of disorders that are characterized by inflammation and fibrosis of the alveolar walls and the perialveolar tissue. The spectrum of ILD ranges from idiopathic diseases to diseases resulting from exposure to pharmacologic, environmental, and occupational substances. The **unifying features** of these conditions are the similarity in:

- Symptoms
- Alteration in pulmonary physiology
- Chest radiograph appearance
- Histologic appearance

Due to the fact that there are a wide range of causes however, management will vary depending on the exact etiology.

ETIOLOGY AND PATHOGENESIS

The central pathophysiologic process in ILD involves chronic inflammation of the alveolar wall and surrounding structures. The inflammatory response can involve polymorphonuclear lymphocytes (PMNs), lymphocytes of B and/or T lineage, and macrophages, depending on the specific etiology. Chronic inflammation eventually leads to scarring and fibrosis. The resulting fibrosis leads to the following **disturbances in lung function**:

- Decreased transalveolar gas diffusion
- A restrictive respiratory pattern (resulting in decreased lung volumes)
- Variable obstructive respiratory pattern (depending on the underlying etiology)

There are close to 200 described causes of ILD. However, the majority of them can be grouped into four **major divisions**:

- Pneumoconioses
- Hypersensitivity pneumonitis
- Drug-induced disease
- Idiopathic/primary lung diseases

PNEUMOCONIOSES

The pneumoconioses are a group of disorders characterized by pulmonary exposure to inorganic and organic dusts and gases. Chronic inflammation develops, characterized by mucous hypersecretion, scarring, and fibrosis. As compared with other causes of ILD, the mucous hypersecretion can result in a prominent obstructive picture. The list of **dusts and gases that can result in ILD** is extensive and includes the following.

Dusts
- Asbestos
- Coal
- Rock (talc, silica, cement)
- Metals (beryllium, antimony, tin, silver, iron)
- Graphite
- Cotton
- Grain

Gases
- Acid fumes
- Chlorine
- Nitrogen dioxide
- Phosgene

HYPERSENSITIVITY PNEUMONITIS

Hypersensitivity pneumonitis (HP) is a condition in which the inflammation is immunologically mediated. Deposition of antigen (again, usually in the form of dusts) in the alveoli results in the formation of antigen-antibody complexes. There is early infiltration by PMNs and later by mononuclear cells and mast cells. Granuloma formation, in a classic delayed-type hypersensitivity reaction, can result.

Exposure to a variety of antigens can result in the development of HP. These **antigens** can be from various microorganisms (fungi and bacteria), plants, or animals:

- Thermophilic *Actinomycetes* (farmer lung, bagassosis or sugar cane worker lung, potato riddler lung)
- *Aspergillus* species (malt worker lung, tobacco worker lung, compost lung, allergic bronchopulmonary aspergillosis)
- *Botrytis cinerea* (winegrower lung)
- Bird proteins (e.g., feathers, droppings; bird fanciers/bird breeder lung)
- Animal fur dust (furrier lung)
- Wood dust (woodworker lung)
- *Bacillus subtilis* enzymes (detergent worker lung)

The **appearance of HP** is influenced by a number of variables, including:

- The degree and length of antigen exposure
- The specific antigen
- Host factors

DRUGS

A large number of drugs can cause diffuse pulmonary injury.

Cytotoxic Drugs
- Bleomycin
- Vinblastine
- Alkylating agents (cyclophosphamide, melphalan)
- Antimetabolites (methotrexate, azathioprine, cytosine arabinoside)

Noncytotoxic Drugs
- Antibiotics (nitrofurantoin, amphotericin, penicillins, sulfas)
- Nonsteroidal anti-inflammatory agents
- β-Blocking agents
- Antiarrhythmic agents (lidocaine, amiodarone)

For the cytotoxic agents, the pathophysiology is felt to be direct pulmonary toxicity. For noncytotoxic drugs, a combination of direct pulmonary toxicity as well as immunologic injury may be involved.

OTHER CAUSES (IDIOPATHIC)

ILD can develop in the setting of a number of **collagen vascular disorders**:

- Systemic lupus erythematosus (SLE) (ILD less common than pleural disease and acute pneumonitis)
- Rheumatoid arthritis
- Ankylosing spondylitis (upper lobe fibrosis)
- Progressive systemic sclerosis
- Polymyositis
- Goodpasture syndrome (pulmonary hemorrhage and glomerulonephritis because of antibasement membrane antibodies)
- Wegener granulomatosis

Sarcoidosis and the group of diseases referred to as histiocytosis X can also result in ILD.

Idiopathic pulmonary fibrosis (IPF) is a well-defined disease in which there is typical immunologic damage to the lung without identification of a causative antigen as in HP. The disease is characterized by an alveolar infiltrate composed of PMNs and activated macrophages. Fibrosis results, but without granuloma formation (which can distinguish it from some forms of HP).

CLINICAL MANIFESTATIONS

HISTORY

The typical history in ILD is one of months or years of gradually **progressive dyspnea** (early on, dyspnea may only be encountered on exertion) and a **nonproductive cough**. Some patients can have a more acute onset, as in HP, where it occurs several hours after allergen exposure. If no further allergen exposure occurs, symptoms will diminish over several days. Patients with occupational HP may give a history of relatively symptom-free weekends, with an increase in symptoms associated with return to work on Monday.

A detailed history of possible environmental and occupational exposures, both past and present, must be obtained when evaluating possible ILD.

PHYSICAL EXAMINATION

Initially, the physical examination in patients with ILD may be unremarkable, but as the disease progresses the classic finding of **fine expiratory crackles** appears. With progressive fibrosis and resultant pulmonary hypertension, signs of right heart overload and failure develop (accentuated pulmonary component of the second heart sound, right-sided heave, hepatic congestion, lower extremity edema).

If ILD is associated with a systemic illness such as SLE, physical finding of these diseases may be present. In most cases, however, physical examination can help identify a patient with ILD but rarely suggests an underlying etiology.

DIFFERENTIAL DIAGNOSIS

The major differential diagnosis is among the illnesses that comprise ILD, but the pulmonary symptoms of dyspnea and cough can also be seen in:

- Congestive heart failure (CHF)
- Asthma
- Chronic obstructive pulmonary disease (COPD)

DIAGNOSTIC EVALUATION

The initial diagnostic test in suspected ILD is the chest radiograph. The typical **chest radiograph** findings in ILD are **reticular** or **reticulonodular infiltrates** with diminished lung volumes (Fig. 17-1). A variety of abnormalities, including alveolar infiltrates, hilar and mediastinal adenopathy, pleural disease, and honeycombing, can also be seen. Larger nodules are more common in granulomatous diseases such as sarcoidosis and Wegener granulomatosis, as well as in silicosis and asbestosis.

The **anatomic location of the infiltrates** can suggest different etiologies:

Upper Lung Zones
- Sarcoidosis
- Silicosis
- Berylliosis
- Hypersensitivity pneumonitis

Lower Lung Zones
- IPF
- Collagen vascular disease–associated ILD
- Asbestosis

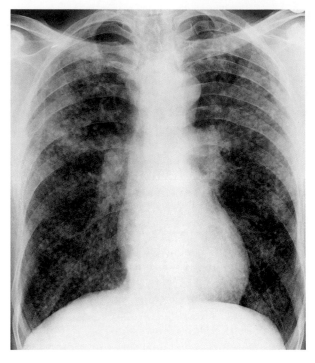

Figure 17-1 • Chest radiograph from a patient with interstitial lung disease caused by exposure to coal dust. There are multiple nodular densities involving both lung fields. Lung volume is preserved in this case.

Note that up to 10% of patients with biopsy-proven ILD have a normal or near-normal chest radiograph. **High-resolution computed tomography** (CT) (Fig. 17-2) provides added sensitivity and specificity in diagnosis and in assessing disease extent and severity. It can detect disease early on, even before pulmonary function testing becomes abnormal.

Pulmonary function tests (see Chapter 12) typically reveal **restrictive physiology** with decreased lung volumes. There may be a small degree of airway obstruction. The **diffusion capacity is reduced**, often with an **increased alveolar-arterial oxygen gradient** that increases further with exercise.

Fiberoptic bronchoscopy combined with **bronchoalveolar lavage** (BAL) can be useful. Endobronchial nodules can be seen in sarcoidosis. BAL can reveal infectious agents and/or specific antigens or small molecules. Characterization of the inflammatory cells present can suggest a specific etiology. For example, HP generally yields BAL fluid with a predominance of lymphocytes and mast cells, whereas eosinophils are more common in IPF and collagen vascular disorders.

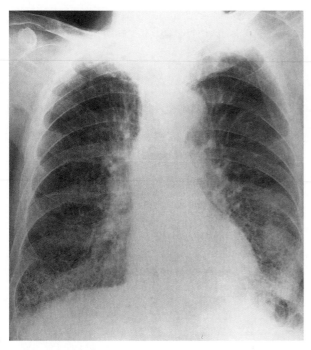

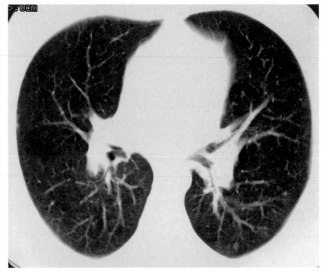

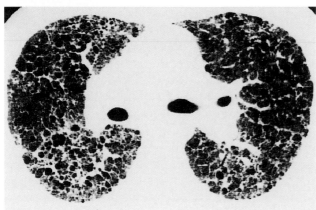

Figure 17-2 • Idiopathic pulmonary fibrosis. **(A)** Chest radiograph reveals reticulonodular shadowing (honeycomb lung) with basilar predominance. **(B)** High-resolution CT scan of a different patient showing the honeycomb pattern in the lungs. **(C)** Normal chest CT is shown for comparison.

Lung biopsy is the gold standard for making the diagnosis of ILD. Biopsy can be obtained by the transbronchial route during bronchoscopy, but this yields small pieces of tissue that may be insufficient for diagnosis. Thoracoscopic and open biopsy allow direct visualization of abnormal lung and provide the most tissue but at the risk of increased morbidity.

TREATMENT

Once the diagnosis of ILD is suspected by history, physical, and chest radiograph, the physician must search aggressively for an etiologic agent while confirming the diagnosis. This is often done in consultation with a pulmonary specialist, particularly if invasive diagnostic procedures are to be done.

For HP and the pneumoconioses, **eliminating or preventing exposure to the offending agent** is the first priority. This recommendation cannot be taken lightly because it can result in a severe alteration in lifestyle and livelihood. In some cases of occupational exposure involving larger particles, proper masks may be sufficient to eliminate exposure. Conditions such as Wegener granulomatosis and SLE may require immunosuppressive treatment.

In cases where removal of a specific etiology is insufficient and for diseases where treatment of the underlying condition is not possible (e.g., IPF, ankylosing spondylitis), the treatment options are limited. **Corticosteroids**, initially high dose and then tapered for response, can provide benefit in a number of patients. Corticosteroids may also hasten recovery in patients with hypersensitivity pneumonitis.

For patients who present early with hypersensitivity pneumonitis, prompt withdrawal of the offending agent, with steroid treatment if necessary, results in a complete normalization of pulmonary status. In patients with a pneumoconiosis, damage often results from years of exposure. Removal of the offending agent may stop the decline in respiratory function, but fixed defects often remain. Other patients, including those with IPF who fail to respond to corticosteroid therapy, have continued decline in respiratory function, eventually leading to death from pulmonary failure. For a limited number of these patients, lung transplantation is an alternative.

 KEY POINTS

- ILD refers to a group of disorders characterized by inflammation of the alveolar and perialveolar structures.

- The majority of cases of ILD are secondary to direct or immunologic lung injury caused by inhaled or ingested substances.

- The cardinal clinical features of ILD are a history of progressive dyspnea on exertion accompanied by a nonproductive cough. Physical examination generally reveals fine crackles, whereas reticular or reticulonodular infiltrates are seen on chest radiograph.

- Treatment of ILD involves removal of any underlying etiologies and corticosteroid therapy for selected conditions. Treatment options are limited beyond this.

Pleural Effusions

The **pleural cavity** exists between the mesothelial layers of visceral and parietal pleura. The **visceral pleura** completely covers the lung except at the hilum, where the bronchus, pulmonary vessels, and nerves enter the lung parenchyma. The opposing **parietal pleura** lines the inner surface of the chest wall, mediastinum, and diaphragm and becomes continuous with the visceral pleura at the hilum.

The parietal and visceral pleura are normally separated by a very thin layer of fluid. A **pleural effusion** is an accumulation of excess fluid in the space between the parietal and visceral pleura. When a patient presents with a pleural effusion, the nature of the underlying etiology needs to be determined. Although many etiologies are benign, the possibility of infection and malignancy needs to be considered.

ETIOLOGY AND PATHOGENESIS

The pleural fluid is normally formed as an ultrafiltrate of plasma across the capillaries of the parietal pleura and is removed by lymphatics also located in the parietal pleura. The rate formation of the pleural fluid is determined by the **Starling law**, which describes the balance of hydrostatic and oncotic pressures between the microvasculature and the pleural cavity. The normal volume of the pleural fluid is 0.1 to 0.2 mL per kg, or <15 mL in a 70-kg person. Despite this small volume of fluid, the rate of pleural fluid filtration and reabsorption can exceed 1 L per day. Formation of a pleural effusion thus reflects either an **increase in production** or **decrease in removal** of the pleural fluid. Excess production of fluid can arise from the parietal pleura, the interstitial spaces of the lung, or the peritoneal cavity (the latter via defects in the diaphragm

or lymphatics). Decreased removal because of blockage of the pleural lymphatics most commonly occurs secondary to malignant invasion of the mediastinal lymph nodes but can also be caused by inflammation from processes such as an empyema.

A pleural effusion can be classified either as a **transudate** or an **exudate**. The formation of a **transudate** reflects an alteration in the disturbance in the Starling forces such that the rate of formation of pleural fluid exceeds the maximal rate of lymphatic clearance. The pleural capillary endothelium remains intact, and the protein content of the fluid is low. The development of an **exudate**, however, implies a loss of integrity of the pleural membrane and/or disruption of the lymphatic drainage. Exudative effusions are characterized by an elevated protein concentration.

The **causes of pleural effusions**, both transudative and exudative, reflect the pathophysiology just outlined.

Transudates are caused by:
- Congestive heart failure (CHF) (increased capillary hydrostatic pressure)
- Cirrhosis (decreased plasma oncotic pressure)
- Nephrotic syndrome (decreased plasma oncotic pressure)
- Pulmonary embolism (altered hemodynamics)

Exudates are caused by:
- Bacterial pneumonia (damage to pleural membrane)
- Metastatic disease, most commonly lung, breast, and lymphoma (blockage of lymphatic drainage via lymph node infiltration)
- Pulmonary embolism (damage to pleural membrane)

- Tuberculosis (damage to pleural membrane and blockage of lymphatic drainage)
- Collagen vascular diseases, for example, rheumatoid arthritis, systemic lupus erythematosus (SLE) (damage to pleural membrane from inflammation)
- Mesothelioma (altered pleural membrane because of primary tumor of mesothelial cells)
- Viral infection (damage to pleural membrane)

Overall, the vast majority of transudates are caused by heart failure, whereas the combination of pneumonia, metastatic disease, and pulmonary embolism accounts for approximately 80% of exudates. Note that pulmonary embolism can result in either a transudate or exudate.

CLINICAL MANIFESTATIONS

HISTORY

Symptoms in the setting of a pleural effusion often reflect the underlying cause rather than respiratory compromise because of the effusion itself:

- Pleuritic chest pain (bacterial pneumonia, pulmonary embolism, viral infection, tumor)
- Cough (pneumonia, tumor)
- Sputum production (pneumonia)
- Hemoptysis (pulmonary embolism, tumor, tuberculosis)
- Shortness of breath (heart failure, pneumonia)

Symptoms directly related to the effusion itself can be minimal, but if the effusion becomes large enough, dyspnea, chest pain, and cough can result. This is often seen in the large pleural effusions associated with malignancy.

PHYSICAL EXAMINATION

A large pleural effusion can result in the following **physical findings**:

- Decreased tactile fremitus
- Dullness to percussion
- Absent or diminished breath sounds
- Shift of trachea and heart away from affected side

In addition, findings related to the underlying etiology may be present:

- Adenopathy (malignancy, tuberculosis)
- Elevated neck veins, peripheral edema (heart failure)
- Ascites (cirrhosis)

DIAGNOSTIC EVALUATION

Large pleural effusions are readily seen on routine **chest radiographs**. Smaller effusions can be seen by obtaining bilateral **decubitus films** in addition to the routine upright films (Fig. 18-1).

Chest computed tomography (CT) is useful in detecting small pleural effusions and is also more

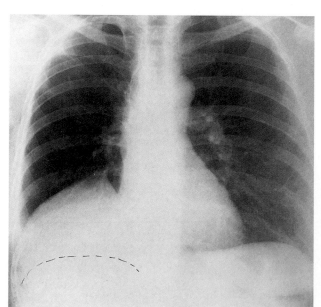

A

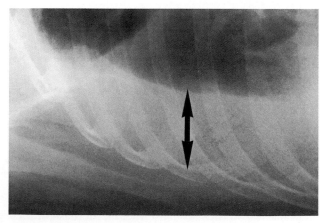

B

Figure 18-1 • Large right subpulmonary effusion (the patient has had right mastectomy). **(A)** In the upper position, almost all the fluid is between the lung and the diaphragm. The right hemidiaphragm cannot be seen. Its estimated position has been penciled in. **(B)** In the lateral decubitus view, the fluid moves to lie between the lateral chest wall and the lung edge (*arrows*).

sensitive in detecting parenchymal masses and enlarged lymph nodes in cases of suspected malignant pleural effusion.

Once a pleural effusion is detected by examination and radiographic studies, a sample should be obtained by **diagnostic thoracentesis** to determine if it is an exudate or transudate. For large, free-flowing effusions, this can be done blindly with guidance based on physical examination (via percussion to determine the extent of the effusion). Smaller effusions and loculated effusions may need to be sampled under US guidance.

A number of criteria have been proposed to differentiate transudates from exudates, but the most commonly used **criteria** were proposed by Light and colleagues:

- Pleural fluid-to-serum protein (albumin) ratio more than 0.5
- Pleural fluid lactate dehydrogenase (LDH) more than 200 IU (or greater than two thirds of the upper limit of the laboratory's normal serum LDH).
- Pleural fluid-to-serum LDH ratio more than 0.6

If **any one** of the critical values is exceeded, the effusion is judged to be an **exudate**.

An effusion occurring in the setting of a bacterial pneumonia or lung abscess (so-called parapneumonic effusion) needs further evaluation. The diagnosis of a **complicated parapneumonic effusion** is made if any of the following conditions are found:

- Gross pus present in the pleural space
- Organisms visible on Gram stain of the pleural fluid (defines an empyema)
- Pleural fluid glucose <50 mg per dL (this can also be seen in malignant effusions)
- Pleural fluid pH <7.00 (with an arterial pH >7.15)

Culture of a suspected empyema should be done as well as a Gram stain.

If a **malignant pleural effusion** is suspected, the pleural fluid should be sent for **cytology**. If this is negative, a needle biopsy of the pleura should be performed. If this is also negative, thoracoscopic or open biopsy of the pleura may be needed. These latter procedures are often needed to make the diagnosis of **malignant mesothelioma**.

TREATMENT

The management of pleural effusions varies between transudates and exudates. **Transudative effusions** are managed simply by correcting the underlying problem.

Because the pleural membranes are intact, restoring the normal Starling forces permits reabsorption of the excess fluid. Management of an **exudate** may require local control of the effusion (drainage or sclerosis) as well as correction of the underlying disorder.

For **transudates**, **diuretic treatment** is the mainstay of therapy, reducing the intravascular hydrostatic pressure. In rare cases, a therapeutic thoracentesis is required to relieve dyspnea until the Starling forces are in proper balance and further accumulation stops.

A **complicated parapneumonic effusion** requires drainage with **tube thoracostomy**. This is to prevent loculation of the effusion and also because antibiotics penetrate and perform poorly in such effusions. If loculation has already occurred, multiple tubes may be required. Alternately, streptokinase or urokinase can be instilled via the chest tube in an attempt to dissolve the loculations. In severe cases, **surgical decortication** may be required.

The management of **malignant pleural effusions** is often problematic. Treatment of the underlying malignancy is generally not possible. Malignant effusions are often quite large and reaccumulate after therapeutic needle thoracentesis. Alternatives include:

- Instillation of sclerosing agents such as bleomycin or minocycline via a chest tube
- Application of talc or direct abrasion via thoracoscopy
- Insertion of a pleuroperitoneal shunt

 KEY POINTS

- A pleural effusion is the accumulation of excess fluid between the parietal and visceral pleura.
- Pleural fluid can form because of excess production caused by a disturbance in the Starling forces across the pleural membrane (transudates) or as a result of damage to the pleural membrane and/or the draining lymphatics (exudates).
- Transudates can be distinguished from exudates by measuring the protein and LDH contents in the pleural fluid and comparing them with serum values.
- Treatment of a transudate involves restoration of the normal Starling forces by correction of the underlying condition.
- Treatment of a transudate often requires drainage and, in severe cases, pleural sclerosis in addition to correction of the underlying condition.

Lung cancer is the leading cause of cancer death for both men and women in the United States. Because most of these cancers are caused by **cigarette smoking**, many of these deaths are preventable.

EPIDEMIOLOGY

Approximately 200,000 new cases of lung cancer are diagnosed each year in the United States, and an estimated 160,000 deaths occur annually, exceeding the combined mortality due to colorectal, breast and prostate cancer combined. Formerly, the majority of these cases occurred among men, but with the increased rate of cigarette use among women over the past 50 years, the incidence of lung cancer among women has correspondingly increased, now surpassing breast cancer as the leading cause of cancer-related mortality.

From 80% to 90% of all lung cancers occur among **smokers**. There is a 10% mortality from lung cancer among smokers, whereas the mortality among non-smokers is <1%. The major determinants of risk among smokers are the number of cigarettes smoked per day as well as the total number of years smoked (usually expressed as **pack years**, that is, the number of packs smoked per day multiplied by the number of years a patient has smoked).

If a person quits smoking, risk declines, and by 10 years the lung cancer risk is only slightly above that of someone who had never smoked. However, the risk never returns to baseline.

Other exposures that increase a person's risk of developing lung cancer, generally in a cocarcinogenic manner along with smoking, are as follows:

- Radon gas (a naturally occurring radioactive gas)
- Asbestos
- Environmental pollutants (e.g., automobile exhaust, metals)

These other carcinogens may be responsible for some of the nonsmoking-related lung cancers that are encountered.

PATHOPHYSIOLOGY

The four major histopathologic types of lung cancers can be separated into **two major groups** based on clinical grounds:

- Small cell cancers (100% of which are associated with smoking)
- Nonsmall cell cancers (further divided into squamous cell, large cell, and adenocarcinoma)

These cancers account for more than 95% of all lung cancers.

Rarer types of lung neoplasms include:
- Primary pulmonary lymphomas
- Carcinoid tumors
- Bronchoalveolar cancers (usually encountered in nonsmokers)
- Mesotheliomas

The grouping of lung cancers into small cell and nonsmall cell cancers is based on clinical characteristics. **Nonsmall cell lung cancers** arise as discrete masses within the lung parenchyma that can spread to regional lymph nodes and then metastasize to distant sites. As such, they are staged with the tumor-node-metastasis (TMN) system used to stage many solid tumors. For patients with limited tumors, surgical resection can result in cure. Unfortunately, these tumors are not very responsive to chemotherapy, limiting treatment options in disseminated disease.

In contrast, **small cell lung cancers** metastasize rapidly to regional lymph nodes and distant sites. As such, the staging of small cell lung cancers is either as **limited disease** (overt disease confined to one hemithorax and the regional lymph nodes) or **extensive disease** (where there is further spread). Only approximately 30% of patients present with limited disease. Because of the early spread of small cell lung cancer, surgery is generally reserved to relieve symptoms from the mass effect of the tumor. Unlike non-small cell cancer, small cell cancers are generally **quite responsive to chemotherapy**.

Approximately half of all patients with limited-stage disease and a third of those with extensive disease have a complete remission, and 90% have at least a partial response. Unfortunately, recurrence is common, leading to overall survival of approximately 5%. Patients with limited disease appear to have an estimated three- to fivefold better long-term survival rate compared with those with extensive disease.

Lung cancers are unusual among neoplasms in that they are relatively more likely to produce active substances that result in a variety of **paraneoplastic syndromes**:

- Hypercalcemia (caused by PTH-like substance)
- Syndrome of inappropriate antidiuretic hormone (SIADH)
- Ectopic adrenocorticotropic hormone (ACTH) secretion (with resultant Cushing syndrome)
- Eaton-Lambert syndrome (a myasthenialike disorder seen in the setting of small cell cancer)
- Hypercoagulable state (including migratory venous thrombophlebitis—Trousseau syndrome)

CLINICAL MANIFESTATIONS

HISTORY

The symptoms of lung cancer can arise from (a) the local mass effect and systemic effects (e.g., constitutional symptoms) of the tumor itself, (b) effects of metastatic disease (local or distant), and (c) effects of products produced by the tumor (paraneoplastic syndromes). The majority (estimated over 90%) of patients with lung cancer present with symptoms, which makes screening of asymptomatic smokers (see below) of questionable utility.

Because most lung cancers arise in patients with a long smoking history, the symptoms of **cough** and **dyspnea** are relatively nonspecific. However, since cough is the most common symptom in patients with lung cancer, an acute change in previously stable symptoms can suggest an underlying malignancy. Other symptoms related to the tumor itself can be **chest pain** and **hemoptysis**. Hemoptysis is generally not massive and can also be seen in patients with chronic obstructive pulmonary disease (COPD). Patients may present with the nonspecific constitutional symptoms of **anorexia**, **weight loss**, and **fevers/night sweats**.

Symptoms attributable to tumor **mass effect** include:

- Cough (because of irritation of nerves, including the phrenic nerve)
- Hoarseness (with tumor compression of the recurrent laryngeal nerve)
- Facial and/or upper extremity swelling (see SVC [superior vena cava] syndrome later)

Lung neoplasms commonly metastasize to the pleura, bone, brain, liver, and adrenal glands, where they can also produce symptoms. Patients may present with symptoms that are caused by a paraneoplastic process.

PHYSICAL EXAMINATION

The physical examination generally provides few clues to the presence of an underlying lung cancer. However, certain classic physical findings are associated with specific lung cancers:

- Horner syndrome (sympathetic ganglion dysfunction with ptosis, miosis, enophthalmos, and anhidrosis)
- A supraclavicular mass caused by a Pancoast tumor (apical tumor involving C8 and T1-2 nerve roots causing shoulder pain radiating down the arm)
- SVC syndrome (upper extremity swelling with or without facial swelling because of vascular obstruction)

In addition, clubbing of the fingers and adenopathy (axillary or supraclavicular) are suggestive (but not pathognomonic) of an underlying malignancy.

DIFFERENTIAL DIAGNOSIS

Lung cancer figures prominently in the differential diagnosis of lung masses as well as the so-called **solitary pulmonary nodule** (defined as a mass of <4 cm that appears on the chest radiograph). The differential diagnosis of lung masses includes:

- Tuberculosis
- Fungal infection (histoplasmosis, coccidioidomycosis, cryptococcus)
- Metastatic cancer to the lung
- Other granulomatous diseases (e.g., sarcoidosis)

The significance of the solitary pulmonary nodule is that approximately half are proven to be malignancies. If a solitary nodule is found to be malignant, it is associated with a 5-year survival rate of 40%, significantly better than all lung cancer patients as a group, which have an overall survival rate of 14%.

DIAGNOSTIC EVALUATION

The diagnosis of a lung cancer is first suggested on routine **chest radiograph**, which can reveal a mass as well as hilar adenopathy (Fig. 19-1). The ability of chest radiography to detect lung cancers has led to attempts to use the test as a screening method for smokers. However, it was shown that detection of asymptomatic masses on yearly chest radiograph **did not** lower mortality, presumably because of the rapid growth rates of the tumors and the relatively advanced stage of disease once a mass is visible on chest film. The use of computed tomography for screening appears to be more sensitive, but it has not yet been determined if this screening modality will serve to decrease mortality.

If a potential mass is found on chest radiograph, imaging with computed tomography (**CT**) can further define the mass and better detect nodal disease (Fig. 19-2). Magnetic resonance imaging (**MRI**) has also been used but is less well studied.

Tissue diagnosis can be obtained in a number of ways. **Sputum cytology** can yield a diagnosis of malignancy. Generally, first-morning sputum samples give the highest yield. **Bronchoscopy** (with bronchial washings, brushings, and/or biopsy) can also yield tissue. The location of a lesion determines accessibility. The flexible bronchoscope can be inserted only as far as secondary branches of the bronchial tree. Peripheral masses can be sampled with CT-guided **transthoracic needle biopsy**. Pneumothorax occurs in approximately a third of patients undergoing the procedure, but usually less than half of these require a chest tube.

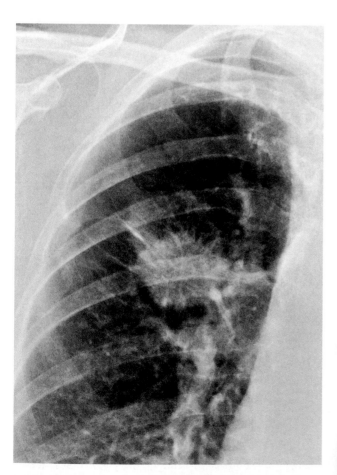

Figure 19-1 • Chest radiograph revealing a solitary pulmonary nodule. The large size and irregular edges are important diagnostic features suggesting a primary carcinoma of the lung.

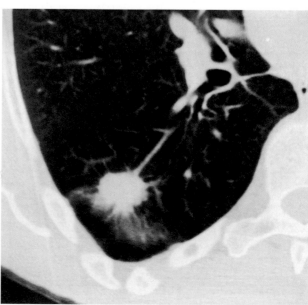

Figure 19-2 • CT revealing a spiculated mass, suggestive of a peripheral lung carcinoma.

Sampling of potentially involved nodes can be performed via the following techniques:

- Transbronchial biopsy via flexible bronchoscopy.
- Mediastinoscopy, where an incision is made in the suprasternal notch and a biopsy is taken via a mediastinoscope.
- Mediastinotomy, where an incision is made along the lower sternal border, allowing access to paratracheal nodes not accessible to mediastinoscopy. However, mediastinotomy is associated with a higher risk of complication.

Thoracoscopy can allow sampling of nodes as well as providing tissue samples of peripheral masses. It requires general anesthesia and the insertion of a chest tube.

TREATMENT

Once a lung cancer has been diagnosed, studies must be done to determine the histologic type as well as the stage of disease. Once this has been determined, therapeutic options can be discussed, generally in consultation with an oncologist.

As mentioned earlier, surgery with removal of the mass can be curative in some patients with nonsmall cell lung cancer. In patients with parenchymal tumors with either no nodal disease or involvement of only ipsilateral peribronchial or hilar nodes (stage I or II disease), surgery can be curative in 30% to 50% of cases. Adjuvant chemotherapy is also often added for stage IB and stage II disease. Once disease has progressed past this, a few selected patients can be cured surgically (with adjuvant therapy including chemotherapy and radiotherapy), but the proportion is much smaller.

Prior to surgery, the ability of the patient to survive the procedure needs to be assessed. Because many patients with lung cancer have underlying COPD, assessment of predicted postsurgical residual lung function must be done, usually with spirometry and/or nuclear perfusion studies.

Radiotherapy alone is generally not as effective as surgery but can be curative in some patients who are unable to tolerate surgery or in some whose disease is more advanced. More often, radiation is used in a palliative manner (see later text).

Chemotherapy in advanced nonsmall cell lung cancer is still experimental. After referral to an oncologist, some patients can be candidates for clinical trials.

Small cell lung cancer is considered to be clinically or subclinically metastatic at the time of diagnosis, and therefore surgery is unlikely to be curative (except when combined with chemotherapy in the rare patient who presents with a solitary pulmonary nodule and small cell cancer). Combination chemotherapy is the standard treatment. In some cases, cranial and/or thoracic irradiation is added. As mentioned previously, the majority of patients have a good response, but most relapse, giving an overall 5-year survival rate of approximately 5% to 10%, depending on the protocol used.

Patients with nonsmall cell cancer who have undergone surgery with the intent of cure need to be monitored for local recurrence as well as for the appearance of metastatic disease. The same applies to patients with small cell cancers who have undergone chemotherapy.

Patients who have advanced disease and/or severe mechanical problems because of their cancer (e.g., airway obstruction, SVC syndrome, tracheal compression) are candidates for palliative therapy involving:

- Radiation therapy (generally in lower doses and for shorter duration compared with curative radiation)
- Laser surgery (for endobronchial obstructing lesions)
- Brachytherapy (local application of radioactive material, generally via an endobronchial catheter)

In palliative care, the main goal is the relief of symptoms for the patient. Use of pain medications and hospice care are generally considered.

 KEY POINTS

- Lung cancer, most of which is associated with cigarette use, is the leading cause of cancer death in the United States.
- Clinically, lung cancers can be divided into small cell lung cancers, which metastasize early and are very responsive to chemotherapy but frequently recur, and nonsmall cell cancers, which in some cases of limited disease can be cured with surgery but are not very responsive to chemotherapy.
- Lung cancers are associated with a number of paraneoplastic syndromes, which in a number of cases are the presenting findings of the cancer.
- In the case of a solitary pulmonary nodule (a mass of <4 cm found on radiograph), approximately half turn out to be malignant; patients with a malignant nodule have a 5-year survival rate of 40%.

Part 3

Renal

Acid–Base Disturbances

Acids are continually produced as a by-product of metabolism. **Acid** is produced in two forms: (a) carbonic acid (H_2CO_3), a volatile acid principally produced by metabolism in the form of carbon dioxide, and (b) nonvolatile acids, such as sulfuric acid from sulfur-containing amino acids, organic acids from partial metabolism of carbohydrates and fats, uric acid from nucleic acid metabolism, and inorganic phosphates and protons from the metabolism of organic phosphorus compounds.

Most of the daily acid load is carbonic acid (approximately 15,000 to 20,000 mmol per day), with nonvolatile acids being produced at the rate of approximately 80 mmol per day. Although nonvolatile acids are produced in a much lower amount on a molar basis, they can have a profound effect on acid–base balance because of the differential elimination of carbonic acid and nonvolatile acids (see later).

Despite the continual metabolic production of acid, the pH of extracellular fluids is normally tightly maintained between 7.35 and 7.45. The primary organs that deal with the acid load are the **lungs** and **kidneys**. The **lungs rapidly eliminate carbon dioxide**, maintaining a concentration of CO_2 in the body fluids of 1.2 mmol per L (PCO_2 of 40 mm Hg). Protons produced by nonvolatile acids are removed by buffering with bicarbonate, converting it to water and carbon dioxide, the latter of which is exhaled. In the process, the bicarbonate buffer is destroyed. The respiratory response to changes in extracellular pH is rapid, with acidosis stimulating ventilation and alkalosis depressing it.

The **kidneys maintain the bicarbonate buffer system**. They do this by retaining existing bicarbonate and generating new bicarbonate to replace that destroyed by the buffering of nonvolatile acids.

Preservation of bicarbonate is accomplished by tubular reabsorption (Fig. 20-1). **New bicarbonate** is generated by secretion of protons into urinary buffers (phosphate and ammonia) that are then eliminated (Fig. 20-2). Proton secretion is stimulated by acidosis and aldosterone secretion. Bicarbonate reabsorption is stimulated by hypercapnia, extracellular volume contraction, and severe potassium depletion. The renal response to changes in extracellular pH is slower than the respiratory response, generally requiring 24 to 48 hours for a maximal response.

PATHOGENESIS

Acidosis is any abnormality that results in addition of acid or removal of alkali from the body fluids, whereas **alkalosis** is any abnormality that removes acid or adds base. If the primary disturbance is in the concentration of bicarbonate, it is referred to as **metabolic**. Conversely, if the primary disturbance is in the concentration of carbon dioxide, it is referred to as **respiratory**. **Mixed** disturbances are possible (e.g., a mixed metabolic acidosis and respiratory alkalosis). The term **acidemia** refers to a decrease in blood pH from normal, whereas **alkalemia** refers to an abnormal increase in blood pH. These terms are particularly useful when referring to mixed acid–base disturbances, when the direction of pH change can be the opposite from what is expected (e.g., a mild respiratory alkalosis in the setting of a severe metabolic acidosis manifests as an acidemia).

Metabolic acidosis can arise via:

- Increased production of nonvolatile acids
- Decreased acid excretion by the kidney
- Loss of alkali (generally from the GI tract)

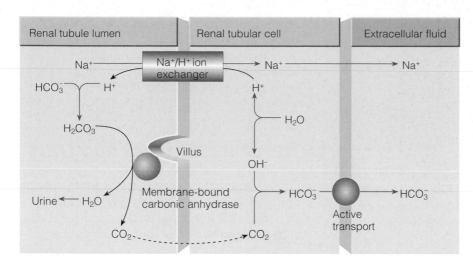

Figure 20-1 • Reclamation of HCO_3^- is driven by Na/H exchange in the proximal tubule and by the proton pump in the distal tubule. Note that there is no net loss of H.

The first mechanism leads to a so-called **increased anion gap** acidosis. The serum anion gap, calculated as

$$[Na^+] - ([HCO_3^-] + [Cl^-])$$

is normally 8 to 12 mEq per L and is the result of unmeasured anions such as serum proteins. Nonvolatile acids contribute to these unmeasured anions and increase the calculated gap. Decreased acid excretion by the kidney and loss of alkali do not increase the anion gap.

Metabolic alkalosis arises by increased loss of acid (generally from the stomach or kidney). Excess intake of base generally does not cause alkalosis unless large amounts are given continuously or in the setting of renal insufficiency.

Primary respiratory abnormalities can either be failure of respiration, leading to accumulation of carbon dioxide and acidosis, or hyperventilation, leading to a reduction in carbon dioxide and alkalosis.

An important aspect of acid–base balance is that the lungs and kidneys attempt to **compensate** for any abnormality that arises. A change in the plasma bicarbonate induces a compensatory change in ventilation that tries to counteract the effect of the bicarbonate change on the extracellular pH. Conversely, a primary change in carbon dioxide results in a renal alteration in bicarbonate handling to offset this. The magnitude of an **appropriate** compensatory response has been determined from empirical observation of the responses in humans and experimental animals.

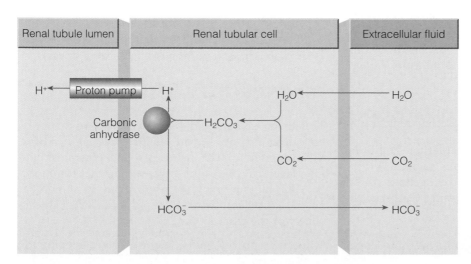

Figure 20-2 • Regeneration of HCO_3^- occurs mainly in the distal tubule. Note that this results in the net secretion of hydrogen ion into the tubule, where it combines with phosphate and ammonia and is eliminated from the body.

The following are the **expected compensations** for a primary acid–base disturbance:

- **Metabolic acidosis:** 1.0 to 1.5 mm Hg fall in Pa_{CO_2} for each 1 mEq per L decrease in HCO_3^- (maximal decrease is to Pa_{CO_2} 12 to 15 mm Hg)
- **Metabolic alkalosis:** 0.25 to 1.0 mm Hg rise in Pa_{CO_2} for each 1 mEq per L rise in HCO_3^-
- **Respiratory acidosis:** Acute, 0.1 mEq per L rise in HCO_3^- for each 1 mm Hg of Pa_{CO_2} rise over 40 mm Hg; chronic, 0.3 mEq per L rise in HCO_3^- for each 1 mm Hg of Pa_{CO_2} rise over 40 mm Hg
- **Respiratory alkalosis:** Acute, 0.1 to 0.3 mEq per L fall in HCO_3^- for each 1 mm Hg of Pa_{CO_2} decrease below 40 mm Hg; chronic, 0.2 to 0.5 mEq per L fall in HCO_3^- for each 1 mm Hg of Pa_{CO_2} decrease below 40 mm Hg

DIFFERENTIAL DIAGNOSIS

It is useful to consider the differential diagnosis of acid–base disorders based on the primary abnormality.

CAUSES OF METABOLIC ACIDOSIS

With **increased anion gap**, causes include:

- Lactic acidosis (from inadequate tissue oxygenation, hepatic failure, neoplasms)
- Ketoacidosis (from diabetes, starvation, alcoholism)
- Poisons/drugs (salicylates, methanol, ethylene glycol)
- Renal failure (chronic, end-stage disease)

With **normal anion gap**, causes include:

- Renal tubular disorders (renal tubular acidosis, potassium-sparing diuretics, hypoaldosteronism)
- Loss of base (diarrhea, carbonic anhydrase inhibitors, ureterosigmoidoscopy, pancreatic fistula)
- Excess acid intake (ammonium chloride, cationic amino acids)

CAUSES OF METABOLIC ALKALOSIS

- Volume loss with chloride depletion (vomiting, gastric drainage, diuretics, villous adenoma)
- Hypermineralocorticoid states (exogenous steroid treatment, primary aldosteronism, Cushing syndrome, renovascular disease)
- Severe potassium deficiency
- Excess alkali intake (milk-alkali syndrome, bicarbonate administration)

CAUSES OF RESPIRATORY ACIDOSIS

- Acute respiratory failure (drug intoxication, cardiopulmonary arrest)
- Chronic respiratory failure (chronic obstructive pulmonary disease [COPD], neuromuscular disorders, obesity)

CAUSES OF RESPIRATORY ALKALOSIS

- Hypoxia stimulating hyperventilation (asthma, pulmonary edema, pulmonary fibrosis, high altitude, congenital heart disease)
- Increased respiratory drive (pulmonary disease, anxiety, salicylate intoxication, cerebral disease, fever)
- Cirrhosis, pregnancy
- Excessive mechanical ventilation

CLINICAL MANIFESTATIONS

There are few specific clinical findings for most acid–base disorders. Diagnosis depends on recognition of the appropriate clinical setting, as described earlier, and appropriate laboratory studies (see Diagnostic Evaluation). Given the role of the pulmonary and renal systems in maintaining acid–base balance, disease of these systems increases the likelihood of developing acid–base abnormalities.

Nonspecific signs such as fatigue and mental status changes can be seen along with findings related to the underlying etiologies. Some **signs and symptoms** that can be suggestive are the following:

- Profound hyperventilation in the setting of acute metabolic acidosis (Kussmaul respiration)
- Papilledema with severe, acute hypercapnia in the setting of acute respiratory acidosis
- Neurologic symptoms in acute respiratory alkalosis (paresthesias, numbness, light-headedness)

DIAGNOSTIC EVALUATION

The diagnosis of acid–base disorders is made by measurement of **serum electrolytes** and **ABGs**. Measurement of the **urine pH** and **plasma creatinine level** can be useful in assessing renal function.

ABG measurement is useful, but it should be noted that several technical aspects can affect the accuracy of the results:

- Delay in processing the sample or not keeping the sample on ice

- Contamination of the sample with excess heparin
- Failure to purge air from the syringe
- A difficult arterial puncture leading to a respiratory alkalosis caused by pain and anxiety
- Sampling of venous blood instead of arterial blood

The last error (sampling venous blood) can result in severe misreadings (usually decreased pH and P_{O_2} and increased P_{CO_2}). This is particularly true in disease states that impair peripheral oxygen delivery and/or increase peripheral metabolism.

TREATMENT

The **evaluation and treatment of acid–base disorders** are linked and proceed through a series of logical steps:

1. Determine the magnitude and direction (i.e., acidemia vs. alkalemia) of the acid–base disturbance through measurement of ABGs.
2. Determine the primary abnormality (in terms of acidosis vs. alkalosis and metabolic vs. respiratory).
3. Determine whether there is an appropriate compensatory response.
4. If the compensatory response is not appropriate, determine whether there is a secondary abnormality.
5. Find and correct the underlying abnormality or abnormalities.

Generally, if the underlying disturbance is corrected, the kidneys and lungs restore acid–base balance. This assumes, of course, that there is normal function of both the renal and respiratory systems or that normal function can eventually be restored. For example, uncorrectable metabolic acidosis can be a manifestation of end-stage renal disease; a chronic respiratory acidosis can be a feature of end-stage lung disease.

Several conditions may require specific therapeutic interventions: metabolic acidosis in the setting of chronic renal failure (administration of oral bicarbonate), severe uncorrectable metabolic acidosis in the setting of acute renal failure (temporary hemodialysis), and metabolic alkalosis from volume and chloride loss (fluid replacement with saline solution).

KEY POINTS

- Metabolic acid exists as either carbonic acid or nonvolatile acids (which are buffered by the blood bicarbonate system).
- The lungs serve to eliminate carbonic acid as CO_2, and the kidneys are responsible for maintenance of the bicarbonate buffer system.
- Acidemia is a decrease in normal blood pH; alkalemia is an abnormal increase in blood pH.
- Disturbance in the acid–base balance can be classified as acidosis (addition of acid or loss of base) or alkalosis (loss of acid or addition of base). If the primary abnormality is related to bicarbonate balance, the disturbance is said to be metabolic. If the primary abnormality is related to CO_2 handing, the disturbance is said to be respiratory.
- For each primary acid–base disturbance, there is an appropriate compensatory response that attempts to counteract the primary change.
- To treat alkalemia or acidemia successfully, the underlying abnormality or abnormalities need to be identified and corrected. This permits the kidneys and lungs to restore acid–base balance.

Fluid and Electrolytes

Water constitutes approximately 50% to 60% of body weight. Approximately two thirds of total body water (TBW) is intracellular fluid (ICF), and the remainder is extracellular fluid (ECF). The plasma volume constitutes approximately 25% of the ECF, and the remaining 75% is interstitial fluid.

All principal electrolytes in the body are asymmetrically distributed across cell membranes. **Sodium** is the **principal extracellular cation**, with **chloride** and **bicarbonate** the main extracellular anions. **Potassium**, **calcium**, **magnesium**, and **organic anions** (e.g., proteins) are the main intracellular electrolytes.

The asymmetric distribution of electrolytes is maintained by a variety of energy-requiring electrolyte "pumps" that move the electrolytes against their electrochemical gradients. The action of these pumps results in the vast majority (more than 95%) of sodium staying in the ECF and a similar majority of potassium staying intracellularly.

Because sodium salts account for more than 90% of the osmolality of the ECF, the plasma sodium concentration generally reflects the osmolality of the ECF. Because water rapidly moves across membranes to dissipate osmotic gradients, the plasma sodium concentration not only reflects the osmolality of the ECF but also is a marker for the relationship between total body solute and TBW.

This chapter discusses the evaluation and management of disorders affecting water balance and levels of the electrolytes sodium and potassium.

REGULATION OF SODIUM AND WATER

The **kidneys** tightly **regulate** the total body **sodium** content. Sodium depletion triggers decreased excretion, whereas sodium overload results in increased excretion. Peripheral receptors in the atria, central arteries, and juxtaglomerular apparatus sense the effective blood volume. These receptors regulate renal sodium handling via the **renin-angiotensin system** and a number of **natriuretic hormones**.

Plasma osmolality is regulated via the action of antidiuretic hormone (ADH), which is produced by the hypothalamus in response to increased plasma osmolality. ADH acts on the kidney to reduce urine volume and increase urine osmolality, thus conserving water. Similarly, in the absence of ADH, the kidneys produce very dilute urine, allowing water diuresis at rates up to 20 L per day.

DISTURBANCES IN SODIUM AND WATER BALANCE

Disturbances in sodium and water balance can reflect an excess or deficit in either one or a combination of abnormalities. Pure sodium or water deficits are uncommon compared with combined deficits. Pure or disproportionate **water excess leads to hyponatremia**, whereas absolute or disproportionate **water deficit leads to hypernatremia**. A **pure excess of sodium** results in edema, as seen in heart failure, cirrhosis, and the nephrotic syndrome.

VOLUME DEPLETION

Extracellular fluid can be lost via renal or extrarenal routes.

Renal loss can occur from:

- Excess diuretics
- Osmotic diuresis (diabetic glycosuria)

- Renal disease (end-stage renal disease, diuretic phase of acute renal failure)
- Adrenal disease (mineralocorticoid deficiency)

Extrarenal loss can occur from:

- Gastrointestinal (GI) losses (vomiting, nasogastric suction, diarrhea)
- Abdominal sequestration (ascites, pancreatitis, ileus, peritonitis)
- Skin (sweating, burns)

Clinical Manifestations

The clinical manifestations of volume loss depend on the magnitude and on the plasma osmolality (see "Hyponatremia" and "Hypernatremia"):

- Fatigue, weakness
- Orthostatic light-headedness and syncope
- Orthostatic hypotension/tachycardia
- Decreased skin turgor, lack of axillary sweat, sunken eyes, dry mucous membranes
- Oliguria

Treatment

Volume depletion requires replacement of the lost fluid and electrolytes. In mild cases, this can be accomplished orally, but in severe cases, IV fluids should be provided. Monitoring of serum electrolytes and avoidance of fluid overload are necessary.

HYPONATREMIA

Hyponatremia is the result of an **excess of water relative to total solute**. Because this results in a dilution of body fluids and hypo-osmolality, there is usually an accompanying defect in production of dilute urine, which is the normal response to hypo-osmolar states. Causes of hyponatremia include:

- Volume depletion with sodium loss in excess of water loss (by mechanisms listed earlier for volume depletion)
- Edematous states (cirrhosis, heart failure)
- Euvolemic hypo-osmolar states (renal failure, syndrome of inappropriate antidiuretic hormone [SIADH], water intoxication, glucocorticoid deficiency)
- Normo-osmolar states (hyperglycemia, hyperlipidemia, hyperproteinemia)

Clinical Manifestations

Most patients with a serum sodium concentration of >120 to 125 mEq per L are asymptomatic. With greater movement of water into brain cells, symptoms can develop and include:

- Lethargy
- Confusion
- Coma
- Hyperexcitability, muscular twitching, and seizures (usually occur only with rapid-onset hyponatremia)

These symptoms are related to the degree of hyponatremia and the rapidity with which it develops.

Treatment

Treatment of hyponatremia generally involves correction of the underlying etiology. When there is severe volume depletion, IV fluid replacement may be needed. If required, normal saline (0.9%) should generally be the standard choice. The use of hypertonic saline is almost never required. Edematous states generally require free water restriction. Care must be taken not to raise the plasma sodium level too rapidly because it can cause neurologic damage (central pontine myelinolysis). Unless severe neurologic symptoms are present, correction should be at a rate of approximately 8 to 12 mEq/L/24 hours.

HYPERNATREMIA

Hypernatremia results from a deficit in water relative to solute. Hypernatremia invariably results in hyperosmolarity. This in turn normally results in ADH secretion that stimulates renal water conservation and thirst. Therefore, sustained hypernatremia usually only occurs in patients who are unable to respond to thirst by drinking (e.g., young children and mentally and/or physically limited adults).

Etiology

The **causes of hypernatremia** can be divided into these categories:

- Pure water deficits (insensible losses via skin and lungs, diabetes insipidus)
- Water loss in excess of sodium loss (sweating, osmotic diuresis)
- Sodium overload (administration of hypertonic oral or IV solutions)

Clinical Manifestations

As with hyponatremia, the **clinical features** of hypernatremia are a result of CNS dysfunction and can manifest as lethargy, confusion, neuromuscular hyperexcitability, and coma. Again, symptoms are usually only encountered with rapid and significant alterations in sodium level (usually >160 mEq per L).

Treatment

Correction of hypernatremia involves oral or IV replacement of water as well as sodium replacement if required. The **free water deficit** (FWD) can be calculated as

$$FWD = 0.6 \times \text{body weight (kg)}$$
$$\times ([Na]_{serum}/140) - 1)$$

As a rule of thumb, **only half of the free water deficit should be replaced in the first 24 hours**, and the remainder of the deficit over the next 24 to 48 hours.

DISORDERS OF POTASSIUM BALANCE

Potassium is the main intracellular anion. The **ratio of intracellular to extracellular potassium** is the **principal determinant of membrane excitability** in nerve and muscle cells. Because the extracellular potassium is low, small absolute changes in concentration can influence this ratio greatly. Similarly, small changes in the plasma potassium level may reflect large changes in the total body potassium level.

Excess potassium is mainly **eliminated by the kidneys**. Aldosterone stimulates renal potassium excretion. Additionally, the balance between intracellular and extracellular potassium is influenced by acid–base balance, with acidosis favoring a shift of potassium out of cells. Hormones also influence this balance. Insulin and β-adrenergic catecholamines promote the movement of potassium into cells.

HYPOKALEMIA

Potassium depletion results from insufficient dietary potassium intake or increased loss. **Potassium loss** can occur via:

- GI loss (diarrhea, vomiting, villous adenoma, ureterosigmoidostomy)
- Diuretic use
- Metabolic alkalosis (renal wasting because of bicarbonate excess)
- Mineralocorticoid excess
- Licorice intoxication (caused by a compound with mineralocorticoid-like activity)
- Glucocorticoid excess
- Renal tubular disease (renal tubular acidosis, certain antibiotics)

In addition, the shift of potassium into the intracellular compartment (from insulin effect, alkalosis) can result in hypokalemia without an actual total body potassium deficit. Hypokalemia manifests as disturbances in the function of excitable tissues:

- Skeletal muscle (weakness, particularly of the lower extremities; rhabdomyolysis)
- Smooth muscle (GI ileus)
- Cardiac muscle (prominent U waves on electrocardiogram; cardiac arrest, with rapid reduction of serum potassium, enhanced digitalis toxicity)
- Peripheral nerves (decreased or absent tendon reflexes)

Potassium replacement is generally done via oral supplementation, with potassium chloride the usual form. Because oral administration of potassium causes slower changes in the serum potassium level (because of slow entry into the circulation), this form of administration is safer. However, severe hypokalemia or hypokalemia in patients who cannot absorb oral supplements may need to be treated with IV supplementation. IV potassium solutions should normally contain at most 60 mEq per L and should be administered no faster than 20 mEq per hour to avoid cardiac toxicity from transient hyperkalemia.

HYPERKALEMIA

Hyperkalemia can occur via a number of mechanisms:

- Inadequate renal excretion (acute renal failure, end-stage renal failure, tubular disorders)
- Adrenal insufficiency
- Administration of potassium-sparing diuretics (spironolactone, amiloride)
- Tissue damage with release of intracellular potassium (muscle crush injury, hemolysis, internal hemorrhage)
- Shift of potassium from the intracellular compartment (acidosis, insulin deficiency, digitalis poisoning, β-adrenergic antagonists)

- Excess potassium intake (usually in the setting of underlying renal insufficiency)

Note that, in most cases, significant hyperkalemia, regardless of underlying cause, generally has a component of decreased or impaired renal potassium excretion because the kidneys can usually rapidly excrete an excess of potassium present in the serum.

The **major toxicity** of hyperkalemia is the **development of cardiac arrhythmias. Electrocardiogram (ECG) manifestations** of hyperkalemia (Fig. 21-1) include:

- Peaking of T waves (earliest sign)
- PR prolongation
- Complete heart block
- Atrial asystole
- QRS widening
- Ventricular fibrillation/standstill

Severe hyperkalemia is a medical emergency, requiring immediate treatment. Note that because the serum potassium represents only a small fraction of the total body potassium load, small changes in serum levels can indicate a significant change in total body potassium. Therefore, the absolute serum potassium level is not a very good indicator of patients who have a life-threatening potassium overload. However, any patient who presents with a potassium level >6.0 mEq per L should be monitored carefully for the development of cardiac arrhythmias.

Treatment

The **therapies for hyperkalemia** can be divided into those that antagonize the toxic effects of excess potassium on excitable membranes, those that immediately lower the serum potassium concentration (by causing shift of potassium from the extracellular compartment to the intracellular compartment), and those that eliminate excess potassium from the body. The first two strategies are used for emergent management, followed by removal of the excess potassium (because the latter generally is a slower process).

Membrane stabilization can be accomplished by:

- Calcium administration (does not lower plasma potassium levels but counteracts the effect of hyperkalemia on excitable membranes—transient effect)

Intracellular shift of potassium is accomplished by:

- Insulin administration (with concomitant glucose administration to avoid hypoglycemia)
- IV bicarbonate

Elimination of excess potassium is accomplished by:

- Use of oral potassium-binding resins to promote GI removal of potassium
- Diuretics and saline infusion
- Dialysis (hemodialysis and peritoneal dialysis—generally in patients with several renal impairments)

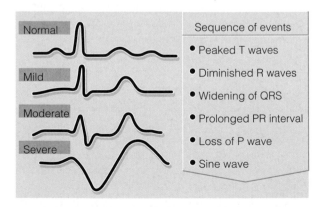

Figure 21-1 • ECGs of increasingly severe hyperkalemia. An individual patient's response cannot be predicted from the plasma potassium level.

 KEY POINTS

- The plasma sodium concentration reflects both extracellular fluid osmolality and total body water.
- Treatment of hyponatremia or hypernatremia requires assessment of the patient's volume status.
- When treating free water deficit in hypernatremia, a maximum of half the water deficit should be replaced in the first 24 hours.
- Potassium levels over 6 may result in peaked T waves and diminished R waves, and require close monitoring for cardiac arrhythmias.

Chapter

22 Acute Renal Failure

The kidneys normally serve many important functions, such as:

- Maintenance of water, volume, and electrolyte balance
- Removal of nitrogenous and other metabolic wastes
- Vitamin D metabolism
- Synthesis of erythropoietin
- Blood pressure regulation (via secretion of renin and prostaglandins)

Acute renal failure (ARF) occurs over hours to days. Often arising in patients with co-morbid conditions, ARF needs to be quickly recognized and the underlying etiology determined.

ETIOLOGY AND PATHOPHYSIOLOGY

The etiologies of ARF can be divided into three major groups based on the anatomic nature of the lesion. **Prerenal** etiologies are conditions that lead to an overall decrease in renal perfusion, including:

- Hypovolemia (e.g., from blood loss, dehydration)
- Decreased cardiac output (e.g., during acute myocardial infarction, cardiac arrest)
- Renovascular disease (e.g., dissection of renal artery, renal artery thrombosis)
- Systemic vasodilation (e.g., from administration of systemic vasodilator agents)
- Renal vasoconstriction (e.g., from administration of vasopressor agents)
- Impairment of renal autoregulation of blood flow (e.g., caused by drugs such as angiotensin-converting enzyme [ACE] inhibitors or non-steroidal anti-inflammatory drugs).

Intrinsic renal etiologies encompass conditions affecting the renal vascular, glomerular, and tubular tissues, such as:

- Vasculitis or microangiopathy
- Glomerulonephritis
- Acute tubular necrosis (can be caused by an ischemic insult or nephrotoxic drugs such as aminoglycoside antibiotics or radiographic contrast agents)
- Interstitial nephritis (often an allergic-type reaction to various drugs such as β-lactam antibiotics)
- Tubular obstruction

Postrenal etiologies are conditions that result in impairment of urine flow from the kidneys:

- Ureteral obstruction (e.g., because of tumor, retroperitoneal hemorrhage, or nephrolithiasis)
- Bladder neck obstruction (e.g., because of tumor)
- Urethral obstruction (e.g., secondary to an enlarged prostate, bladder thrombus, or renal calculus)

RISK FACTORS

ARF occurs in both hospital and ambulatory settings. Among ambulatory patients, it is more frequently seen in patients with co-morbid conditions and a debilitated state. ARF is more commonly encountered in the hospital setting (occurring in up to 5% of all hospitalized patients), where it is associated with:

- Surgery
- Trauma (hemorrhage, muscle injury)
- Administration of nephrotoxic drugs (aminoglycoside antibiotics, contrast agents)
- Bladder catheterization

- Sepsis
- Shock (low cardiac output states and the use of vasoactive drugs)

CLINICAL MANIFESTATIONS

HISTORY

Symptoms of acute renal failure are usually not present until the glomerular filtration rate falls to approximately 10% to 15% of normal, and complications of functional loss become apparent. Oliguria or even anuria is frequently but not invariably seen. Given the normal functions of the kidney listed earlier, **complications and symptoms of ARF** commonly seen are:

- Intravascular volume overload (dyspnea, orthopnea, edema)
- Metabolic acidosis (dyspnea)
- Anemia (fatigue)
- Hyperkalemia
- Uremic syndrome (when BUN is over 60 to 100 mg/dL: anorexia, nausea/vomiting, pruritus, mental status changes, serositis/pericarditis, coagulopathy)

Because symptoms are generally present only with the greatest degrees of renal impairment, the diagnosis of ARF is often made by routine laboratory assessment. History can provide clues to the etiology. A drug history is important, as is a history of recent surgery, trauma, or infection. A history of prior bladder function changes, such as nocturia, hesitancy, or reduced stream, suggest risk for postrenal failure. Intrinsic renal disease caused by Wegener granulomatosis is suggested by a history of otitis, sinusitis, epistaxis, hemoptysis, or nasal septal ulcers. Hemoptysis is also a worrisome symptom suggestive of renal failure due to Goodpasture or antiglomerular basement membrane disease.

PHYSICAL EXAMINATION

The physical examination of a patient with ARF can give an assessment of the degree of renal failure but often fails to yield insight into the underlying etiology. The patient's fluid balance can be assessed by orthostatic vital signs, assessment of skin turgor, and examination of jugular veins. Signs of fluid depletion can indicate a prerenal condition, whereas fluid overload can indicate either severe intrinsic renal failure or a prerenal edematous state such as congestive heart failure (CHF) or cirrhosis. The presence of abdominal bruits suggests renovascular disease. A pelvic or rectal examination can reveal causes of urinary outflow obstruction such as an enlarged prostate or a pelvic mass. The kidneys can be palpable in cases of hydronephrosis or polycystic kidney disease (which generally causes chronic renal failure). Skin rash may indicate vasculitis or other systemic diseases.

The **uremic syndrome** is a constellation of symptoms (described earlier) and **physical findings** that result from the accumulation of toxins normally handled by the kidney:

- Pericarditis (manifested by a cardiac rub)
- Uremic frost (crystals of urea that collect on the skin)
- Asterixis
- Uremic fetor (a urine-like odor to the breath because of accumulating nitrogenous waste products)

DIFFERENTIAL DIAGNOSIS

The main diagnostic challenge in ARF is to determine the underlying cause. However, fluid and electrolyte abnormalities can result in a symptom complex that can mimic a number of other conditions, such as CHF, dehydration, and intoxication. Therefore, it is important to assess renal function in patients who present with such a clinical picture.

DIAGNOSTIC EVALUATION

The diagnosis of ARF is often made by the finding of an elevated BUN level and creatinine level. Once the diagnosis of renal failure is made, measurement of serum electrolytes (sodium, potassium, chloride, bicarbonate, calcium, and phosphate) is important for monitoring the patient because life-threatening abnormalities can develop.

Analysis of urine sediment can provide important information. The presence of red blood cells (RBCs), either alone or in casts suggests glomerular or vascular lesions (see Chapter 24). White blood cells (WBCs) and white cell casts are seen in interstitial nephritis. Granular casts (in particular, "muddy-brown" casts) are often seen in acute tubular necrosis but are generally less specific than the other types of casts.

Assessment of the degree of proteinuria by a 24-hour urine collection can give clues to the etiology.

Generally, nephrotic-range proteinuria (i.e., more than 3 g per 24 hours) indicates a glomerular lesion. Lesser amounts are usually seen in interstitial disorders.

Calculation of the fractional excretion of sodium (FE_{Na}), which is defined as

$$100 \times (\text{urine Na/serum Na} \div \text{urine Cr/serum Cr})$$

can distinguish prerenal azotemia from other etiologies. In prerenal conditions, the FE_{Na} is generally <1 because the kidneys try to preserve intravascular volume by maximally conserving sodium. A low FE_{Na} can however be present in some intrinsic renal diseases as well, such as glomerulonephritis. A confirmatory high urinary osmolality (>500 mOsm/kg H_2O) supports the diagnosis of prerenal failure due to a stimulus to preserve intravascular volume through water retention. If volume deficiency prerenal conditions are suspected, a fluid challenge may be considered both diagnostically and therapeutically.

If a glomerular process (see Chapter 24) is suspected from the clinical context, immune-mediated disease can be screened for by measurement of antinuclear antibodies, antineutrophil cytoplasmic antibodies (antineutrophil cytoplasmic antibodies [ANCAs]; seen in Wegener granulomatosis), antiglomerular basement membrane (anti-GBM) antibodies, complement levels, and cryoglobulins.

Postrenal obstruction may be both diagnosed and treated through bladder catheterization. A large postvoid residual volume of urine emptied by catheterization of the bladder indicates bladder dysfunction or obstruction.

Renal imaging can determine the etiology of ARF. **Renal ultrasound** (US) is commonly used (Fig. 22-1) because it can allow assessment of kidney size and can detect hydronephrosis. If hydronephrosis indicative of obstruction is found, a urologist should be consulted and a search for the precise location of the obstruction can be undertaken with further tests, such as CT (in particular helical CT), retrograde pyelography, and cystoscopy.

The nuclear medicine **renal scan** can detect unilateral renal artery stenosis but is less sensitive in detecting bilateral renal artery disease.

The use of **renal biopsy** has decreased in recent years. Traditionally used in the diagnosis of glomerulopathies, the development of serologic tests such as ANCA and antiGBM has allowed many diagnoses to be made without biopsy. However, in cases where the diagnosis is uncertain, consultation of a nephrologist with possible biopsy can be useful in making a diagnosis or in giving prognostic information.

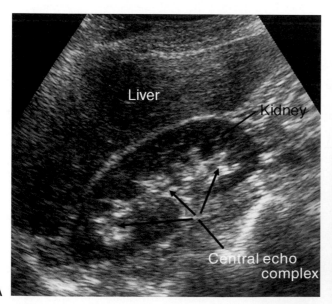

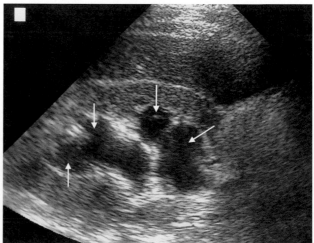

A

B

Figure 22-1 • Ultrasound of the kidney. **(A)** A normal US of the right kidney reveals a smooth outline with the parenchyma surrounding a central echodense region (central echo complex) consisting of the pelvicaliceal system, together with surrounding fat and renal blood vessels. **(B)** Urinary obstruction leads to dilatation of the pelvicaliceal system, which is shown sonographically as a spreading apart of the central echo complex.

TREATMENT

Treatment of ARF involves correction of fluid and electrolyte abnormalities (see Chapter 21) and attempting to find and correct the underlying cause. The search for an etiology is important because it will influence the long-term management. In all cases, drugs that are nephrotoxic (such as radiocontrast dye or certain antibiotics) or that reduce renal blood flow (such as NSAIDs) should be avoided if possible. Hyperkalemia in ARF can be life-threatening, and emergent management is required in patients with extreme elevation (more than 6.0 mmol per L) or in any patient with electrocardiogram (ECG) abnormalities (see Chapter 21). Other fluid and electrolyte abnormalities should be managed using the general principles outlined in Chapter 21.

The presence of prerenal azotemia dictates restoration of intravascular volume and perfusion blood pressure. In prerenal failure secondary to absolute hypovolemia, replacement of fluid depends on the mechanism of loss. Fluid deficit because of hemorrhage should be corrected with both saline and red cells. GI fluid loss is generally hypotonic and should be replaced accordingly.

For intrinsic renal failure, the goal is to prevent hypotension and to try to move the patient toward a nonoliguric state. In many cases of acute tubular necrosis, which is often caused by nephrotoxic agents, once the offending agent is removed, renal function will often return and supportive measures are all that is necessary. Other intrinsic renal diseases, such as glomerulonephritis in Wegener granulomatosis, require treatment (immunosuppression with prednisone and cyclophosphamide) to prevent irreversible renal damage (see Chapter 24). Supportive methods are generally sufficient while waiting for reversal of the underlying problem. In more severe cases, temporary dialysis (see Chapter 23) may become necessary.

The management of postrenal azotemia involves prompt determination of the level and then relief of the obstruction to urinary flow. For patients with urinary outflow obstruction, once the level of obstruction is determined, relief of obstruction (with urologic consultation if needed) usually results in reversal of the renal impairment. For urethral obstruction, bladder catheterization or placement of a suprapubic tube (if catheterization is not possible) is sufficient. If the obstruction is higher (at the vesicoureteral junction or in the ureter or renal pelvis), percutaneous nephrotomy or ureteral stent placement by a urologist will be needed.

Once therapy for ARF has begun, continued monitoring for both complications of renal failure and return of renal function is maintained. One important consideration is dose adjustment of renally excreted drugs, both to avoid systemic drug toxicity and to direct renal toxicity. The need for dialysis can arise later in the course if recovery is delayed or not forthcoming. In some cases (glomerulonephritis in particular), renal function may not return to a sufficient degree, and long-term dialysis is required.

 KEY POINTS

- ARF can be divided into prerenal (related to decreased renal perfusion), intrinsic renal (related to primary defects in the renal parenchyma), and postrenal (related to obstruction of the flow of urine).

- ARF leads to complications because of the dysregulation of fluid and electrolyte balance and the accumulation of toxic waste products.

- Signs and symptoms of ARF generally do not appear until renal function falls to approximately 10% of normal.

- Treatment of ARF involves determining the underlying etiology, addressing that etiology, and providing supportive management of fluids and electrolytes.

- In more severe cases of ARF, temporary or permanent dialysis may be necessary.

Chapter 23

Chronic Kidney Disease

The term *chronic kidney disease* (CKD) was recently adopted as part of a coordinated effort to standardize the detection, evaluation, and treatment of conditions associated with progressive decreases in kidney function. The National Kidney Foundation's Kidney Diseases Outcomes Quality Initiative (KDOQI, see http://www.kidney.org/professionals/KDOQI/) has resulted in a formal definition (Table 23-1) and staging scheme for CKD as well as a definition for end-stage renal disease (ESRD; Table 23-2).

CKD can develop following acute renal failure (ARF; see Chapter 22) but is most commonly a gradual onset complication of diabetes and hypertension. Because evidence suggests that kidney failure can be delayed or even prevented by control of blood sugar levels and blood pressure, there is a push for the early recognition and treatment of CKD.

EPIDEMIOLOGY AND ETIOLOGY

CKD affects approximately 19 million Americans older than 20 years. In addition, almost 450,000 individuals have end-stage renal disease. This burden of disease is increasing at a significant rate, doubling almost every 10 years since 1980. This has been placing an ever-increasing load on the healthcare system and in part has contributed to the increased emphasis on early recognition and treatment of CKD.

Diabetes is the major underlying condition leading to CKD, accounting for more than half of cases. Hypertension contributes to an additional 20% to 30% of cases. Although **diabetes and hypertension** are the major **conditions leading to CKD**, other conditions include:

- Glomerulonephritis (10%)
- Interstitial nephritis (3%)
- Polycystic kidney disease (3%)

PATHOPHYSIOLOGY

Uremia refers to the syndrome resulting from the failure of the kidneys to perform their normal excretory, metabolic, and endocrine functions. Uremia is a complex syndrome that includes a variety of physiologic and clinical abnormalities:

- **Fluid and electrolyte abnormalities:** fluid overload, metabolic acidosis, sodium imbalances, hyperkalemia, hyperphosphatemia, hypocalcemia
- **Endocrine/metabolic abnormalities:** hypertriglyceridemia, vitamin D deficiency, secondary hyperparathyroidism, osteodystrophy, hyperuricemia, impotence
- **Cardiovascular disorders:** hypertension, heart failure, pericarditis, accelerated atherosclerosis
- **GI disturbances:** anorexia, nausea/vomiting, peritonitis, ascites, hemorrhagic colitis
- **Dermatologic abnormalities:** pruritus, uremic frost, hyperpigmentation
- **Hematologic/immunologic abnormalities:** anemia (generally normochromic, normocytic), impaired platelet function, leukopenia, T-cell dysfunction (leading to increased risk of infection)
- **Neurologic/neuromuscular abnormalities:** fatigue, asterixis, headache, myoclonus, seizures, peripheral neuropathy, altered mentation, coma

■ **TABLE 23-1** Kidney Diseases Outcomes Quality Initiative (KDOQI) Definitions

Chronic kidney disease

Kidney damage for ≥3 mo based on findings of abnormal structure (imaging studies) or abnormal function (blood tests, urinalysis)

or

GFR below 60 mL/min/1.73 m² for ≥3 mo with or without evidence of kidney damage

End-stage renal disease (kidney failure)

GFR below 15 mL/min/1.73 m²

or

Need for kidney replacement therapy (dialysis or transplant)

Some abnormalities are caused by an accumulation of toxic metabolites, and others are the result of underproduction (e.g., vitamin D, erythropoietin) or overproduction (e.g., renin) of substances produced by the kidney. For other abnormalities, the exact pathophysiology is unclear. Note that cardiovascular disease is the most common cause of death in patients with CKD.

CLINICAL MANIFESTATIONS

Because of the significant functional reserve of the kidneys, symptoms generally do not appear until renal function (as measured by glomerular filtration rate [GFR]) declines to 10% to 15% of normal. At approximately 30% to 40% of normal GFR, biochemical evidence of renal failure can be seen, but patients are generally asymptomatic. Therefore, it is imperative

■ **TABLE 23-2** Stages of Chronic Kidney Disease Based on Estimated Glomerular Filtration Rate

Stage	GFR (mL/min/1.73 m²)
I	≥90
II	60 to 89
III	30 to 59
IV	15 to 29
V	<15 or dialysis

that patients with historical features that put them at risk for developing CKD (e.g., diabetes, hypertension, family history of CKD, history of glomerulonephritis) be screened for clinically occult CKD (see later).

The **history and physical examination findings** in a patient with advanced CKD are manifestations of the abnormalities associated with uremia:

- Fatigue, shortness of breath, pruritus, headache
- Peripheral edema, ascites
- Auscultatory rales, pericardial rub
- Bruising, uremic frost, hyperpigmentation
- Asterixis, peripheral neuropathy, and altered mental status

DIAGNOSTIC EVALUATION

As with acute renal failure, detection of the underlying etiology is important to determining treatments to slow the progression of disease. While addressing the etiologic factors, monitoring of the **serum creatinine level** can track the progression of CKD. Given the functional reserve of the kidneys, the GFR (normally more than 100 mL/min/1.73 m² and more than 125 mL/min/1.73 m² for men) can fall to 40% to 50% of normal with only a modest change in creatinine level.

GFR can be estimated in a number of ways. Although a 24-hour urine collection can provide an estimate of GFR (creatinine clearance = urine Cr × volume/plasma Cr), it is more common to estimate based on the plasma creatinine level (P_{Cr} in mg per dL). The two most common formulas to provide an estimate of the GFR are the Cockcroft-Gault equation: CCr = ([140–age][weight in kg][0.85 for women])/(72 × serum creatinine [mg/dL]) and the Modification of Diet in Renal Disease (MDRD) study equation:

$$\text{GFR (mL/min/1.73 m}^2) = 186 \times P_{Cr}^{-1.154} \times \text{age}^{-0.203} \times (0.742 \text{ if female}) \times (1.210 \text{ if black})$$

Both of these formulas are not accurate in the setting of rapidly changing renal function.

Routine monitoring of the complete blood count (CBC) can detect anemia secondary to erythropoietin deficiency. Monitoring of urinalysis can detect increasing proteinuria. The detection of proteinuria is associated with more rapid progression of CKD and greater likelihood of the development of ESRD, making detection, quantitation, and treatment of proteinuria key components of the management of CKD. When renal function declines further, closer monitoring of routine laboratory tests to detect dangerous electrolyte imbalances (e.g., hyperkalemia) and acidosis is required.

TREATMENT

The treatment of CKD is based on:

- Determination and control of the underlying etiology
- Monitoring changes in renal function
- Conservative treatment of complications of CKD
- Instituting more aggressive treatment (dialysis and/or renal transplantation) when appropriate

Aggressive control of diabetes, hypertension, and acute glomerulonephritis can delay or prevent the development of CKD. In patients who present with CKD, control of these underlying etiologies can delay or prevent progression to more advanced stages.

Diet modification is a key element in the conservative treatment of CKD. **Restriction of fluid and sodium** can diminish secondary hypertension. In some cases, diuretics may be required. At the same time, **dehydration must be avoided** to prevent prerenal azotemia. As renal function declines further, restriction of dietary phosphate and potassium becomes necessary. **Protein reduction** can relieve uremic symptoms and delay progression of renal failure. Dietary protein intake of 0.55 to 0.6 g/kg/day is sufficient to prevent negative nitrogen balance while relieving uremia.

In patients who have developed proteinuria, treatment with an ACE inhibitor or an angiotensin II receptor blocker can slow the progression of CKD. This applies to both patients with and without diabetes. Response to such therapy is generally monitored by serial quantitation of proteinuria.

The progression of CKD is initially monitored by following the BUN level, creatinine level, and creatinine clearance. As disease progresses to the more advanced stages, conservative management begins to fail and the patient has problems with fluid balance and may experience repeated episodes of hyperkalemia, hypertension, acidosis, and severe uremia. By the time the patient develops stage V disease, the decision for **advanced therapy** may need to be made. Options include hemodialysis, peritoneal dialysis, and renal transplantation.

Hemodialysis involves circulating the patient's blood through a machine that uses diffusion across a semipermeable membrane to remove unwanted substances while adding other desirable materials. The composition of the dialysate (i.e., the solution the blood is equilibrated against) can be altered to increase the amount of solute removed or added. A prerequisite for hemodialysis is vascular access. For emergent (e.g., in severe ARF) hemodialysis, a catheter can be placed, but for long-term dialysis, permanent access is required. This can be a surgically constructed arteriovenous fistula, usually involving the radial artery of the nondominant arm. If the patient's vessels are inadequate, synthetic graft material can be placed, but these tend to be more prone to clotting and infection. An arteriovenous fistula generally needs to mature for 1 to 2 months before it can be used, making it important to place it before dialysis is imminent or to use temporary access while it matures.

Chronic hemodialysis is typically performed three times a week. Each session lasts approximately 3 to 4 hours, during which time the patient remains attached to the dialysis machine.

Peritoneal dialysis is a procedure in which the dialysate is placed via a specialized permanent catheter directly into the peritoneal cavity of the patient. In this case, fluid and toxic solutes are transferred across the mesenteric capillary bed into the dialysis fluid. The fluid is then removed via the catheter. The most common method, **continuous ambulatory peritoneal dialysis** (CAPD), involves having the patient continually carry approximately 2 L of dialysis fluid in the peritoneal cavity. The fluid is then exchanged four times a day. Because exchange is accomplished by gravity flow, no machinery is required and dialysis can be performed virtually anywhere.

In **renal transplantation**, kidneys for transplantation are either **cadaveric** or from **living related donors**. The best success rates involve organs from living related donors who are HLA identical. Close to 100,000 renal transplants have been performed in the United States, with approximately 9,000 new transplants performed each year. The best candidates for renal transplants are younger patients who have minimal co-morbid disease.

The decision to move to dialysis and/or transplantation is usually made in consultation with a nephrologist. Patient characteristics often determine which modality is appropriate. Hemodialysis requires several periods a week of being hooked up to a dialysis machine, which can make travel and scheduling problematic, but between dialysis sessions, patients only have to continue their conservative treatment measures. CAPD allows more lifestyle freedom but requires a much greater degree of patient responsibility to manage the dialysate changes and to maintain the dialysis catheter. Transplantation offers the best treatment option for relieving the various manifestations of renal failure, but patients must be able to adhere to and tolerate their immunosuppressive regimen. As with all organ transplants, organ supply is limited.

Patients who are on hemodialysis generally tolerate the procedure well. Hypotension during the procedure is a common complication but is generally easily managed by adjusting the flow rates and dialysate. Psychiatric problems related to the loss of independence and altered self-image can arise. Long-term hemodialysis has been associated with a dementia that may be related to aluminum contamination of dialysate water. Failure of the vascular access can occur.

The major complication of peritoneal dialysis is the development of peritonitis. A patient on CAPD who develops fever and abdominal pain and/or who notices a change in the clarity of the dialysate should be evaluated for possible peritonitis. Treatment of peritonitis generally involves administration of antibiotics, which can be given on an outpatient basis to a patient who is not systemically ill. CAPD can usually be continued during treatment. In severe cases, catheter removal and temporary hemodialysis are required.

Patients who undergo a successful renal transplant usually have normalization of most abnormalities associated with renal failure. The major complications are caused by either the immunosuppression required or rejection of the transplanted organ.

KEY POINTS

- CKD most often occurs as a complication of a chronic systemic illness. In the United States, the leading conditions are diabetes and hypertension.

- Early detection and treatment of CKD can delay or prevent the progression to more advanced stages and to end-stage renal disease.

- Monitoring of CKD involves serial calculation of estimated GFR (based on the plasma creatinine) and monitoring for the development of proteinuria.

- Progressive CKD can lead to the syndrome of uremia, which is manifested as signs and symptoms related to the loss of the excretory, metabolic, and endocrine functions normally performed by the kidneys.

- When conservative treatment (fluid and electrolyte management, dietary modification) fails, patients require more aggressive treatment and advanced planning for dialysis may be indicated.

Glomerular Disease

The glomerulopathies are a heterogeneous group of disorders characterized by direct injury to the glomerulus, as opposed to other intrinsic renal pathologies such as tubulointerstitial diseases or primary vascular diseases. Because the glomerulus provides primary filtration for the urinary system, glomerular disease should be suspected when urine contains findings consistent with abnormal filtration: dysmorphic red cells, red cell casts, significant proteinuria, or lipiduria.

ETIOLOGY AND PATHOGENESIS

The etiologies of glomerular injury are varied and give rise to a number of distinct clinical syndromes. A particular etiology can give rise to more than one clinical syndrome, making classification of the glomerulopathies difficult. Glomerular injury can be divided into two major categories based on pathology: nephritis and nephrosis. These two forms of injury are not mutually exclusive, and a single etiology can produce both forms of injury. We will however approach them separately for clarity.

Nephritis, characterized by glomerular inflammation and/or necrosis, leads to hematuria with proteinuria. The immunologic injury that characterizes **glomerulonephritis** can be subdivided into **focal nephritic** (less than half of glomeruli affected) or **diffuse nephritic** pathologies. Focal nephritic diseases tend to present with less severe proteinuria, while diffuse nephritis may lead to severe proteinuria such as that seen in nephrosis. The most commonly found glomerulonephritic pathology (though rare in black individuals) is **IgA nephropathy**, which is caused by deposition of IgA immunoglobulins with resultant inflammation and mesangial cell proliferation. In **poststreptococcal glomerulonephritis**, deposits of antigen are found humped in the subepithelial region. This pathology may develop 2 to 3 weeks following a bout of pharyngitis or cellulitis.

A particularly severe form of diffuse and rapid onset nephritis is known as **rapidly progressive glomerulonephritis** (RPGN, see below). The key pathologic finding in RPGN is extensive formation of extracapillary **crescents** in more than half of glomeruli (see Color Plate 2), giving rise to the synonym **crescentic glomerulonephritis**. All of the following conditions may present with mild focal nephritis or more aggressive diffuse nephritis, including RPGN:

- **Antiglomerular basement membrane disease** (anti-GBM disease, a.k.a. **Goodpasture** disease), which is caused by direct glomerular damage occurring as a result of inflammation triggered by antibodies directed against components of the glomerular basement membrane. **Linear** deposits of immunoglobulin are seen by immunofluorescence microscopy (IF) of renal tissue. The circulating antibodies may also lead to pulmonary hemorrhage, causing a constellation of pathology known as Goodpasture syndrome.
- **Immune complex disease**, which is glomerular deposition of immune complexes (composed of antibody bound to a variety of circulating antigens) that result in an inflammatory response. IF reveals **granular** immunoglobulin deposits.
- **Pauci-immune (antineutrophil cytoplasmic antibody) disease** is a group of disorders characterized by the presence of antineutrophil cytoplasmic antibodies (ANCAs) that are associated with multisystemic disease. Minimal or no immunoglobulin

is seen by IF, hence the name "pauci-immune." Despite this name, the glomerular injury is still believed to be immunologic. This pathology is considered to be part of the **Wegener granulomatosis** spectrum of diseases, and patients with such pathology should be watched carefully for evidence of systemic vasculitis.

Nephrosis, characterized by abnormal permeability of the glomerular membrane, allows macromolecules such as albumin to pass, with resultant heavy proteinuria and lipiduria. The pathogenesis is less inflammatory than in nephritis; hematuria and cellular casts are generally not seen (but can be present). In classic forms, the nephrotic syndrome (see later) develops, but lesser degrees of proteinuria can be seen. Nephrosis commonly results from:

- **Diabetes mellitus**
- **Systemic lupus erythematosus** (SLE)
- **Amyloidosis**
- **Membranous nephropathy** is one of the most common causes of nephrotic syndrome in nondiabetics, characterized by diffuse thickening of the glomerular basement membrane. The membrane thickening is caused by formation of in-situ immune complexes against a deposited antigen. In some cases, medications trigger this pathology, and it may also be triggered by underlying infections (hepatitis B) or malignancies (breast, colon, other solid tumors).
- **Minimal change disease** is characterized by lack of abnormality on light microscopy or IF, with electron microscopy showing flattening of glomerular epithelial cells. While minimal in detectable pathology, the resultant proteinuria can be massive, even rising above 8 to 9 g daily.
- **Focal glomerulosclerosis** results in focal scarring involving only scattered glomeruli and segments of the glomerular tufts, with microscopy showing immunoglobulin deposits and obliteration of the foot processes.

CLINICAL MANIFESTATIONS

Glomerular diseases can present with symptoms related to the underlying etiology or may simply manifest as a number of clinical syndromes:

- Acute nephritis (a.k.a. acute glomerulonephritis), including rapidly progressive glomerulonephritis (RPGN)
- Nephrotic syndrome
- Chronic kidney disease (CKD) including end-stage renal disease (ESRD)

Acute nephritis is characterized by the abrupt onset of **hematuria**, **hypertension**, **edema**, **oliguria**, and **azotemia**. These symptoms may be preceded by insidious and nonspecific symptoms of fatigue with edema. **RPGN** refers to acute glomerulonephritis that advances to end-stage renal disease in days to weeks. Of patients with acute nephritis who progress to RPGN, approximately 20% have anti-GBM disease. The remaining cases are evenly divided between immune-complex and pauci-immune (ANCA) disease.

Nephrotic syndrome is defined as proteinuria in excess of 3 g per day. Secondary findings caused by this extreme proteinuria include **hypoalbuminemia**, **edema**, **hyperlipidemia**, and **coagulation abnormalities** with increased risk for deep vein thrombosis (DVT) and renal vein thrombosis. The onset of nephrotic syndrome can be insidious. Gross hematuria is rare, and patients may present without azotemia.

Chronic kidney disease (CKD; see Chapter 23) refers to slowly progressive disease that can lead to end-stage renal disease over a period of years. Any acute glomerular disease can lead to CKD. Advanced CKD can lead to volume overload, hyperkalemia, metabolic acidosis, hypertension, anemia, and bone disease. The onset of end-stage renal disease results in signs and symptoms of uremic syndrome. The most important cause of chronic kidney disease in the United States is diabetes mellitus.

One notable clinical presentation of glomerular disease is the concurrent presence of hemoptysis. This pulmonary-renal presentation is most commonly caused by antiGBM (Goodpasture) disease due to pulmonary alveolar hemorrhage. ANCA-associated vasculitis with glomerulonephritis and pulmonary capillaritis (Wegener disease) can also lead to this clinical presentation, though upper respiratory tract involvement is more common in this syndrome. These syndromes can be differentiated based on serology and biopsy findings (see below.) Also in the differential but less common as causes of pulmonary-renal syndrome are SLE and Henoch-Schonlein purpura.

Renal-dermal syndromes include SLE, **Henoch-Schönlein purpura** (HSP), cryoglobulinemia, and ANCA-associated vasculitis. In these syndromes, dermal involvement may include palpable purpura (HSP), necrotic dermal inflammation, ulcers, or nodules.

DIAGNOSTIC EVALUATION

Workup of a patient with possible glomerular disease should start with:

- Measurement of electrolytes and creatinine to detect and quantify renal insufficiency and associated electrolyte abnormalities.
- Urinalysis to detect proteinuria and hematuria.
- Microscopic examination of the urine sediment can reveal the presence of **dysmorphic** RBCs or **RBC casts** (highly suggestive of glomerulonephritis), and lipiduria.

In patients who present with acute nephritis or RPGN, **serology** has become an important part of the workup. Screens for **anti-GBM antibodies** and **ANCA** are readily available in many hospitals and can diagnose Goodpasture syndrome, Wegener granulomatosis, and microscopic polyarteritis. Immune complex disease is often associated with low **serum complement levels**. Several antistreptococcal antigen antibodies (e.g., antistreptolysin O, anti-DNase B) can develop in poststreptococcal glomerulonephritis.

Renal biopsy with examination by light microscopy, immunofluorescence, and electron microscopy is often useful for establishing a diagnosis in the setting of acute nephritis, RPGN, and nephrotic syndrome. It is usually reserved for patients who have negative serology and an unclear clinical diagnosis. Performed in consultation with a nephrologist, it is a relatively safe procedure.

TREATMENT

For most glomerular disease, supportive care with fluid and electrolyte management (as outlined in Chapters 20 and 21) is the initial intervention. For diseases that are usually self-limited (e.g., poststreptococcal glomerulonephritis), this supportive care is sufficient. Additionally, for poststreptococcal glomerulonephritis, suppression of the infectious agent with antibiotics (to limit antigen load) is a treatment measure.

For conditions that present primarily as nephrosis (particularly in patients who develop the nephrotic syndrome), **control of proteinuria** can be accomplished by nonspecific treatments such as **ACE inhibitors and angiotensin II receptor blockers**. For diabetic patients, control of blood pressure and glycemic control will delay or prevent progression of renal disease. Severe edema is treated with moderate salt restriction (1 to 2 g per day) and the careful use of loop diuretics (taking care to avoid volume depletion and prerenal azotemia).

Treatment with **immunosuppressive agents** (e.g., steroids, cyclophosphamide, mycophenolate mofetil) is usually recommended in diseases such as Goodpasture syndrome, Wegener granulomatosis, and polyarteritis. In addition, it can limit disease in idiopathic nephrotic syndrome, lupus nephritis, and idiopathic RPGN. Immunosuppression may be considered in other diseases such as IgA nephropathy and amyloidosis when their presentations are particularly progressive or severe. In still other diseases, such as poststreptococcal glomerulonephritis and acute nephritis in the setting of infections such as endocarditis, the use of immunosuppression is not useful.

Once fluid and electrolyte balance is achieved and any specific treatment is initiated, close monitoring should be maintained, awaiting return of normal renal function.

PROGNOSIS

Prognosis in the glomerular diseases varies. In general, for a given disease, patients who develop RPGN have a poorer chance of preservation of renal function than those who manifest with less aggressive acute nephritis. For nephrotic syndrome, prognosis varies by histologic subtype, with approximately 95% of patients with minimal change disease maintaining baseline renal function.

Patients who develop chronic kidney disease from glomerular disease are managed as outlined in Chapter 23. Patients who develop end-stage renal failure may be candidates for long-term dialysis or renal transplantation.

KEY POINTS

- Causes of glomerular injury can be divided into those that cause inflammation (nephritis) and those that alter the permeability of the glomerular membrane (nephrosis).

- The most common glomerular diseases in adults include diabetic kidney disease, IgA nephropathy, rapidly progressive glomerulonephritis, minimal change disease, and membranous nephropathy.

- The major clinical syndromes of glomerular disease are acute glomerulonephritis (including rapidly progressive glomerulonephritis) and nephrotic syndrome. Either can lead to chronic kidney disease.

- A given etiology of glomerular disease can manifest as one or more clinical syndromes.

- In addition to maintenance of fluid and electrolyte balance, control of proteinuria and immunosuppression are important for specific glomerular diseases.

Nephrolithiasis

Calcium and oxalate are normally present in the urine in amounts exceeding their solubility (supersaturated solution). However, most people do not form kidney stones, in part because of the kidney's natural inhibitors such as citrate or kidney proteins (Tamm-Horsfall mucoprotein and nephrocalcin).

This supersaturated balance can be disturbed by either increased excretion of solutes or a change in urine volume. When this occurs, calcium and oxalate may precipitate on their own (homogeneous nucleation) or, more commonly, crystallize on another source such as urate crystals, epithelial cells, or urinary casts (heterogeneous nucleation).

EPIDEMIOLOGY

Nephrolithiasis is common, affecting about 5% of women and 12% of men. The peak incidence is between 20 and 30 years of age. Struvite stones are more common in women because of the association with urinary tract infections.

RISK FACTORS

Modifiable **dietary factors** that can increase risk for nephrolithiasis include:

- low fluid intake
- grapefruit juice intake
- high sodium intake, with increased sodium excretion accompanied by increased passive calcium excretion
- high protein intake, with associated rise in acid and uric acid production

- low dietary calcium intake, which reduces gut binding of dietary oxalate therefore increasing oxalate absorption.

Medical conditions that increase risk for nephrolithiasis include hyperparathyroidism, obesity, gout, diabetes, and renal tubular acidosis.

ETIOLOGY AND PATHOGENESIS

Nephrolithiasis may be grouped into four categories on the basis of stone composition. First, **calcium** constitutes 75% to 85% of all stones. Calcium oxalate predominates, but stones may occur as calcium phosphate or even mixed salts. The following metabolic abnormalities lead to calcium stones:

- **Hypercalciuria** is the most common urinary abnormality (more than 50% of patients). It is important to exclude secondary causes, such as malignancy, hyperparathyroidism, sarcoidosis, or Cushing syndrome, but most patients have idiopathic hypercalciuria (caused by increased intestinal absorption, renal leak of calcium, or both).
- **Hypocitruria** is a deficiency of this natural inhibitor, found in approximately 30% of patients. It is usually idiopathic but may be caused by distal renal tubular acidosis (type 1) or chronic diarrhea, both of which create a non–anion gap acidosis.
- **Hyperoxaluria**, found in 8% of stone formers, is caused by high dietary oxalate, malabsorption, or ileal disease. The latter two conditions increase oxalate absorption by two mechanisms: Malabsorbed fat binds calcium, leaving oxalate free for absorption, and colonic mucosa injured from bile acids absorbs more oxalate.

- **Hyperuricosuria** may serve as the nucleating agent for calcium.

The second category of stones, **uric acid**, occurs as a predominant crystal in 5% to 10% of stones. Patients often have gout (50%), myeloproliferative disease, or a family history of nephrolithiasis. **Struvite**, the third category, constitutes 10% to 20% of all stones, composed of magnesium ammonium phosphate crystals. This type is associated with urease-producing bacteria (e.g., *Proteus*) and may grow quite large. Finally, **cystine**, which is an uncommon cause (1%) of stones, occurs only in patients with cystinuria, an inherited defect of amino acid transport.

CLINICAL MANIFESTATIONS

HISTORY

Acute flank pain with hematuria is the hallmark presentation. Pain begins gradually and then escalates to a severe pain in 20 to 60 minutes. Pain radiating to the groin or testicle (labia in women) may indicate migration of the stone into the lower third of the ureter. There can be associated nausea and vomiting. The hematuria may produce pink or grossly bloody urine.

PHYSICAL EXAMINATION

The physical examination is often unrevealing. There can be tenderness to palpation or costovertebral tenderness. The presence of peritoneal signs suggests an alternate diagnosis. Fever is also not typical and may indicate a complicating infection.

DIFFERENTIAL DIAGNOSIS

In the clinical presentation of **acute flank pain**, the following diseases may have similar pain and radiation:

- Aortic dissection
- Lumbar disk disease
- Renal infarct
- Intestinal disease/ischemia
- Ectopic pregnancy

If **gross hematuria** predominates the picture, the following diagnoses should be considered as well:

- Renal malignancy
- Pyelonephritis
- Glomerulonephritis
- Trauma

DIAGNOSTIC EVALUATION

The **urinalysis** is the key to diagnosis, with hematuria as the predominant feature. Urine sediment will reveal nondysmorphic cells and the absence of red cell casts, in contrast to glomerulonephritis (see Chapter 24). The urine should also be examined for crystals and tested for pH. Table 25-1 lists the typical findings for each stone. A **plain film of the abdomen** can be obtained in patients to look for radiopaque stones (90% of all stones).

Noncontrast **helical computed tomography (CT) scan** is now the confirmatory radiologic test of choice. In addition to its high sensitivity and specificity for stones as small as 1 mm, this test requires no IV contrast (as compared with intravenous pyelogram, the prior gold standard) and may also diagnose alternative pathology responsible for the patient's symptoms (e.g., appendicitis, diverticulitis). Renal ultrasonography detects stones and urinary tract obstruction but is less sensitive for smaller stones. Intravenous pyelography remains highly sensitive and specific but the requirement for IV contrast dye has lessened its use.

TREATMENT

Initial treatment should focus on adequate hydration, pain relief, and evaluation for possible urologic procedure. Patients often require narcotic analgesia, but those patients who can maintain adequate oral fluid intake may use oral medication. Patients who have had a kidney stone should ensure an adequate daily urine volume (more than 2 L) by **increasing fluid intake** (6 to 8 glasses a day).

Stone retrieval is desirable because further workup and treatment are dictated by type of stone. Patients should be instructed to strain urine at home or in the hospital, then return collected stones for analysis.

All hospitalized patients should receive **IV fluids** and adequate **analgesia**. Stones that are smaller than 5 mm usually pass on their own. Larger stones may require one of the following procedures. **Extracorporeal shock wave lithotripsy (ESWL)** has greatly diminished the need for invasive procedures. Shock waves fragment the stone into smaller pieces that can then pass.

	TABLE 25-1 Clinical Features of Kidney Stones			
Type of Stone	**Urine pH (normal 5.5 to 6.0)**	**Crystals**	**Radiograph Findings**
Calcium	Increased	Color Plate 3	Radiopaque
Uric acid	Decreased	Rhomboid	Radiolucent
Struvite	Increased	Color Plate 4	Radiopaque
Cystine	Decreased	Hexagonal	Radiopaque

Adapted from Coe FL, Parks JH, Asplin JR. The pathogenesis and treatment of kidney stones. *N Engl J Med* 1992;327:1142.

Referral for this procedure should be considered in the following situations:

- Stone fails to progress
- Infection, severe bleeding, or intractable pain is present
- Stone is larger than 0.5 cm and smaller than 2 cm

Stents may be used to assist passing the stone.

Retrograde ureteroscopy is a more invasive method but highly successful. It has emerged as first-line therapy for midureteral stones, for which ESWL is less effective (because of interference from pelvic bones). In **percutaneous nephrolithotomy**, stones are extracted manually under fluoroscopy by a percutaneous approach. It may be used for stones not well treated by the methods just described, including stones larger than 2 cm diameter.

Struvite stones often grow quite large, but complete removal is essential. These stones are usually colonized with bacteria and recur unless adequately removed. Treatment options include percutaneous nephrolithotomy in combination with ESWL. This treatment is often followed by a repeat percutaneous nephrolithotomy (the "sandwich" method). Open lithotomy is reserved for the most difficult cases.

Following removal of the stone, treatment focuses on prevention of recurrent stones. Some experts recommend a minimal workup for first-time stone formers, consisting of serum **electrolytes**, **creatinine**, **calcium**, **phosphorus**, and **urinalysis**. Only hypercalcemic patients should be tested for hyperparathyroidism. Uric acid and urine cystine may be ordered if clinically suspected. However, there is continued debate over what workup (if any) a patient should receive after the first stone.

Recurrence of a kidney stone occurs in most patients within a decade (14% at 1 year, 35% at 5 years, 50% to 60% at 10 years). Patients with an inherited defect, such as cystinuria, may have a malignant course, leading to renal failure. More extensive workup, involving **24-hour urine collection**, is indicated in recurrent stone formers. Some advocate this workup in first-time stone formers, given the high rate of recurrence. Urine should be sent for sodium, creatinine, calcium, uric acid, citrate, and oxalate. Cystinuria, a rare cause of kidney stones, may be screened for with the **nitroprusside test**. This sensitive test may also detect asymptomatic heterozygotes; therefore, a positive test should be followed up with a quantitative cystine analysis. Almost all patients (97%) have some detectable abnormality on the urine test, and most have more than one.

Alkalinization of urine with potassium citrate may be useful for stones that form in acid urine. These include uric acid stones, cystine stones, and those calcium stones associated with normocalciuria, renal tubular acidosis, and hypocitraturia.

For **calcium stones**, sodium restriction and thiazide diuretics, both of which decrease calcium excretion, are used for hypercalciuria. Thiazide diuretics decrease serum potassium and urinary citrate, so potassium citrate should be given to these patients as well. A calcium-restricted diet is not recommended because it will encourage continued calcium wasting (from bone). In **hyperoxaluria**, decreased dietary oxalate, calcium supplements to bind oxalate (not to be used by patients with concurrent hypercalciuria), or cholestyramine to bind fatty acids, bile salts, and oxalate is used.

Treatment for **uric acid stones** includes alkalinization of the urine to pH >6 using potassium citrate, dietary restriction (avoid meats, fish), and allopurinol.

Following surgical removal of struvite stones, a course of antibiotics is targeted against the offending organism.

For **cystine stones**, aggressive fluid intake (more than 4 L per day), alkalinization, and sodium restric- tion is mandatory. The drug penicillamine forms a soluble complex with cystine to prevent stones, but its toxic side effects limit its use to patients who fail routine therapy. Tiopronin and captopril are alterna- tive medical treatments.

KEY POINTS

- Calcium stones, specifically calcium oxalate, are the most common type of kidney stone.
- The clinical picture of nephrolithiasis consists of flank pain, often radiating to the groin, and hematuria. Urine sediment reveals nondysmorphic red cells. An abdominal plain film shows kidney stones (except for radiolucent uric acid stones), and diagnosis is con- firmed with a helical CT scan or intravenous pyelo- gram (IVP).
- Treatment is hydration and pain control, with shock- wave lithotripsy used for more complicated cases, and invasive stone removal reserved for large or stru- vite stones.

- Systemic conditions often predispose to nephrolithi- asis. Calcium stones may be caused by hyperparathy- roidism, sarcoidosis, or Cushing syndrome. Uric acid stones are associated with myeloproliferative disor- ders, chemotherapy (tumor lysis syndrome), or gout. Patients with intestinal malabsorption and ileal dis- ease usually have calcium oxalate stones.
- Dietary factors such as low fluid intake, high protein intake, low calcium intake, and high sodium intake are all modifiable risk factors for nephrolithiasis.
- Alkalinization of the urine using potassium citrate and allopurinol reduce recurrence of uric acid stones.

Hematuria (the presence of blood in the urine) is a very common disorder and can be classified as **gross** or **microscopic** depending on whether or not blood is visible to the naked eye. Normal individuals excrete up to 2 million red blood cells (RBCs) into the urine each day; more than this is considered to be abnormal hematuria. Gross and microscopic hematurias share a common differential diagnosis.

In many instances, hematuria is benign and patients have no evidence of renal or systemic disease. In other cases, hematuria may be a manifestation of a systemic disease such as vasculitis or urologic pathology such as bladder cancer. Determination of the cause of hematuria is important because up to 10% of patients with hematuria are found to have an underlying malignancy.

ETIOLOGY AND PATHOGENESIS

The **causes of hematuria** can be divided based on the anatomic site of the blood source (asterisks indicate the most common causes):

Kidney
- Infection (pyelonephritis, tuberculosis, parasites)*
- Nephrolithiasis*
- Malignancy (renal cell carcinoma)
- Trauma
- Glomerular disease (vasculitis, idiopathic)
- Cysts (single and polycystic disease)
- Allergic interstitial nephritis (drug induced)
- Ischemia (embolism, thrombosis, papillary necrosis)

Ureters
- Nephrolithiasis
- Tumor
- Endometriosis

Bladder
- Infection (bacterial cystitis, parasites)
- Calculus*
- Interstitial cystitis
- Tumor
- Vascular malformations (hemangiomas, telangiectasias)
- Endometriosis
- Drugs (e.g., hemorrhagic cystitis from cyclophosphamide)

Prostate/Male Reproductive Tract
- Infection (prostatitis, epididymitis)
- Benign prostatic hypertrophy (BPH)
- Tumor

Urethra
- Urethritis (gonococcal, nongonococcal)
- Stricture
- Calculus
- Trauma

Systemic Illnesses/Other
- Intense exercise*
- Coagulopathy
- Thrombocytopenia
- Hemoglobinopathy

CLINICAL MANIFESTATIONS

HISTORY

Although many times microscopic hematuria is found in asymptomatic patients, hematuria may present with other **symptoms** suggestive of particular etiologies:

- Flank pain (pyelonephritis, nephrolithiasis, neoplasms, ischemia, glomerulonephritis, hemorrhagic cyst)
- Dysuria (cystitis, pyelonephritis, prostatitis, BPH, urethritis)
- Urethral discharge (urethritis)
- Weight loss (tumor)
- Fever (pyelonephritis, neoplasms, tuberculosis)
- Nocturia (cystitis, BPH, pyelonephritis)

In women, the **menstrual history** is important. Hematuria can be caused by urologic endometriosis, but more commonly blood in a clinical urine specimen is vaginal in origin.

Other historical findings are associated with specific causes of hematuria and should be sought:

- Recent streptococcal infection (poststreptococcal glomerulonephritis)
- Gross painless hematuria (bladder cancer, glomerulonephritis)
- Recent heavy exercise (exertional hematuria)
- History of nephrolithiasis
- Medication history (allergic interstitial nephritis, hemorrhagic cystitis)
- Travel (parasitic infections)

Family history of hematuria suggests polycystic kidney disease or three common causes of isolated glomerular hematuria:

- IgA nephropathy (the most common cause of nephritis in adults)
- Alport syndrome (a.k.a. hereditary nephritis)
- Thin basement membrane disease (a.k.a. benign familial nephritis)

PHYSICAL EXAMINATION

The physical examination can provide important clues regarding the origin of hematuria:

- Skin lesions, for example, ecchymoses, petechiae (coagulopathy, vasculitis)
- Costovertebral angle tenderness (pyelonephritis, tumor, glomerulonephritis)
- Abdominal mass (polycystic kidneys, renal cell cancer)
- Urethral discharge (urethritis)

- Suprapubic tenderness (cystitis)
- Enlarged prostate (BPH)
- Tender prostate (prostatitis)
- Prostatic nodule (prostate cancer)

DIAGNOSTIC EVALUATION

The **initial diagnosis** of microscopic hematuria is commonly made with either a urine dipstick or microscopic examination of spun urine sediment. The **urine dipstick** detects the presence of hemoglobin and can detect free hemoglobin or hemoglobin contained in RBCs. The **microscopic examination** detects only intact RBCs but provides additional information. Normally performed on a spun urine sediment (obtained by centrifuging approximately 10 mL of fresh urine), it can detect the presence of 1.2×10^6 RBCs per 100 mL. This corresponds to the presence of 2 to 3 RBCs per high-power field (hpf). Most nephrologists accept up to 2 to 3 RBCs per hpf as normal in a routine urinalysis. Microscopic examination can also reveal the presence of **bacteria** in the setting of urinary tract infections. The presence of **RBC casts** indicates a renal origin for the hematuria.

Examination of the **morphology** of RBCs present in the urine using **phase-contrast microscopy** can provide clues about the etiology of hematuria. RBCs originating from **glomerular disease** are often **dysmorphic**, whereas nonglomerular disease is associated with normomorphic RBCs (Fig. 26-1). It is important to examine a fresh urine sample because changes in RBC morphology can occur if the urine is allowed to sit.

Routine chemistries, such as CBC, platelet count, BUN, and creatinine, should be performed in the initial evaluation of hematuria.

In many cases, an asymptomatic patient is found to have hematuria on a routine screening urinalysis, but no clear source is found by history and physical examination. Such patients are said to have **isolated asymptomatic hematuria**. The challenge for the clinician is to determine the cause for the hematuria with a minimum of invasive testing while detecting potentially malignant causes.

The initial test for isolated asymptomatic hematuria should be urine culture. If positive, appropriate treatment should be instituted and then culture and urinalysis repeated. If hematuria is still present, further evaluation is necessary.

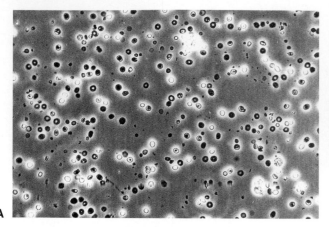

A

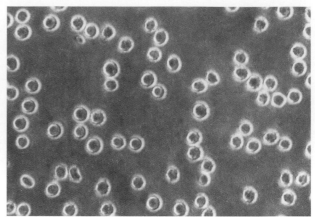

B

Figure 26-1 • Appearance of RBCs in urine using phase-contrast microscopy. Dysmorphic RBCs **(A)** seen in the setting of glomerular disease compared with nondysmorphic RBCs **(B)** caused by lower urinary tract bleeding (**B**, higher magnification).

Patients with isolated asymptomatic hematuria who are older than 50 years (or younger in those with risk factors) should be evaluated extensively because the incidence of urologic tumors is much higher in this group. In younger patients, a 3-month period of "watchful waiting" with repeat urinalyses performed **at least monthly** is acceptable. If hematuria is still present after this time, evaluation should be continued as with patients older than 50 years.

The next step in evaluation is **structural examination of the urinary system**. A **helical computed tomography** (CT) is generally the initial test due to its ability to detect small tumors. Helical CT can also detect the presence of stones, soft-tissue masses, hydronephrosis, and cysts. **IV intravenous pyelogram** may be considered instead for younger patients in whom tumor is less likely, dye load is more tolerable, and detection of medullary sponge kidney is a priority. **Ultrasonography** can be used to further evaluate possible cystic lesions and also as the initial study in the case of a patient in whom the use of contrast is contraindicated. At the same time that structural evaluation is undertaken, additional laboratory tests may be performed, including:

- Assessment for bleeding diathesis (PT, PTT, platelet count)
- Tuberculosis screening (purified protein derivative followed by urine acid-fast bacilli stains and cultures if PPD is positive)
- Malignancy and infection screening (ESR, urine cytology)

- Glomerulonephritis assessment labs if indicated (complement levels, ESR, serologies, antistreptolysin O, ANA, cryoglobulin, etc.; see Chapter 24)

Urine cytology is performed on three consecutive first-voided urine samples. While urine cytology is fairly sensitive for bladder cancer, it is relatively insensitive for detection of upper urinary tract tumors.

If the source of bleeding is still not apparent, referral to a urologist for **cystoscopy** is indicated for high risk individuals. Smokers, men over age 50, and individuals exposed to certain dyes, cyclophosphamide, phenacetin, and high dose chronic analgesics are at increased risk for bladder or renal cancer. In addition, cystoscopy is often performed as part of the initial evaluation of **gross hematuria**. At this point, if the etiology is still elusive, further evaluation can involve CT or magnetic resonance imaging (MRI) (if not already performed) or angiography to detect small structural abnormalities or arteriovenous malformation. Renal biopsy can be considered. For persons with isolated glomerular hematuria without evidence of renal failure, biopsy may be deferred because it will not generally affect decision making for these benign conditions.

If, after exhaustive evaluation, no etiology is found, long-term follow-up at 6-month intervals is generally recommended for high risk individuals. This consists of repeat history and physical examination, urinalysis, complete blood count (CBC), and BUN and creatinine. In patients older than 40 years, repeat cytology should be done. Imaging (radiologic and cystoscopic) is repeated as indicated by results of follow-up testing.

KEY POINTS

- Hematuria is detected by the presence of hemoglobin on a urine dipstick or by a finding >2 to 3 RBCs per hpf on examination of a spun urine sediment.

- Up to 10% of patients with hematuria have an underlying malignancy.

- Determining the source of hematuria involves a stepped approach, starting with assessment of history for clues to specific disorders and determination of glomerular v. nonglomerular bleeding.

- Men over age 50, smokers, people treated with cyclophosphamide, and those using high dose analgesics are at increased risk for urinary tract malignancy.

- Helical CT is the usual first-line imaging technique due to its sensitivity to detect tumor.

- Referral for consideration of cystoscopy is indicated when nonglomerular bleeding persists.

Part 4

Infectious Disease

27 Fever and Rash

A patient who presents with fever and rash poses a diagnostic challenge to the clinician. The causes of this combination form a broad differential diagnosis that includes a **wide variety of infectious and noninfectious conditions**. Some of these conditions are trivial, whereas others can be life-threatening.

Rashes can be classified according to their appearance (see Color Plates 5 to 10):

- **Maculopapular:** A **macule** is a spot with a change in normal skin color without elevation or depression of the surrounding skin. A **papule** is a raised area of skin (i.e., a "bump"). Therefore, a maculopapular rash is an outbreak of pigmented bumps.
- **Petechial/purpuric:** Petechiae are small red or brown spots formed by extravasation of blood into the skin. When these lesions coalesce, they are often referred to as **purpura**. When pressure is applied with a glass slide (diascopy), these lesions **do not** blanch.
- **Vesicular and bullous:** These are small and large blisters. If the fluid within a vesicle is cloudy (purulent), it is referred to as a **pustule**.
- **Erythematous:** Diffuse erythema can be a manifestation of a number of systemic illnesses. Generally, diascopy results in blanching because extravasation of red blood cells (RBCs) is not occurring.
- **Urticarial:** Urticaria (wheals or "hives") are rounded or flat-topped raised areas. They may have a slight pale red discoloration or may have normal coloration. They are characteristically evanescent, disappearing within several hours.

DIFFERENTIAL DIAGNOSIS

See Table 27-1 for a list of conditions presenting with fever and rash.

CLINICAL MANIFESTATIONS

When a patient presents with fever and rash, the clinician must determine if empirical treatment needs to be started along with diagnostic tests. As a rule of thumb, patients who present with a **petechial rash and fever**, particularly if there are other systemic signs of illness, are most likely to have a **potentially life-threatening illness**. Among the potential fatal "do-not-miss" diagnoses that present with fever and rash are:

- Meningococcemia
- Bacterial sepsis (e.g., staphylococcal sepsis)
- Endocarditis
- Rocky Mountain spotted fever
- Gonococcemia
- Typhoid fever

If any of these life-threatening illnesses are suspected, proper diagnosis and immediate treatment (see Treatment) should be initiated.

HISTORY

A number of **important historical features** should be sought:

- Food and water history
- Drug ingestions
- Recent travel
- Animal exposure
- Insect bites/exposure
- Ill contacts
- Sexual history
- Prior rashes/illnesses

■ TABLE 27-1 Conditions Presenting with Fever and Rash

Disease	Type of Rash	Epidemiology	Clinical Findings
Infectious			
Endocarditis	P	Abnormal heart valves	Cardiac murmur, mucosal lesions, retinal findings
Meningococcemia	P, MP, VB	Outbreak of *Neisseria*	+/− meningitis, septic shock (hypotension, oliguria), pustules may be present, organisms visible on Gram stain
Gonococcemia	P, VB	Sexual activity, esp. with prostitutes or multiple partners	± urethritis, joint pain/effusions
Typhoid fever	MP ("rose spots")	Poor sanitation (fecal/oral spread), contact with asymptomatic carriers	Prolonged, persistent fever; constipation; relative bradycardia during febrile episodes
Staphylococcal sepsis	VB	IVDU, poor skin hygiene	Evidence of dermatologic staphylococcal infection
Vibrio vulnificus	VB	Ingestion of raw seafood, exposure to seawater	Patients with cirrhosis are most susceptible; septic shock; lesions on extremities, legs > arms
Folliculitis	MP, VB	Hot tubs (*Pseudomonas*), freshwater exposure (swimmer's itch from avian schistosomes)	Diffuse rash, marked pruritus in swimmer's itch
Streptococcal infection	E	Outbreaks of scarlet fever	Diffuse erythematous rash with "sandpaper" texture, well-circumscribed cellulitis (erysipelas)
Staphylococcal infection	MP, VB, E	Tampon use (toxic shock), poor skin hygiene	Shock, with diffuse erythema and later palmar desquamation (toxic shock), folliculitis, pustules (staphylococcal bacteremia)
Ehrlichiosis	E	Endemic area in summer, tick bite, outdoor exposure, LFT, rash variable	Headache, leukopenia, abnormalities
Rocky Mountain spotted fever	P	Endemic area in summer, tick bite, outdoor exposure	Severe headache, rash starts in extremeties and spreads centripetally
Secondary syphilis	MP	Sexual activity, esp. with prostitutes or multiple partners	Involves palms and soles
Mycoplasma	MP, U	Younger patients	Bullous myringitis, pneumonia
Lyme disease	MP	Endemic area in summer, tick bite, outdoor exposure	Erythema migrans rash, joint effusions, headache
Enteroviral infection	P, MP, VB, E, U	Winter months	Myalgia, diarrhea, headache, meningitis
Rubella	P, MP	No history of immunization	Viral prodrome, rash starts on forehead and spreads downward to feet, adenopathy
Rubeola	MP	No history of immunization	Viral prodrome with conjunctivitis; small, irregular mucosal lesions (Koplik spots); rash starts on forehead and spreads downward to feet
Adenovirus	MP, U	Year-round occurrence, but greatest in winter months	Upper respiratory illness, conjunctivitis, adenopathy

continued

■ TABLE 27-1 Conditions Presenting with Fever and Rash *(continued)*

Disease	Type of Rash	Epidemiology	Clinical Findings
Primary HIV infection	MP	Sexual activity, esp. with prostitutes or multiple partners; IVDU	Viral syndrome with fever, malaise, headaches and myalgia
HIV (established infection)	VB, U	Sexual activity, esp. with prostitutes or multiple partners; IVDU	Often with no other symptoms
Varicella-zoster	VB	No history of disease (primary infection)	Reactivation in dermatomal distribution
Herpes simplex virus	VB	Multiple sexual partners, other STD	HSV-1 typically oral; HSV-2 typically genital
EBV	U	Outbreaks occur among college students and military recruits	Mononucleosis (fever, adenopathy, pharyngitis, malaise, spelnomegaly); 5% incidence of rash in mononucleosis, almost 100% if ampicillin is administered
Hepatitis	U	IVDU, multiple sexual partners	Urticaria may occur during acute hepatitis, but also during chronic disease
Noninfectious			
Allergy	P, MP, VB, E, U	Exposure to various drugs, foods, animals	Manifestations vary greatly
Thrombocytopenia	P	Previous viral syndrome, known idiopathic thrombocytopenia	Easy bruising as well as spontaneous petechiae
Henoch-Schönlein purpura	P	Mostly in children	Abdominal pain, arthralgias, glomerulonephritis, IgA deposits in skin and kidneys
Hypersensitivity vasculitis	P	Antigen exposure (infectious agent, drug)	Biopsy reveals leukocytoclastic vasculitis with antigen/antibody immune complex deposition
Vasculitis (e.g., SLE, polyarteritis nodosum, dermatomyositis)	P, MP	Known history of vasculitis	Manifestations vary as to type of vasculitis
Erythema multiforme	MP	Drug exposure	Characteristic "target" lesions, can have mucosal involvement (Stevens-Johnson syndrome)
Plant dermatitis (poison ivy, poison oak)	VB	Known exposure to plants	Weepy, vesicular/bullous lesions in areas of contact, pruritus
Vasodilation	E	Shock, vigorous exercise	Blanching, bright erythema
Psoriasis	E	Known history	Silvery scale present over diffuse erythema, pustular variant seen
Lymphoma	E	Peak incidence 55 to 60 years old; 2:1 male:female (cutaneous T-cell lymphoma)	Diffuse erythema can occur in all lymphomas, T-cell lymphoma of skin (mycosis fungoides and Sezary syndrome)
Kawasaki disease	E	Generally children	Resembles scarlet fever, but without evidence of streptococcal infection

E, erythematous; IVDU, intravenous drug use; MP, maculopapular; P, petechial/purpuric; U, urticarial; VB, vesicular/bullous.

The presence of a prodrome (fatigue, malaise, myalgias) prior to the appearance of rash is often suggestive of an infectious illness (viral, Rocky Mountain spotted fever, bacterial). The pattern of appearance and spread of the rash also have diagnostic significance (see Table 27-1).

PHYSICAL EXAMINATION

On physical examination, the extent and morphology of the rash need to be determined carefully. Mucosal surfaces, genitalia, scalp, palms, and soles all need to be examined. Patients may not be aware of the full extent of the lesions, and a careful examination is important. Examination of the fundi can reveal embolic phenomena indicative of an intravascular bacterial infection (e.g., endocarditis).

Signs of severe systemic illness (e.g., hypotension, meningismus) suggest a potentially life-threatening condition (meningococcemia, toxic shock, endocarditis, Rocky Mountain spotted fever, Kawasaki disease).

Table 27-1 lists other important physical examination findings.

DIAGNOSTIC EVALUATION

When history and physical examination narrow the differential diagnosis to a group of relatively benign illnesses, extensive diagnostic testing is unnecessary. In cases where the diagnosis is unclear, **routine laboratory tests** (complete blood count [CBC], creatinine, liver function tests [LFTs], UA, chest radiographs) can provide useful information.

The overall diagnostic test strategy is to limit the differential diagnosis based on history and physical examination and then use selected tests to confirm potential diagnoses. Certain test results (e.g., serology and pathology) can take days to become available and thus are used only to confirm a diagnosis and not to guide therapy.

If the patient is systemically ill, **blood cultures** should be obtained. Pustules can be sampled and the material subjected to **Gram stain and culture**. Vesicles can be unroofed and material sent for **Tzanck test**, direct **antibody stain**, and **viral culture** to identify varicella-zoster and herpes viruses.

Patients with meningeal signs should have a **lumbar puncture** with Gram stain, culture, and cell count performed on the fluid.

Serology can be useful to identify diseases such as syphilis, Rocky Mountain spotted fever, Lyme disease, and ehrlichiosis. Paired acute and convalescent serology is often more helpful. Again, note that serology is generally used to confirm a suspected diagnosis, but treatment of potentially serious conditions should not be delayed while waiting for results.

In patients with severe systemic illness, **empirical antibiotic therapy** is often initiated to cover meningococcemia, Rocky Mountain spotted fever, and typhoid fever. A third-generation cephalosporin such as ceftriaxone and a tetracycline provide broad empirical coverage pending culture results.

Skin biopsy and culture may be necessary. Special stains for certain organisms and for vasculitis (e.g., IgA in Henoch-Schönlein purpura) can be done.

Skin testing for possible allergic reactions can be useful in selected cases.

KEY POINTS

- The combination of fever and rash can indicate a variety of benign and life-threatening diseases.
- The nature of the rash coupled with the history and physical examination play a key role in narrowing the differential diagnosis.
- In cases of severe systemic illness, empirical antibiotic treatment is initiated at the same time as the diagnostic workup.

Pneumonia

Pneumonia can occur among otherwise healthy (from an immunologic standpoint) individuals. This clinical entity is referred to as **community-acquired pneumonia** (CAP). Organisms, management, and outcome vary between patients based on host characteristics. The physician must be able to identify pneumonia and, based on host characteristics and a variety of physical and laboratory findings, start empiric antimicrobial therapy when indicated.

EPIDEMIOLOGY

Pneumonia is the sixth leading cause of death in the United States; among infectious causes of death, it ranks number one. An estimated 4 million cases of CAP occur each year in the United States. Approximately 20% of these cases require hospitalization, and, among these patients, mortality averages 15%, compared to <1% of patients who can be managed as outpatients.

ETIOLOGY

The microbial agents responsible for pneumonia range from bacteria to fungi to viruses. Specific etiologic agents of pneumonia occur with different frequencies depending on specific **host factors**:

- Age
- Socioeconomic status
- Prior antibiotic use
- Underlying medical conditions (e.g., alcohol abuse, chronic obstructive pulmonary disease [COPD], DM, chronic liver disease, chronic renal insufficiency, congestive heart failure [CHF],

underlying neoplastic disease, use of immunosuppressive drugs)

These host factors not only influence the **etiology** of pneumonias in patients but also have an impact on the **prognosis**.

CLINICAL MANIFESTATIONS

HISTORY

Patients presenting with pneumonia may present with pulmonary or extrapulmonary **symptoms**:

- Fever, chills, rigors
- Cough
- Sputum production
- Chest pain
- Shortness of breath

Other important historical points are the presence of underlying disease (see preceding list), history of recent travel, and exposure (sick individuals, animals, environmental irritants).

PHYSICAL EXAMINATION

The physical examination can aid in establishing the diagnosis and extent of a possible pneumonia and to assess the severity of disease. It should be noted that the clinical exam alone lacks sensitivity and specificity for the diagnosis of CAP.

Classically, pneumonias present with signs of **consolidation**:

- Bronchial breath sounds
- Egophony ("e" to "a" changes)

- Dullness to percussion
- Increased tactile fremitus

Even if evidence of frank consolidation is not present, most patients with pneumonia have **crackles** on lung examination. The presence of a **pleural effusion** (Chapter 18) can present with dullness to percussion, with decreased tactile fremitus and decreased breath sounds.

Physical findings in patients with CAP that are associated with **increased morbidity and mortality** include:

- Tachypnea (respiratory rate ≥30)
- Temperature <95°F (35°C) or ≥104°F (40°C)
- Hypotension (diastolic ≤60, systolic ≤90)
- Pulse ≥125
- Evidence of extrapulmonary disease (meningitis, septic arthritis)
- Confusion/altered mental status

DIFFERENTIAL DIAGNOSIS

A number of **infectious illnesses** can present with symptoms (especially cough, fever, and sputum production) that are seen in patients with pneumonia:

- URI
- Sinusitis
- Pharyngitis
- Bronchitis

Noninfectious conditions that can mimic pneumonia include:

- Pulmonary embolus
- CHF
- Lung cancer
- Inflammatory lung disease (e.g., Wegener granulomatosis, eosinophilic pneumonia)

DIAGNOSTIC EVALUATION

A number of tests can be useful in detecting the presence and extent of pneumonia. A **standard posteroanterior (PA) and lateral chest radiograph** (Fig. 28-1) can differentiate pneumonia from conditions such as bronchitis (which is associated with a normal chest radiograph) and detect other conditions such as lung abscesses, pleural effusions, and masses. Differences in the radiographic findings in pneumonia (lobar vs. diffuse) are not specific enough to allow

diagnosis of a specific etiology of a pneumonia but can be suggestive.

Gram stain and sputum culture can help define the etiologic cause of a pneumonia. The exact usefulness of a Gram stain has been debated, but it may add information helpful in determining empirical antibiotic therapy, pending results of culture.

In addition to sputum cultures, blood cultures (both anaerobic and aerobic) should be collected from those patients who require hospitalization. Although positive in only a minority of cases (in particular, in cases of pneumococcal pneumonia), they can provide useful information about the etiologic agent, and, if positive, they are also predictive of a more severe clinical course.

Urinary antigen tests for *Legionella pneumophila* group 1 and *S. pneumoniae* are available for rapid diagnosis. These tests have the advantage in that they are unaffected by the initiation of antibiotic therapy (at least for the first 48 to 72 hours), but may suffer from a lack of sensitivity and specificity in patients without bacteremia. Additionally, if relied on for diagnosis, there is no pathogen isolate available for antimicrobial sensitivity testing.

In a manner similar to certain physical findings (see earlier), certain laboratory results are predictive of **higher morbidity and mortality**:

- Total WBC count $<4 \times 10^9$/L or $>30 \times 10^9$/L, or absolute neutrophil count $<1 \times 10^9$/L
- Pa_{O_2} <60 mm Hg or Pa_{CO_2} >50 mm Hg (Fi_{O_2} 0.21)
- Arterial pH <7.35
- Hematocrit <30% or hemoglobin <9 g per dL
- Serum creatine >1.2 mg per dL or BUN >20 mg per dL
- Certain unfavorable chest radiograph findings (e.g., multilobar consolidation, pulmonary effusion, cavity formation)

TREATMENT

Once the diagnosis of pneumonia has been established, there are **two main management questions**:

1. Does the patient require admission to the hospital?
2. What is appropriate initial antibiotic therapy?

A number of **prediction rules** for the outcome in CAP have been developed, most notably by the British Thoracic Society (BTS) and the Pneumonia Patient Outcomes Research Team (PORT). Although these

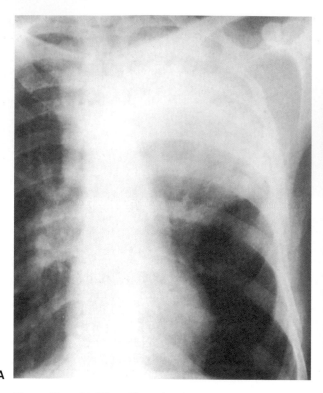

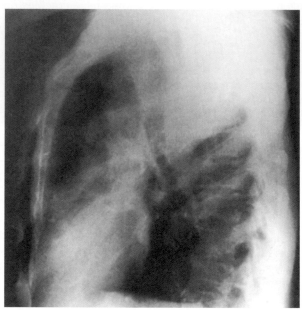

A

B

Figure 28-1 • PA **(A)** and lateral **(B)** chest radiographs showing left upper lobe consolidation in a patient with pneumonia caused by *Streptococcus pneumoniae*.

prediction rules could potentially determine which patients with CAP require admission, most experts believe **these rules should be used to support, but not replace, physician decision making**. Overall, the severity of the illness plus social factors (homelessness, support services, etc.) play a role in determining the need for hospitalization. In general, if multiple risk factors coexist, hospitalization should strongly be considered, at least long enough to monitor clinical status and determine response to therapy. These prediction rules often require the measurement of multiple clinical variables, so in an attempt to simplify this process, one model named CURB-65 (based on the factors mentioned) was recently developed:

- Confusion
- Blood **u**rea nitrogen >20 mg/dL
- **R**espiratory rate >30 breaths per minute
- **B**lood pressure (systolic <90, diastolic <60)
- Age >**65** years

Using the CURB-65 model, 30-day mortality increased with increasing score (1 point given for each positive factor) thus leading to the recommen-

dation that patients with a score of 0 to 1 can be treated as outpatients, those with a score of 2 be admitted and patients with a score >3 may require ICU care.

With regard to antimicrobial therapy, certain epidemiologic conditions are related to specific pathogens (Table 28-1).

Additionally, attempts have been made to guide initial antimicrobial therapy in CAP based on patient characteristics. The **American Thoracic Society** and the **Infectious Diseases Society of America** have published joint guidelines based on patient characteristics to guide empirical therapy for CAP (Table 28-2).

The presence of a pleural effusion on chest radiograph may indicate a possible empyema (Chapter 18). Consideration should be given to sampling the pleural fluid to determine if it is infected; and if an empyema is diagnosed, placement of a chest tube is indicated.

Once empirical antimicrobial therapy is initiated, the patient's response needs to be carefully monitored. Generally, therapy should not be altered in

TABLE 28-1 Epidemiologic Conditions and Associated Pathogens	
Condition	**Commonly Encountered Pathogens**
Alcoholism	*Streptococcus pneumoniae* and anaerobes
Smokers and/or COPD	*S. pneumoniae, Haemophilus influenzae, Moraxella catarrhalis, Legionella*
Nursing home resident	*S. pneumoniae*, gram-negative bacilli, *H. influenzae, Staphylococcus aureus*, anaerobes, *Chlamydia pneumoniae*
Poor dental hygiene	Anaerobes
Exposure to bats	*Histoplasma capsulatum*
Exposure to birds	*Chlamydia psittaci, Cryptococcus neoformans, H. capsulatum*
Exposure to rabbits	*Francisella tularensis*
Travel to southwestern United States	*Coccidioides* spp.
Exposure to farm animals or parturient cats	*Coxiella burnetii* (Q fever)
Influenza active in community	Influenza, *S. pneumoniae, S. aureus, Streptococcus pyogenes, H. influenzae*
Recent antibiotic therapy	Drug-resistant *S. pneumoniae, Pseudomonas aeruginosa*
Injection drug use	*S. aureus, S. pneumoniae*, tuberculosis, anaerobes
Suspected large-volume aspiration	Anaerobes (chemical pneumonitis, obstruction)

the first 72 hours. **Early change in therapy is indicated if**:

- Initial diagnostic studies identify a pathogen not covered by original empirical therapy (e.g., tuberculosis, fungal pneumonia)
- A resistant organism is isolated from blood or other sterile site (e.g., pleural fluid)
- There is marked clinical deterioration

When determining clinical response, signs and symptoms can persist even if appropriate therapy is being given. Fever may last for several days, although the magnitude should decrease each day. Leukocytosis may also persist for 2 to 4 days. Physical findings (e.g., crackles, egophony) can persist beyond a week, and chest radiograph changes can be present for several weeks.

If a patient does not improve or worsens on empirical therapy, consideration must be given to several causes:

- Inadequate antimicrobial selection (e.g., because of resistance, presence of a viral pathogen)
- Undrained infection (i.e., pulmonary abscess or empyema)
- Unusual pathogens (e.g., fungal pneumonias, psittacosis)
- Noninfectious illness

If a patient is failing initial therapy, consideration should be given to **further diagnostic testing**, including:

- Bronchoscopy with sampling of respiratory secretions
- Computed tomography (CT)
- Pulmonary arteriogram (if pulmonary embolism is suspected)
- Serology (not usually useful in the acute setting)

 KEY POINTS

- Pneumonia is the leading infectious cause of death in the United States.
- Etiologic agents differ depending on various host factors, including age and coexisting illness.
- Empirical therapy for pneumonia should be based on patient characteristics as well as data from sputum Gram stain.
- Failure of initial therapy may be because of resistant organisms, unusual organisms, or a noninfectious cause and may warrant further diagnostic testing, including bronchoscopy.

■ Table 28-2 Classification and Empirical Therapy for Community-Acquired Pneumonia

Patient Group	Major Pathogens	Miscellaneous Pathogens	Empirical Therapy
Outpatient (previously healthy and no use of antimicrobials within the previous 3 months)	S. pneumoniae M. pneumoniae C. pneumoniae H. influenzae Respiratory viruses	Legionella spp. M. tuberculosis Endemic fungi	Advanced-generation macrolide (e.g., azithromycin or clarithromycin)[a] or doxycycline
Outpatient (with comorbidities)[b]	S. pneumoniae (including DRSP) M. pneumoniae C. pneumoniae Mixed infection (bacterial plus atypical pathogen or virus) H. influenzae Respiratory viruses	M. catarrhalis Legionella spp. M. tuberculosis Endemic fungi Aspiration (anaerobes)	Respiratory fluoroquinolone (moxifloxacin, gemifloxacin, levofloxacin) or Beta-lactam plus a macrolide
Inpatients (non-ICU treatment)	S. pneumoniae (including DRSP) H. influenzae M. pneumoniae C. pneumoniae Mixed infection (bacteria plus atypical pathogen or virus) Enteric gram-negative organisms Respiratory viruses Aspiration (anaerobes) Legionella spp.	M. tuberculosis Endemic fungi Pneumocystis jirovecii	Respiratory fluoroqinolone (moxifloxacin, gemifloxacin or levolfoxacin) or Beta-lactam plus a macrolide
Inpatients (ICU treatment)	S. pneumoniae (including DRSP) H. influenzae M. pneumoniae C. pneumoniae Mixed infection (bacteria plus atypical pathogen or virus) Enteric gram-negative organisms Respiratory viruses Aspiration (anaerobes) Legionella spp.	M. tuberculosis Endemic fungi Pneumocystis jirovecii	A beta-lactam (cefotaxime, ceftriaxone, or ampicillin-sulbactam: aztreonam for penicillin-allergic patients) plus either azithromycin or respiratory fluoroquinolone If Pseudomonas is a concern:[c] Change beta-lactam to an antipneumococcal, antipseudomonal (piperacillin-tazobactam, cefepime, imipenem, or meropenam: aztreonam for penicillin-allergic patients) plus either ciprofloxacin or levofloxacin or aminoglucoside and azithromycin or animoglycoside plus respiratory fluoroquinolone If community-acquired MRSA is a consideration: add vancomycin or linezolid

Recommendations are based on both the American Thoracic Society and the Infectious Diseases Society of America published guidelines and updates.
[a]In regions with a high rate (>25%) of high-level macrolide-resistant S. pneumoniae, consider use of alternative agents listed as with patients with comorbidities).
[b]Co-morbidities include chronic heart, lung, liver, or renal disease; diabetes mellitus; alcoholism; malignancies; asplenia; immunosuppressing conditions or use of immunosuppressing drugs; or use of antimicrobials within the previous 3 months (in which case an alternative from a different class should be selected).
[c]Risks for P. aeruginosa infection include chronic or prolonged (i.e., >7 days within last month) broad-spectrum antibiotic use, bronchiectasis, malnutrition, therapies associated with neutrophil dysfunction (e.g., ≥10 mg of prednisone per day).
DRSP, drug-resistant Streptococcus pneumoniae; ICU, intensive care unit.

Sexually Transmitted Diseases

EPIDEMIOLOGY

Sexually transmitted diseases (STDs) are among the most common infections. In the United States, there are an estimated 8 to 12 million cases of STDs each year. Accurate estimation is made difficult by the fact that not all STDs are reported because of social stigma. Many health organizations have adopted the term *sexually transmitted infection* (STI) to replace STD because many affected individuals do not exhibit symptoms and in part because of the social stigma attached to the term STD. However, we continue to use the term STD because it is still common in the medical literature.

The rates of many STDs are influenced by:

- Socioeconomic class
- Drug use
- Sexual practices (number of partners, rate of partner change, prostitution, oral–fecal exposure)

In the United States, STDs are most prevalent among young individuals of low socioeconomic class. The notable exception is infection with *Chlamydia trachomatis*, which is more evenly distributed across the population.

Human immunodeficiency virus (HIV) infection is discussed separately in Chapters 35 and 36.

ETIOLOGY AND PATHOGENESIS

A variety of organisms can be transmitted by sexual contact, including bacteria, viruses, and arthropods. Annually, the most **common STD agents** encountered in the United States are:

- *Chlamydia trachomatis* (4 to 5 million cases)
- *Neisseria gonorrhoeae* (620,000 cases)
- *Treponema pallidum* (35,000 cases)

- Human papilloma virus, or HPV (~500,000 new cases; 40 million chronic cases)
- Herpes simplex virus type 2, or HSV-2 (~400,000 new cases; 30 million chronic cases)
- Hepatitis B virus, or HBV (~250,000 cases)
- HIV infection (~50,000 new cases; 1.5 million chronic infections)

Most nonviral STDs can induce **acute inflammation** when the organisms colonize the mucosa. This inflammation leads to the symptoms associated with infection (see later). In addition, infection of the upper female reproductive tract (endometrium, fallopian tubes, and pelvic peritoneum), also known as **pelvic inflammatory disease** (PID), can lead to a variety of **sequelae**:

- Ectopic pregnancy
- Tubal infertility
- Chronic pelvic pain

PID can also be completely asymptomatic. This is important in maintaining a reservoir of infection.

Infection with HPV and HSV is lifelong. Recurrences (which may be asymptomatic) are common and responsible for continued spread of the viruses. In addition, chronic infection with certain types of HPV (e.g., types 16 and 18) is associated with the development of a premalignant lesion (cervical intraepithelial neoplasia) and frank cervical cancer.

CLINICAL MANIFESTATIONS

A number of distinct **clinical syndromes** can arise from STDs (Table 29-1):

- Urethritis
- Epididymitis

■ TABLE 29-1 Clinical Syndromes Seen in Sexually Transmitted Diseases

Clinical Syndrome	Common Etiologies	Clinical Findings	Laboratory Findings	Treatment
Urethritis (male)	*Neisseria gonorrhoeae, Chlamydia trachomatis, Ureaplasma urealyticum*	Dysuria, urethral discharge, fever, arthritis, Reiter syndrome	Gram-negative diplococci inside PMNs (*N. gonorrhoeae*); PMNs without organisms (NGU)	Third-generation cephalosporin (*N. gonorrhoeae*); doxycycline or azithromycin (NGU)*
Urethritis (female)	*N. gonorrhoeae, C. trachomatis, E. coli*	Dysuria (without frequency and urgency) ± cervicitis	Pyuria	Third-generation cephalosporin (*N. gonorrhoeae*); doxycycline or azithromycin (NGU)*
Epididymitis	*C. trachomatis, N. gonorrhoeae,* Enterobacteriaceae	Testicular pain and tenderness (usually unilateral)	None specific	Third-generation cephalosporin (*N. gonorrhoeae*), *plus* doxycycline (*C. trachomatis*), quinolone (Enterobacteriaceae)
Vulvovaginitis	*Trichomonas vaginalis, Candida albicans*	Vulvar itching, "cottage cheese" discharge (candidiasis); vulvar itching, purulent, malodorous discharge, mucosa visibly inflamed (*T. vaginalis*)	PMNs, budding yeast on KOH prep or Gram's stain (candidiasis); PMNs with motile organisms seen (trichomoniasis)	Intravaginal azoles (e.g., clotrimazole, miconazole) (candidiasis); metronidazole (trichomoniasis)
Bacterial vaginosis	*Gardnerella vaginalis, Mycoplasma hominis,* anaerobic bacteria	Malodorous, thin discharge (clear to white)	"Clue cells" on wet prep, replacement of *Lactobacilli* with mixed organisms of Gram stain, few PMNs	Metronidazole (either orally or intravaginally)
PID	*C. trachomatis, N. gonorrhoeae*	Abdominal pain, purulent vaginal discharge, cervicitis (purulent); nausea/vomiting, fever, cervical motion tenderness	Elevated WBCs, PMNs in vaginal discharge, gram-negative diplococci seen within PMNs (*N. gonorrhoeae*)	Inpatient: Third-generation cephalosporin or clindamycin and gentamicin *or* ampicillin/sulbactam *plus* doxycycline Outpatient: Third-generation cephalosporin × 1 *plus* doxycycline, *or* quinolone *plus* metronidazole*
Genital ulcers	Herpes simplex virus (HSV); *Treponema pallidum* (syphilis); *Haemophilus ducreyi* (chancroid)	Painful ulcers (HSV, chancroid); painless ulcers (syphilis); painful ulcers and inguinal adenopathy with overlying erythema (chancroid)	Multinucleated giant cells/positive DFA/viral culture (HSV); spirochetes seen on dark-field microscopy (syphilis); isolation of *H. ducreyi* from lesion or lymph node aspirate	Acyclovir (HSV); benzathine penicillin G (syphilis): single IM does for early disease, three doses for late disease (neurosyphilis requires IV therapy), doxycycline for penicillin allergy; ceftriaxone or azithromycin (chancroid)

■ **TABLE 29-1** Clinical Syndromes Seen in Sexually Transmitted Diseases *(continued)*

Clinical Syndrome	Common Etiologies	Clinical Findings	Laboratory Findings	Treatment
Genital warts	Human papilloma virus	Visible papillomas, associated with the development of epithelial cancers	Molecular typing is available, but not usually needed to make the diagnosis	Local wart removal (cryosurgery, laser surgery, podophyllin); Vaccine is available for prevention
Hepatitis	Hepatitis B virus, possibly hepatitis C virus, hepatitis A (fecal–oral contact)	Fever, hepatomegaly, abdominal pain (see Chapter 41)	Elevated liver transaminases; serologic testing available	None available

*When treating presumed *Neisseria gonorrhoeae* infection, empirical treatment for *Chlamydia trachomatis* is also added unless ruled out by definitive (e.g., DNA) testing.
DFA, direct fluorescent antigen; NGU, nongonococcal urethritis.

- Vulvovaginitis/cervicitis
- Acute PID
- Genital ulcers
- Genital warts
- Hepatitis

Although the specific clinical syndromes manifest with typical symptoms and physical findings, STDs can be clinically silent, particularly in women.

HISTORY

Most patients who seek medical attention for a possible STD do so because of **symptoms** such as:

- Dysuria
- Discharge
- Genital lesions (ulcers, warts)
- Abdominal pain
- Fever

Other patients may seek attention because of a high-risk sexual exposure (e.g., prostitutes) or because they were notified by a sexual partner of possible infection. A thorough **sexual history** can identify patients who are risk of infection and should include:

- Number of sexual partners (both lifetime and recent)
- Details of sexual practices (anal–oral, oral–genital, anal receptive, vaginal)
- Condom use (specifically frequency of use)
- High-risk sexual contacts (prostitutes, IV drug users)

- Past history of STDs
- History of abnormal Papanicolaou smears

Because many infections can be asymptomatic, a detailed sexual history to identify patients who may be at risk is an important part of *routine* patient care.

PHYSICAL EXAMINATION

When evaluating a patient with a possible STD, the physical examination should include a close examination of the genitalia (including a speculum and bimanual examination for women and testicular and prostate examination for men) and other mucosal surfaces (conjunctiva, oral cavity, and rectum). Lymphadenopathy should be sought, as well as skin lesions such as rashes and ulcers. Certain findings are suggestive of specific etiologies (see Table 29-1).

DIFFERENTIAL DIAGNOSIS

Certain STD syndromes can mimic other conditions:

- **Urethritis:** Urinary tract infection, prostatitis
- **PID:** Ectopic pregnancy, appendicitis, pyelonephritis, cystitis
- **Vulvovaginitis/cervicitis:** Normal cyclical changes in vaginal secretions during menstrual cycle, dysfunctional uterine bleeding

DIAGNOSTIC EVALUATION

Diagnosis of specific STDs can be made by culture and a variety of nonculture methods, including direct microscopy, immunofluorescence, serology, and deoxyribonucleic acid (DNA) diagnosis (e.g., polymerase chain reaction). Nonculture methods are useful for organisms that cannot be cultured (e.g., *Treponema pallidum*) or are difficult or expensive to culture (HSV, HPV, *Chlamydia*). Nonculture methods are sometimes much more rapid than culture.

Evaluation of specific STDs varies with the particular clinical entity encountered. In a man, the presence of urethritis should be confirmed by examination for discharge, which may require milking the urethra after the patient has not voided for several hours. If no discharge is found, an endourethral sample should be obtained by inserting a small urethral swab approximately 2 to 3 cm into the urethra. The sample should be examined by Gram stain, looking for the presence of PMNs or organisms or both (see Color Plate 11). Further workup and treatment (Table 29-2) can then be based on these findings. Because of greater patient acceptance and willingness to undergo testing, nucleic acid testing for *Chlamydia* and gonorrhea using a urine sample is widely used.

For women with presumed urethritis, the workup is similar. However, it is important first to rule out cystitis, pyelonephritis, and vulvovaginitis. For **vulvovaginitis/bacterial vaginosis** in a woman who presents with abnormal vaginal discharge (with or without malodor) and/or vaginal discomfort (pruritus, burning, dyspareunia, with or without dysuria), it is again important to rule out a urinary tract infection. In addition, vaginal discharge can be a sign of infection higher in the reproductive tract (cervicitis or PID). A careful pelvic examination is thus indicated, with collection of samples for microscopic examination and culture (see Table 29-2). Note that,

unlike the situation with men, testing of a urine specimen for gonorrhea in a woman has much lower sensitivity, and thus the test needs to be performed on an endocervical swab.

Because of the severe sequelae that can result from PID, particularly when not treated in a timely fashion, prompt evaluation and empirical treatment are necessary when evaluating a woman who presents with cervical discharge and/or abdominal pain and fever. As mentioned previously, the important distinction is between PID and surgical emergencies such as appendicitis and ectopic pregnancy. Gram stain and culture should be performed, and empirical treatment for chlamydia and gonorrhea instituted.

TREATMENT

The treatment of most STDs is accomplished on an outpatient basis. Specific or empirical therapy can be initiated based on clinical findings while waiting for the results of specific laboratory diagnosis. In certain populations (e.g., young individuals of low socioeconomic status), empirical treatment is important because of the likelihood of poor follow-up. Similarly, simple (preferably single-dose) drug treatment is preferable.

In cases of suspected PID, consideration should be given to hospitalization when the diagnosis is uncertain, surgical emergencies must be ruled out, severe systemic illness is present (severe emesis, high fever, hypotension), close outpatient follow-up cannot be arranged or the patient is judged to be unable to complete or tolerate outpatient management, or the patient has failed outpatient management.

■ TABLE 29-2 Gram Stain Evaluation of Suspected Cases of PID or Urethritis	
Findings	**Further Workup and Treatment**
<5 PMNs per high-powered field and no organisms	Culture/probe for *Neisseria gonorrhoeae* and *Chlamydia trachomatis* without treatment.* If negative, assess for prostatitis, cystitis.
PMNs with intracellular gram-negative diplococci	Culture/molecular probe for *N. gonorrhoeae*. Treat for gonorrhea (see Table 29-1)
PMNs with atypical gram-negative diplococci (extracellular or with abnormal morphology)	Culture/probe for *N. gonorrhoeae* and *C. trachomatis*. Treat for gonorrhea and *Chlamydia* infections.
PMNs and no gram-negative diplococci	Culture/probe for *N. gonorrhoeae*. Treat for presumed chlamydial infection

*Empirical treatment in patients at high risk for infection who are unlikely to return for follow-up evaluation.

For nonviral STDs, antimicrobial therapy is the mainstay of therapy (see Table 29-1). Generally, empirical therapy based on the clinical picture and preliminary diagnostic tests is started pending definitive diagnosis by culture or other nonculture methods.

Acyclovir and other similar antiviral agents (e.g., famciclovir) are used for the treatment of HSV. Even though HSV infection cannot be cleared, acyclovir can shorten the course of outbreaks, shorten viral shedding time, and shorten healing time. Patients who have frequent outbreaks may be candidates for chronic acyclovir suppression.

From the public health standpoint, the screening and treatment of sexual partners of patients diagnosed with an STD are a critical part of management. Practices vary widely, from supplying medication for partner treatment to requiring the partner to appear in person for assessment. The risks of treating partners without the opportunity to assess for possible drug allergies and provide education need to be balanced against the public health risk of not treating a partner at all.

Primary prevention, mainly through latex condom use and avoiding high-risk contacts, should be encouraged in all sexually active patients, particularly those who have had a previous diagnosis of an STD. Vaccination for hepatitis A and B should also be offered. Additional vaccines for STDs are in development. Routine screening of certain patient groups (e.g., pregnant women, women with multiple sexual partners, or men who have sex with men) for particular STDs is also recommend by the Centers for Disease Control and Prevention (CDC) and the U.S. Preventive Services Task Force (see the CDC or USPSTF Web sites for current recommendations). A recent development in the prevention of STDs is the availability of a vaccine against certain types of HPV (types 6, 11, 16, and 18 L1, which are most commonly associated with genital warts and squamous intraepithelial lesions).

SYPHILIS

Infection with *T. pallidum* deserves separate attention because of its varied clinical manifestations, serious late complications, and diagnostic difficulties. Syphilis is characterized by stages of active clinical disease separated by periods of asymptomatic latent infection. The duration of each stage may vary, the stages may overlap, and a given patient may not progress through each stage. All patients, however,

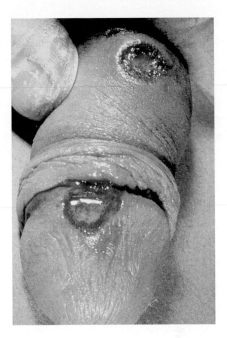

Figure 29-1 • Chancres on the penis of a patient with primary syphilis.

manifest the initial or *primary stage*, which is a painless, indurated ulcer (known as a chancre; Fig. 29-1) at the inoculation site. If untreated, approximately half the patients progress to a *disseminated* (hematogenous) *stage*, and the rest go directly to a stage of *latent disease*. In the disseminated (also known as secondary) stage, the organisms are widely dispersed throughout the body.

Physical findings in **secondary syphilis** commonly include:

- Generalized maculopapular rash (characteristically involves palms and soles; Color Plate 10)
- Mucous patches (silver gray erosions with an erythematous periphery that are generally painless)
- Condylomata (wartlike enlarged papules that are moist and pink to gray white; these lesions are highly infectious)
- Generalized nontender lymphadenopathy
- The primary chancre (present in approximately 15% of cases)

Patients with secondary syphilis can also have a variety of nonspecific constitutional symptoms (fever, sore throat, malaise, and headache). Syphilis has been called the "great imitator" because there is a wide variety of less common manifestations, including hepatitis, nephropathy, arthritis, iridocyclitis, nephrotic syndrome, gastritis, and ulcerative colitis.

Patients in the latent stage, which is defined as *early latent* in the first year after infection and *late latent* thereafter (or operationally, disease of unknown duration), have serologic evidence of infection (see later) but no clinical manifestations. This stage can last for the rest of the patient's lifetime or end with spontaneous clearance of infection or progression to late syphilis.

Late syphilis is marked by end-organ damage, involving:

* Nervous system (general paresis; tabes dorsalis; paresthesias, loss of position, pain, and temperature sensation)
* Cardiovascular system (syphilitic aortitis)
* Gumma formation (granulomas with central necrosis, most commonly involving the skin, skeletal system, mouth, larynx, liver, and stomach, but all organs have been reported to be involved)

The **laboratory diagnosis of syphilis** can be performed by:

* Dark-field microscopy of lesions (to demonstrate the presence of spirochetes)
* Direct immunofluorescence microscopy
* Serology (both nontreponemal tests such as rapid plasma reagin [RPR] and Venereal Disease Research Laboratory [VDRL], which are used for screening, and direct treponemal tests such as immunofluorescence and hemagglutination to detect antibodies specific for *T. pallidum*)

The VDRL can be used to monitor response to therapy, using as the guideline a fourfold decline in titer within 6 to 12 months after treatment as indicative of cure.

KEY POINTS

* STDs are among the most common infections, with an estimated 8 to 12 million new cases a year in the United States.

* Because many infections can be asymptomatic, especially in women, clinicians need to have a high index of suspicion, and a thorough sexual history (coupled with appropriate screening tests) needs to be a part of routine medical care.

* A number of viruses and bacteria are responsible for the most commonly encountered STDs.

* STDs can manifest a number of clinical syndromes, including urethritis, genital ulcers/warts, and upper reproductive tract disease in women (PID).

* PID can result in a number of serious sequelae, including tubal infertility, ectopic pregnancy, and chronic pelvic pain.

Urinary Tract Infections

Urinary tract infections (UTIs) are often divided into lower tract infections involving the urinary bladder (cystitis) and upper tract infections that also involve the kidneys and collecting system (pyelonephritis). In practice, the precise determination of upper tract involvement in a UTI is difficult but is not always necessary for successful treatment.

EPIDEMIOLOGY AND PATHOGENESIS

UTIs are much more prevalent among women than among men, presumably because women have a shorter urethra. Among hospitalized patients, the presence of an indwelling urinary catheter is a major risk for the development of a UTI.

The majority (>90%) of UTIs are caused by **aerobic gram-negative bacteria**. Approximately 80% of community-acquired and 50% of nosocomial UTIs are caused by *Escherichia coli*, with most of the remainder caused by gram-negative bacteria such as *Enterobacter*, *Klebsiella*, *Proteus*, and *Pseudomonas*. Gram-positive bacteria only cause an estimated 10% of UTIs, most notably *Staphylococcus saprophyticus* among sexually active women and enterococci among men and women with indwelling urinary catheters. Another etiologic agent in patients with an indwelling urinary catheter is yeast (most often *Candida* species).

Some of the organisms that commonly cause UTIs have particular **virulence factors** that allow them to colonize the urinary tract successfully:

- Pili/fimbriae (hairlike bacterial appendages that allow adherence to urinary tract epithelial cells)
- Hemolysin (often with strains that produce pyelonephritis)
- Aerobactin (an iron-scavenging molecule)
- Urease

RISK FACTORS

As mentioned earlier, most community-acquired UTIs occur among women. **Risk factors** that increase the incidence of UTIs **among women** are:

- History of recent UTI
- Sexual activity
- Use of diaphragm and/or spermicide
- Failure to void after intercourse

Among men, the presence of an anatomically abnormal urinary tract (e.g., benign prostatic hypertrophy) is the major factor that predisposes to UTIs.

Among hospitalized patients, the presence of a urinary catheter is a significant risk for the development of a UTI.

CLINICAL MANIFESTATIONS

HISTORY

Lower tract infection (cystitis) usually presents with **symptoms of bladder irritation**:

- Frequency
- Urgency
- Dysuria

Gross hematuria may sometimes be present but is not a common feature.

Upper tract infections (pyelonephritis) may present with **symptoms of bladder irritation**, but features that tend to distinguish them from lower tract infections are:

- Fever
- Flank pain
- Abdominal symptoms of pain, nausea, and vomiting

Note that there can be much overlap in symptoms between upper and lower tract disease.

PHYSICAL EXAMINATION

In a patient presenting with classic symptoms of a UTI, the physical examination often does not add much information. Other than the finding of a fever and flank tenderness that raises suspicion of upper tract disease, diagnosis is usually suggested by the history. In women, possible concurrent pelvic inflammatory disease needs to be considered and a pelvic examination performed with collection of appropriate diagnostic specimens (see Chapter 29) if there is evidence of urethritis or vaginitis.

DIFFERENTIAL DIAGNOSIS

A number of **other conditions** may produce signs and symptoms that can mimic a bacterial UTI, including:

- Vulvovaginitis
- Gonococcal and nongonococcal urethritis
- Bladder calculi
- Bladder tumor
- Chemical- or drug-induced cystitis
- Prostatitis

A pelvic examination in women (with vaginal or cervical cultures as noted earlier) and a prostate examination in older men may help distinguish a UTI from other conditions that can produce symptoms suggestive of a UTI.

DIAGNOSTIC EVALUATION

Urinalysis and **urine culture** are the most important laboratory tests used in diagnosis and as a guide to treatment. Examination of a cover-slipped slide of unspun urine can reveal leukocytes and organisms (Fig. 30-1) and the presence of white blood cell (WBC) casts is suggestive of pyelonephritis.

In practice, it is often not feasible or practical to examine all urine samples under a microscope. However,

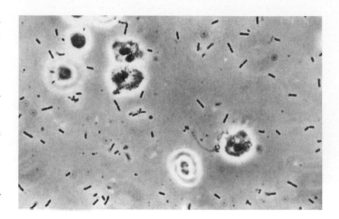

Figure 30-1 • Leukocytes and bacteria in urine in bacterial cystitis.

the presence of both WBC and nitrites on a urine dipstick correlates with the presence of a UTI in approximately 90% of cases.

Except in uncomplicated cases of lower UTI (where the causative agents and their antibiotic susceptibility is predictable), urine culture with susceptibility testing can be important to determine if empirical antibiotic therapy is appropriate for the isolated organism. Patients for whom culture is indicated include:

- Patient with possible upper tract disease
- Patients with known or suspected anatomic abnormalities of the urinary tract
- Patients with recent antibiotic treatment (within 4 weeks) for UTI and recurrent symptoms
- Patients with persistent symptoms following empirical treatment
- Patients with atypical symptoms

TREATMENT

WOMEN

In most cases of community-acquired UTIs, including those with upper tract involvement, treatment as an outpatient with oral antibiotics is adequate. Factors that could lead toward inpatient (i.e., IV antibiotic) treatment include severe nausea and vomiting (which could interfere with oral administration of antibiotics) and signs of sepsis (including high fever and signs of hemodynamic compromise).

In the setting of catheter-related UTI, removal of the urinary catheter, if possible, is the most important consideration. If removal is not possible, directed antibiotic therapy for an isolated organism may be effective, but reinfection with different organisms is common.

Uncomplicated cystitis can be treated with an empirical **3-day course of antibiotics**. This length of treatment can give cure rates equivalent to more traditional 7-day courses and is more effective than one-dose therapy. If upper tract disease is suspected, the length of therapy should be extended to 7 to 14 days, reflecting the increased difficulty in clearing upper tract infections.

Standard oral drugs to treat UTIs include:

- Trimethoprim-sulfamethoxazole
- Quinolones
- Beta-lactams such as ampicillin and amoxicillin

All of these drugs have good activity against most gram-negative bacteria, although increased resistance to beta-lactams among community isolates has led to recommending that these agents not be used as first-line therapy. However, beta-lactams remain important for pregnant patients where other drugs carry the risk of fetal injury. Initial empirical therapy with trimethoprim-sulfamethoxazole is usually recommended, although recent increases in resistance to this therapy have also been noted.

Along with antibiotics, symptomatic relief can be given with a short course of the bladder analgesic phenazopyridine.

The standard 3-day regimen of oral antibiotics is usually effective in most cases of UTI. The most common **causes of treatment failure** are lack of patient compliance and infection with a resistant microorganism. It is important to obtain culture and sensitivity results for patients who fail to respond to empirical therapy so the therapy can be altered based on microbial resistance.

Other complications of UTIs that must be watched for are the development of perinephric abscesses, formation of renal calculi (particularly with recurrent infections with *Proteus*), and the development of sepsis by bloodstream seeding.

For women who have problems with **recurrent UTIs**, a number of **preventive measures** can be tried, including:

- Voiding after intercourse
- Alternative contraception other than diaphragm
- High fluid intake early after symptoms occur
- Prophylactic antimicrobials (often trimethoprim-sulfamethoxazole, nitrofurantoin, or cephalexin) at bedtime or after sexual intercourse if other methods fail.

The latter treatment is usually used for limited time periods (3 to 6 months) before discontinuing and observing but may need to be extended if frequent UTIs recur after prophylaxis is stopped. If there is suspicion of anatomic abnormalities of the urinary tract (e.g., isolation of *Proteus* species or clinical evidence of nephrolithiasis), examination with renal US or CT should be considered.

MEN

The treatment of UTIs in men is less well studied and defined. Because the major risk factor for the development of a UTI in a male patient is the presence of urinary tract abnormalities, evaluation and treatment by a urologist is often indicated. Antibiotic treatment is similar to women except that extended (e.g., 10 to 14 days) treatment is generally prescribed as the urologic workup is initiated.

KEY POINTS

- UTIs most often present with symptoms of bladder irritation: frequency, urgency, and dysuria.
- Most community-acquired UTIs are caused by gram-negative bacteria.
- Urinalysis (dipstick and/or microscopic) and culture are the most important laboratory tests.
- Empirical 3-day courses of antibiotics for lower tract disease and 7- to 14-day courses for upper tract infections are usually sufficient.
- Treatment failure may suggest antimicrobial resistance, and recurrent UTIs may be an indication to check for anatomic abnormalities of the urinary tract.
- Prophylactic use of antimicrobials may be needed to prevent recurrent UTIs.

Tuberculosis

Tuberculosis (TB) is the chronic infection with the organism *Mycobacterium tuberculosis*. The characteristic pathology of *M. tuberculosis* infection is the formation of granulomas via cell-mediated immunity. Although TB can affect virtually any organ system, pulmonary tuberculosis remains the most important manifestation, especially from the public health point of view, and is the focus of the discussion here.

PATHOGENESIS

M. tuberculosis is usually spread via inhalation of droplets, setting up the initial site of infection in the lungs and then spreading via lymphatics to regional (i.e., mediastinal) lymph nodes. Approximately 90% to 95% of immunocompetent individuals control the initial infection via a cellular immune response involving *M. tuberculosis* ingestion by macrophages, both in the lung and the lymph node. Granuloma formation results, with eventual control of the infection. This effective cellular response takes approximately 3 to 9 weeks to develop, at which time the tuberculin skin test becomes positive.

In a minority of patients, the early immune response is so robust that severe necrosis occurs, leading to cavity formation or local extension of disease. In still others, dissemination occurs very early in the course, with systemic spread to **extrapulmonary sites** including the pericardium, extrapulmonary lymph nodes (scrofula), kidneys, epiphyses of long bones, vertebral bodies, and meninges.

In most cases, the initial infection is walled off by granuloma formation, but viable organisms may persist within the granuloma. With waning cellular immunity (e.g., with age, advancing HIV, malignancy, or corticosteroid administration), these organisms may escape from the granuloma, resulting in **reactivation tuberculosis**.

EPIDEMIOLOGY

After falling since the middle part of the 20th century, the incidence of TB in the United States has been rising since 1985. A number of factors (see Risk Factors) have led to this increase; major among these are the HIV epidemic and the appearance of multidrug-resistant *M. tuberculosis*.

M. tuberculosis is most commonly spread from person to person by the **respiratory route** via droplets formed by coughing. Most people with TB shed relatively few bacteria, with the exception of those with endobronchial or cavitary disease. Therefore, transmission usually requires several months of close (e.g., household) contact.

RISK FACTORS

In the United States, important **risk factors** for the development of active TB include:

- Older age (often thought to be reactivation TB)
- Lower socioeconomic status (via crowding, homelessness, poor nutrition, etc.)
- Recent (<5 years) immigrant from area of high prevalence (e.g., Eastern Europe, Latin America, Asia, and Africa)
- HIV seropositivity

CLINICAL FINDINGS

HISTORY

Early pulmonary TB is usually asymptomatic, often discovered by chance on routine chest radiograph. When **symptoms** do develop later in the disease, they are usually **nonspecific** and **constitutional**:

- Fevers, chills, night sweats
- Anorexia
- Weight loss
- Fatigue
- Cough

Development of **hemoptysis** denotes advanced disease.

Because the symptoms just listed are nonspecific, clinical suspicion for TB must be raised in patients with the appropriate risk factors who present with these features.

PHYSICAL EXAMINATION

Physical examination findings depend on the nature of disease present and in general may underestimate its severity. Pulmonary findings of **dullness with decreased fremitus** may be present with pleural effusions or pleural thickening. Signs of consolidation may be present. A cavity may produce distant hollow breath sounds that suggest the sound of blowing across the mouth of a jar (**amphora**).

Extrapulmonary TB is manifest by signs of the particular organ system involved, for example, spine pain and tenderness with skeletal TB and cervical adenopathy (scrofula) in tuberculous adenitis.

DIFFERENTIAL DIAGNOSIS

A number of different diseases may present with the clinical findings found in TB, including:

- Fungal diseases (histoplasmosis, coccidioidomycosis)
- Sarcoidosis
- Malignancy

DIAGNOSTIC EVALUATION

The **chest radiograph** is important in determining the presence and extent of pulmonary disease in TB.

Important radiographic patterns that can be seen in pulmonary TB include:

- Primary parenchymal lesion and mediastinal node (Ghon complex) (Fig. 31-1A)
- Apical pleural scarring (Fig. 31-1B)
- Cavitary disease (Fig. 31-1C)
- Lobar consolidation (Fig. 31-1C)
- Diffuse (miliary) disease (Fig. 31-1D)

Note that in early disease the chest radiograph may be completely normal.

Evaluation of sputum, when present, may be useful. *M. tuberculosis* stains positive in an acid-fast stain (see Color Plate 12). Acid-fast positivity requires a heavy organism burden in the patient, and early disease may be missed. Culture is more sensitive but time consuming because of the slow growth of *M. tuberculosis*.

Skin testing is important for the diagnosis of TB. The administration of the intermediate (5-TU) skin test is useful in documenting exposure and infection with *M. tuberculosis*. Population studies have determined **levels of skin test reactivity** that help identify infected individuals with sufficient sensitivity and specificity:

- **>15 mm** in a normal host from a low-risk group (i.e., no risk factors—it should be noted that it is recommended that persons with no risk factors NOT be routinely tested for TB by skin testing)
- **>10 mm** in a moderate-risk individual (non-HIV–associated risk factors, e.g., recent immigrant from high prevalence area, injection drug users that are HIV-negative or HIV-known status, residents of high-risk group housing settings, patients with underlying conditions that increase risk for active disease such as chronic kidney disease, silicosis, certain malignances)
- **>5 mm** in an HIV-infected individual or individual with high likelihood of infection (e.g., a person with recent close contact with a person with documented TB or a person with known findings on chest radiograph suggestive of old TB) or patients with organ transplants or who are receiving the equivalent of >15 mg prednisone/day for one month or more.

A newer test for the diagnosis of tuberculosis is the whole-blood interferon-gamma assay that detects the presence of T cells that have been previously been sensitized to *M. tuberculosis* antigens and thus will release interferon-gamma upon re-exposure to the antigens. The test appears to have sensitivity and specificity

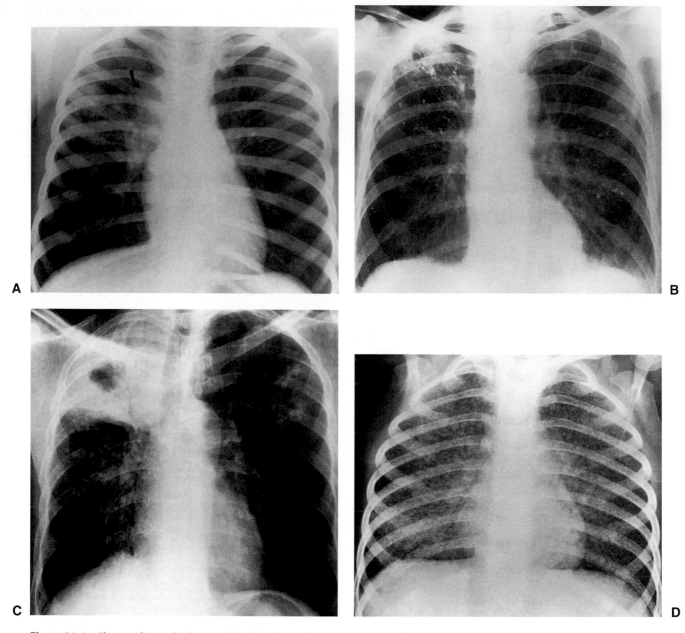

Figure 31-1 • Chest radiograph abnormalities in tuberculosis. **(A)** Primary (Ghon) complex in a 7-year-old child shows an ill-defined consolidation in the right upper lung field together with enlargement of the draining lymph nodes (*arrow*). **(B)** Thickening of the pleura in the right upper lobe. There are multiple calcified nodules in both lung fields. Active disease cannot be excluded in a patient with this radiographic appearance. **(C)** Right upper lobe consolidation and cavitation caused by active tuberculosis. **(D)** Multiple nodular densities throughout the lungs of a child with miliary tuberculosis.

equivalent to the skin test for most indications, and may have greater ability to distinguish between *M. tuberculosis* and nontuberculous *Mycobacteria* infections.

Other laboratory findings (anemia, LFT abnormalities) may be found in TB, particularly with extrapulmonary disease, but are not specific.

TREATMENT

Management of TB is closely tied to the diagnosis of the disease. It is crucial to determine if the patient has **active disease** (i.e., with symptoms and positive physical findings and/or chest radiograph).

Immunologically normal patients with only a newly reactive skin test have approximately a 3% chance of going on to symptomatic disease within the first year after conversion. Patients with a positive skin test but no evidence of active disease are defined as having **latent tuberculosis infection** (LTBI) are treated with **chemoprophylaxis**. Previously, distinction for treatment was made of "recent" TB skin test converters, but current recommendations are to treat all patients with a positive tuberculin skin test. This principle of "a decision to test is a decision to treat" is meant to discourage the routine skin testing of patients who are low risk (see above).

Patients with active disease require more intensive therapy than patients with LTBI. Therefore active TB is treated with various combinations of the so-called **first-line TB drugs**:

- Isoniazid (INH)
- Rifampin
- Pyrazinamide
- Ethambutol
- Streptomycin

The standard treatment regimens for tuberculosis have been evolving with the spread of drug-resistant strains. One commonly used standard treatment regimen currently consists of 2 months of INH, rifampin, pyrazinamide, and ethambutol for an initial induction phase. If testing of the patient's isolate confirms susceptibility to INH, rifampin, and pyrazinamide, induction is followed by INH and rifampin daily for an additional 4 months. Previously, the standard therapy was to give only INH, rifampin, and pyrazinamide for the induction phase, but recent increases in resistance have put the vast majority (approaching 90%) of the U.S. population at risk of exposure to drug-resistant organisms.

Chemoprophylaxis of recent skin test converters is usually administered by giving daily INH for 9 months although alternative regimens exist such as using twice weekly directly observed therapy (DOT).

Compliance with therapy is the major determinant of successful treatment of active TB. Extended periods of therapy are needed to eliminate all of the viable slow-growing bacteria. These long periods of therapy, especially among populations of patients with poor medical follow-up (homeless, poor), are difficult to adhere to. Early stoppage of therapy, es-

pecially as symptoms resolve, is common. It is recommended that smears and cultures be reassessed after 3 months of therapy to monitor for possible nonadherence or infection with drug-resistant bacilli. DOT plays a crucial role in ensuring compliance among patients at risk.

Management of TB in an HIV-positive patient is more complex because of the multiple possible interactions between TB medications and antiretroviral therapies. Consultation with an infectious disease specialist should be considered. Because of the high rate of coinfection with TB and HIV, the Infectious Diseases Society of America has recommended that all patients with active TB be tested for HIV infection within 2 months of diagnosis.

Resistance to one or more anti-TB drugs is becoming more of a problem, especially among the highest risk patients. Resistance is thought to arise by incomplete courses of treatment with insufficient numbers of drugs. The treatment of patients with multidrug-resistant TB (**MDR-TB**, defined as resistance to at least isoniazid and rifampin) and extensively drug-resistant tuberculosis (**XDR-TB**, defined as resistance to at least isoniazid, rifampin, fluoroquinolones, and either aminoglycosides or capreomycin) is very difficult and would represent a significant public health problem if these organisms increase in prevalence.

The drugs themselves have toxic **side effects** that may also limit compliance. With INH, rifampin, and pyrazinamide, this toxicity is mainly hepatic, requiring monitoring of liver function during therapy.

KEY POINTS

- TB has an increased incidence among poor, homeless, immigrant, and HIV-infected populations.
- Spread of TB occurs most commonly via the respiratory route.
- Early infection is often asymptomatic and in most patients is fully controlled.
- Long courses of multidrug therapy are required for treatment of symptomatic disease.
- The therapy of TB has been complicated by the recent emergence of strains with resistance to commonly used drugs.

32 Gastroenteritis

Gastroenteritis refers to inflammation of the stomach and intestinal tract, usually secondary to an infectious agent. Gastroenteritis most commonly presents with **diarrhea** as the primary symptom (see Chapter 38) but also with **nausea**, **vomiting**, and **abdominal pain**. Gastroenteritis is a common health problem in the general population, with approximately 200 million cases in the United States each year. Gastroenteritis is also frequently encountered in the international traveler.

EPIDEMIOLOGY

Acute gastroenteritis can follow the ingestion of pathogenic microorganisms or toxins produced by these agents. **Ingestion of contaminated food or drink** is most common, but swimming or bathing in contaminated water can also result in exposure, particularly among travelers.

Travel to areas of the world where safe food handling practices are not commonly observed is often associated with development of gastroenteritis, but **lapses in food handling** also occur in the home and in restaurants under a number of circumstances:

- Undercooking of foods, in particular ground meats
- Failure to refrigerate foods properly (both prior to preparation and during storage of prepared foods)
- Incorporation or cross contamination of raw ingredients (e.g., eggs) into foods that are not cooked further
- Failure to clean contaminated kitchen equipment properly (e.g., mixing bowls, cutting boards)
- Contamination of food by food handlers who practice poor personal hygiene

Outbreaks of gastroenteritis have occurred from environmental sources (e.g., contaminated lakes) or other point sources (e.g., a single restaurant or food packaging plant).

ETIOLOGY AND PATHOPHYSIOLOGY

Bacteria, viruses, and **protozoans** can cause acute gastroenteritis. The most commonly encountered **viral** pathogens are **norovirus** (a calicivirus), **rotavirus**, **astrovirus** and the **enteric adenovirus**. Rotavirus is an important pediatric cause of gastroenteritis; norovirus is of particular importance in the adult population, responsible for the vast majority of nonbacterial outbreaks of gastroenteritis. Norovirus outbreaks have occurred in restaurants, hospitals, nursing homes, and schools. These enteric viruses directly infect cells of the small intestine, resulting in alteration of the mucosal architecture (notably shortening or loss of the microvilli), causing diarrhea on the basis of malabsorption. The infection is readily controlled, causing a short-lived (24- to 48-hour) illness.

Protozoan infections are most commonly found in travelers and people who may be exposed to untreated water (e.g., hikers). *Entamoeba histolytica* and *Giardia lamblia* are two of the most commonly encountered protozoan pathogens. The former invades the colon, causing a bloody diarrhea, whereas *Giardia* colonizes the small intestine, causing a malabsorptive syndrome and an osmotic diarrhea.

The major bacterial pathogens identified in the United States by the FoodNet surveillance system (http://www.cdc.gov/foodnet) are *Salmonella* species and *Campylobacter jejuni* and *Shigella* species. Among travelers who develop diarrhea, enterotoxigenic *E. coli* is the most common bacterial pathogen identified. Bacterial pathogens can cause gastroenteritis via several distinct **mechanisms**:

- Direct invasion of the mucosa with tissue destruction and inflammation
- Growth of the bacteria within the bowel lumen with toxin production and release
- Adherence (but not invasion) of the bacteria to the mucosal surface with interference of the normal absorptive process without tissue destruction
- Production of a toxin during bacterial growth in food or water, which is then ingested preformed

CLINICAL MANIFESTATIONS

HISTORY

In taking the history, it is useful to obtain **epidemiologic information** that can help determine an etiology. **Food history** should cover at least the 48 hours prior to the onset of symptoms. Any changes from the usual dietary habits, such as eating at restaurants or picnics, should be elicited. **Travel history** should pertain not only to travel to other countries, but also to a history of camping, swimming, or other recreational activity where there can be exposure to untreated water. **History of a similar illness in others**, in particular family members or others who may have shared a particular exposure, should be taken. A complete **history of antibiotic exposure** must be taken because, although *Clostridium difficile*–associated diarrhea is most commonly encountered in the hospital setting, many people take courses of antibiotics as outpatients and may not associate the onset of diarrhea with these drugs. A history of **known infection with human immunodeficiency virus** (HIV) or **HIV risk factors** should be determined because diarrhea is a common symptom in HIV-infected individuals. Some of the etiologic agents seen in these patients are unique and require specific methods of diagnosis and treatment (see Chapter 36).

Once a possible exposure is elicited, the **incubation period** prior to the onset of symptoms can provide a clue to the nature of the etiologic agent. Ingestion of preformed toxin (e.g., *Staphylococcus aureus* food poisoning) is followed by onset of symptoms within 8 hours. Infection with a pathogenic bacterium that needs to replicate to cause disease (e.g., *Campylobacter* or *Salmonella*) does not generally result in symptoms until 24 to 48 hours after exposure. Parasitic infections (e.g., *Giardia*) may not become symptomatic for days to weeks after exposure.

Despite a history of possible exposures to infectious agents of gastroenteritis, note that in many cases, no specific etiology is found. This is particularly true for sporadic cases.

PHYSICAL EXAMINATION

The physical examination generally does little in helping determine a specific etiologic agent. Fever and **abdominal pain** are more suggestive of an invasive pathogen, particularly if **gross or occult blood** is found in stool.

The severity of the illness can be indicated by signs of dehydration such as **orthostatic hypotension, dry mucosal membranes**, and **decreased skin turgor**.

DIFFERENTIAL DIAGNOSIS

Chapter 38 discusses the differential diagnosis of diarrhea.

DIAGNOSTIC EVALUATION

In most cases of acute gastroenteritis, **hydration and watchful waiting** are all that is necessary. However, certain patient variables can trigger a more extensive workup:

- High fever
- Evidence of dehydration
- Prolonged (>48 hours) or profuse (≥6 unformed stools per day) diarrhea
- Severe abdominal pain
- Systemic toxicity
- Bloody stool
- Immunocompromise
- Overseas or outdoor (e.g., hiking) travel
- Male homosexuality
- Recent antibiotic use

The presence of **stool leukocytes** generally suggests a bacterial pathogen. Gram stain can reveal the "gull-winged" shape characteristic of *Campylobacter*. Culture is the gold standard for identifying pathogenic bacteria. However, it is expensive and usually reserved for cases of severe disease in patients with an underlying illness that either increases the likelihood of complications or the presence of unusual pathogens (e.g., HIV-infected individuals). Additionally, certain infections require administration of antimicrobials for clearance (see later and Table 32-1), making attempted isolation of the etiologic agent important if these illnesses are suspected. Note that certain organisms (*Campylobacter jejuni*, *Yersinia*, *Escherichia coli* O157:H7) can require special media and isolation techniques to improve yield; the clinician should be aware of what specific testing needs to be requested of the microbiology laboratory and which tests are "standard" in the workup of stool samples.

If a protozoan etiology is suspected, examination of the stool for **ova and parasites** is indicated. Generally, fresh stool samples have the highest yield, but in some cases this is inconvenient and special containers with stool preservatives can be used. Generally, several samples from consecutive days are needed to increase yield.

In a patient with recent antibiotic use and diarrhea, an assay for the presence of C. *difficile* toxin can be diagnostic.

TREATMENT

The **primary therapy in gastroenteritis is supportive**, with replacement of fluid and electrolytes lost via vomiting and diarrhea. In the majority of cases, the condition resolves on its own with symptomatic therapy. For most patients, as noted earlier, culture and specific antimicrobial treatment is generally reserved until symptomatic therapy fails or if unusual pathogens are suspected.

In most cases of acute gastroenteritis, fluid and electrolyte management can be accomplished with **oral replacement**. For otherwise healthy patients with mild to moderate diarrhea, oral fluids high in sugar content to facilitate passive absorption (water, fruit juices, soda, etc.) are generally sufficient, along with solid food as tolerated. For more severe cases of diarrhea, especially if there are symptoms of dehydration, and for patients with co-morbid conditions **oral rehydration solutions** may be necessary. Premixed pediatric solutions can be used as well as packaged commercial rehydration packets. If there is marked dehydration, particularly in patients with

underlying conditions, or if there are conditions such as intractable vomiting that make oral replacement difficult, administration of **IV fluids** may become necessary.

Antimotility agents such as **loperamide-** and **atropine**-containing compounds (Lomotil) can be used symptomatically, particularly in cases where diarrhea can interfere with the functioning of an otherwise healthy individual. Care must be taken, however, when administering these agents. In cases of invasive organisms (e.g., *Salmonella*) or organisms that produce toxins (e.g., C. *difficile* or enterohemorrhagic E. *coli*), antimotility agents can be harmful.

Bulk agents such as **Kaopectate** can give more form to stools but do not decrease the fluid content and thus do not prevent fluid and electrolyte loss. **Bismuth subsalicylate** (Pepto-Bismol) can decrease the volume of stool in certain cases of bacterial gastroenteritis. In addition, it possesses antibacterial activity.

The use of antibiotics in patients with suspected or documented bacterial gastroenteritis remains controversial. In most cases, these illnesses resolve with conservative treatment. Studies have demonstrated that for certain organisms, administration of antibiotics (generally quinolones or TMP-SMZ) can shorten the length of the diarrheal illness. Concerns about routine antibiotic use include the widespread appearance of antibiotic resistance, adverse drug reactions, and the appearance of C. *difficile*. In patients with *Salmonella* infection, the use of antibiotics can actually prolong the carrier state in some individuals whose only manifestation is gastroenteritis. For this reason, many experts recommend treatment of documented *Salmonella* infections only when there are signs of systemic illness (severe dehydration, fever). Evidence shows that treatment of E. *coli* O157:H7 infection with certain antibiotics may *increase* the incidence of subsequent thrombotic thrombocytopenic purpura and/or hemolytic uremic syndrome. The use of nonabsorbable antibiotics (e.g., rifaximin) has been evaluated for treatment (and prevention) of traveler's diarrhea. This needs further study before standard use of these agents (particularly for prophylaxis) can be widely recommended.

Nonantimicrobial methods for prevention of gastroenteritis are important in effective management. This includes adherence to proper guidelines for the safe handling of food and water at home and while traveling. Travelers should be advised to

■ TABLE 32-1 Causes of Gastroenteritis

Agent	Pathogenesis	Clinical/Epidemiologic Features	Therapy
Bacillus cereus	Preformed toxin	Generally causes vomiting; may also produce diarrhea; classic association with fried rice	None
Staphylococcus aureus	Preformed toxin	Vomiting with some diarrhea; found in high-protein foods (meats, cream-filled cakes), also in those with high sugar contents (custards)	None
Clostridium difficile	Toxin production in colon	Fever, abdominal pain, diarrhea, toxic megacolon; association with previous antibiotic use	Metronidazole, vancomycin
Escherichia coli			
Enterotoxigenic	Enterotoxin formation in small intestine	Voluminous watery diarrhea; fever generally absent; fecal/oral transmission	None
Enteropathogenic	Localized adherence to intestinal mucosa	Watery diarrhea; can occur in outbreaks among newborns	Antibiotics
Enteroinvasive	Invasion of the colonic mucosa	Fever, bloody diarrhea; fecal/oral transmission	Antibiotics
Enteroadherent	Adherence to small intestinal mucosa	Diarrhea, can be prolonged; fecal/oral transmission	Antibiotics
Enterohemorrhagic (e.g., *E. coli* O157:H7)	Production of a cytotoxin (Shiga toxin) in colon	Causes hemorrhagic colitis; colitis can be followed by TTP/HUS; from contaminated meats (especially ground meat)	Diarrhea: none; treatment of TTP/HUS is generally supportive (treatment of diarrhea may *increase* the risk of TTP/HUS; see text)
Campylobacter jejuni	Colonization (invasion) of large and small bowel	Fever, watery or bloody diarrhea with fecal leukocytes, abdominal pain	Antibiotics
Salmonella typhi	Invasion of small intestine; can then disseminate systemically (via bloodstream)	Protracted illness with fever, headache, malaise, splenomegaly; constipation is more common than diarrhea; fecal/oral transmission	Antibiotics
Salmonella (nontyphi)	Invasion of small and large intestine	Fever, diarrhea with fecal leukocytes; animal reservoirs, also in eggs	Antibiotics (see note in text)
Shigella spp.	Invasion of colon	Fever, bloody diarrhea with fecal leukocytes; fecal/oral spread	Antibiotics
Vibrio cholerae	Enterotoxin	Profuse watery diarrhea; fever is rare; fecal/oral spread (often via water contamination)	Doxycycline
Entamoeba histolytica	Invasion of colonic mucosa	Diarrhea, often bloody; fecal/oral spread	Metronidazole
Giardia lamblia	Colonization of small intestine	Diarrhea, secondary to malabsorption; abdominal pain; waterborne ("beaver fever")	Metronidazole
Viruses (e.g., norovirus, rotavirus)	Invasion of mucosa	Can occur in outbreaks, generally watery diarrhea	None

TTP/HUS, thrombocytopenic thrombotic purpura/hemolytic uremic syndrome. See text for description of antibiotics used for treatment of gastroenteritis.

avoid undercooked foods and any foods prepared with unpasteurized milk. Fresh fruits should be peeled by the consumer just prior to consumption.

Ensuring safe drinking water is important. In hotels in large cities the water may be safe, but if there is any uncertainty, the water should be boiled (for at least 10 minutes) prior to drinking. Bottled beverages (carbonated beverages, beer, wine, and water) are generally safe, but particularly in the case of bottled water, travelers should ask to remove the top themselves to ensure that an empty bottle has not been simply filled with tap water.

KEY POINTS

- Many cases of acute diarrhea are caused by infectious agents ranging from bacteria to viruses and parasites

- Microbes can cause diarrhea by damaging the mucosa directly, by producing enterotoxin during growth in the bowel lumen, or by producing a toxin that is then ingested in the form of contaminated food.

- The primary therapy for most cases of gastroenteritis in normal hosts is supportive, with fluid and electrolyte replacement.

- Antibiotics are indicated for certain parasitic infections but are generally not routinely administered for bacterial pathogens unless there are signs of severe infection.

Infective Endocarditis

Infective endocarditis (IE) is the invasion of the endothelial lining of the heart (predominantly the valvular structures) by microorganisms. Originally known as bacterial endocarditis, it can also be caused by fungi, rickettsia, and chlamydia. Prior to the introduction of antibiotics, it was generally a uniformly fatal disease. The introduction of antibiotics and, later, the development of cardiac surgery have decreased overall mortality, but IE is still associated with an estimated 25% mortality.

EPIDEMIOLOGY AND CASE DEFINITION

In the United States, there are approximately 10,000 to 15,000 new cases of IE each year, making it the most common form of endovascular infection. With the decrease in incidence of acute rheumatic carditis, IE has become more frequent in older patients, with a majority of patients older than 50 years. IE has a higher incidence among men than among women.

IE can be **divided into three major groups** based on host characteristics:

- Native valve endocarditis (NVE)
- Prosthetic valve endocarditis (PVE); further subdivided into **early** (i.e., in the first month after valve surgery) and **late** (occurring thereafter)
- Endocarditis in IV drug users

The etiologic organisms, management, and outcome of patients vary in each of these subdivisions.

Traditionally, the gold standard for the diagnosis of endocarditis was pathologic. The **Duke criteria** are useful for the *clinical diagnosis* of IE.

The **major Duke criteria** are:

- Persistently positive blood cultures with microorganisms consistent with IE (more than two positive cultures separated by at least 12 hours or more than three cultures at least 1 hour apart or 70% of blood cultures positive if four or more are drawn)
- A single positive blood culture for *Coxiella burnetii* or IgG antibody titer >1:800
- Echocardiographic evidence of endocardial involvement (see later)

The **minor Duke criteria** are:

- Predisposing heart condition (see later)
- Fever
- Vascular phenomena (arterial emboli, septic pulmonary emboli, mycotic aneurysm, Janeway lesions)
- Immunologic phenomena (glomerulonephritis, Osler nodes, Roth spots, rheumatoid factor)
- Positive blood cultures (not meeting major criteria)

Definitive diagnosis of IE requires two major criteria *or* one major plus three minor criteria *or* five minor criteria. Patients with one major criteria and one minor criteria *or* three minor criteria are classified as **possible IE**. Patients with possible IE may require additional testing (see later).

ETIOLOGY

IE can be caused by a wide variety of microorganisms, but the majority (80%) of cases are due to streptococci and staphylococci.

Most cases of NVE are caused by *Streptococcus viridans* (50%) and *Staphylococcus aureus*, whereas most cases of IE in IV drug users are caused by *S. aureus*. Early PVE is thought to be caused by intraoperative contamination with nosocomial pathogens, in particular coagulase-negative *Staphylococcus*. Late PVE is believed to be community acquired and resembles NVE in microbiology.

RISK FACTORS AND PATHOGENESIS

The major risk factor for the development of IE is the presence of a **structurally abnormal heart**. Generally, this is valvular disease, but any **structural abnormality** (including iatrogenic) that leads to **turbulent blood flow within the heart increases the risk of IE**, including:

- Mitral valve prolapse
- Rheumatic heart disease (aortic and mitral valve)
- Degenerative heart disease (calcifications)
- Congenital heart disease (bicuspid aortic valve, patent ductus arteriosus, ventricular septal defect, coarctation of the aorta, tetralogy of Fallot)
- Hypertrophic cardiomyopathy
- Foreign material (pacemakers, prosthetic valves, pulmonary artery catheters)
- Previous history of endocarditis

Diabetes mellitus and IV drug abuse are also important risk factors for the development of IE. The pathogenesis of IE is a complex interaction among damaged vascular endothelium, local hemodynamic abnormalities (both a result of structural cardiac abnormalities), circulating bacteria, and the host immune system. Damage to the vascular endothelium can lead to the deposition of fibrin and platelets, which form a sterile endocardial mass. This mass can subsequently be colonized by bacteria when organisms gain access to the bloodstream via a loss of skin or mucosal integrity. **Bacteremia** can occur following the manipulation of the **oropharyngeal** (dental work, tonsillectomy), **GI** (upper and lower endoscopy), and **GU tracts** (transurethral resection of the prostate, cystoscopy, urethral catheterization). Of these, dental work is most commonly associated with the highest incidence of bacteremia. Additionally, the presence of intravenous catheters, particularly long-term catheters such as ports increase the risk of bacteremia and thus IE. Transient bacteremia can also occur with daily activities such as tooth brushing, bowel movements, and eating. In fact, it is felt that most cases of IE result secondary to bacteremia occurring in the setting of daily activities rather than iatrogenic causes. This realization has recently resulted in a major revision in the recommendations for IE prophylaxis in the setting of dental and medical procedures (see below).

CLINICAL MANIFESTATIONS

HISTORY

Patients with IE may present with either an **acute** or **subacute** course. The majority of patients present with **systemic**, **constitutional symptoms**:

- Fevers, chills, night sweats
- Fatigue, malaise
- Anorexia
- Weight loss

These constitutional complaints are generally more pronounced in patients with a subacute course, with the exception of fever, which is prominent in both clinical pictures.

When evaluating a patient with possible IE, it is important to inquire about possible risk factors as listed earlier. In particular, a history of known valvular disease, rheumatic fever, or dental work should be elicited.

PHYSICAL EXAMINATION

Because IE often produces destruction and perforation of valve leaflets, patients generally are found to have regurgitant **murmurs**. A new or changing murmur is particularly suggestive of IE. Other cardiac manifestations include heart block from valve ring abscesses and congestive heart failure (CHF) due to severe regurgitant lesions.

A variety of skin and peripheral manifestations of IE have been described (see immunologic and vascular phenomena in the Duke criteria, earlier). These are caused either by microemboli or macroemboli or a local, immune-mediated vasculitis. Note that none of these lesions are pathognomonic of endocarditis, and they can be seen in other disease states.

DIFFERENTIAL DIAGNOSIS

The differential diagnosis of a patient who fulfills the Duke criteria for IE is limited to IE and other endovascular infections (septic thromboembolism, mycotic aneurysm, infected venous catheter). IE itself is a major consideration in the differential diagnosis of fever of unknown origin.

DIAGNOSTIC EVALUATION

The diagnosis of IE is generally suspected on clinical grounds, with confirmation by isolation of the causative organism by **blood culture** and **echocardiographic evidence of endocarditis** (Fig. 33-1):

- Vegetations (defined as a mass of abnormal echoes attached to the endocardial surface of a valve, which displays motion independent of the cardiac structures and is seen in multiple views)
- Ring abscess (defined as an abnormal echodense or echolucent area within the valvular annulus or perivalvular tissue)
- New partial dehiscence of a prosthetic valve
- Mycotic aneurysms
- Perforation of valve leaflets

The Duke criteria were originally developed using two-dimensional and M-mode transthoracic echocardiography (TTE). Transesophageal echocardiography (TEE) is more sensitive for the detection of vegetations and myocardial abscesses than TTE. Current recommendations are to perform TEE in all patients with suspected prosthetic valve IE, with suspected complicated IE (generally a paravalvular abscess), or in patients classified with "possible IE" by other clinical criteria. In other patients, TTE is still considered to be the appropriate initial diagnostic modality.

Other **laboratory abnormalities seen in IE** include:

- Elevated ESR
- Elevated WBC (more in acute IE)
- Anemia (in subacute IE)
- Hematuria and proteinuria (because of immune-mediated glomerulonephritis)
- Positive rheumatoid factor (usually in subacute IE)

TREATMENT

Empirical antibiotic therapy (following the drawing of initial blood cultures) is the initial step in treatment of suspected endocarditis. One major decision to be made early in the treatment course is the need for cardiac surgery. There are several **indications for early cardiac surgery in IE** (i.e., prior to completion of a course of antibiotics):

- Severe **refractory** CHF because of valvular regurgitation
- Severe aortic or mitral regurgitation with evidence of abnormal hemodynamics (assessed by echocardiography or intravascular hemodynamic monitoring)
- Refractory infection (lack of clearance of blood culture after 1 week of appropriate antibiotics) or infection with highly resistant organisms (e.g., fungi)
- Progressive intracardiac spread of infection (ring abscess, heart block, mycotic aneurysm rupture)
- Prosthetic valve dysfunction (major dehiscence or obstruction from vegetation)

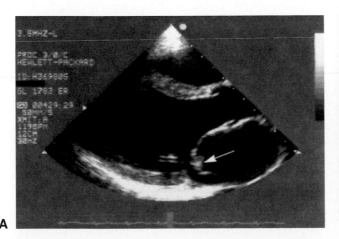 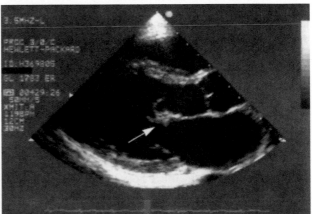

A **B**

Figure 33-1 • Two-dimensional echocardiograms showing parasternal long-axis views of a vegetation (*arrows*) attached to the anterior leaflet of the mitral valve in (**A**) systole and (**B**) diastole.

- Recurrent systemic emboli
- The presence of large (>10 mm), mobile vegetations

The main objective of antibiotic treatment of IE is to sterilize the valvular vegetations. Despite susceptibility of the infective microorganism to antimicrobials, IE is often difficult to cure, requiring long courses of high-dose IV antibiotics. The main reason for this difficulty in cure is the high concentration of organisms that are usually found within vegetations (10^9 to 10^{10} microorganisms per gram). Organisms within the vegetation may have reduced metabolic activity and may produce an exopolysaccharide layer, both of which can reduce susceptibility to antimicrobials.

Because most cases of IE are caused by gram-positive organisms (usually *Staphylococcus* species and *Streptococcus* species), initial empirical treatment is usually with a beta-lactam antibiotic with anti-staphylococcal activity (such as nafcillin), in some cases combined initially with an aminoglycoside. This combination synergistically kills *S. aureus* both in vitro and in experimental in vivo models of endocarditis. Clinically, the major benefit is an enhanced rate of bloodstream sterilization. No benefit in the rate of occurrence of other complications of IE has been shown for *S. aureus* IE, so aminoglycoside therapy is usually only given for the first 5 to 14 days, to avoid aminoglycoside toxicity. If methicillin-resistant *S. aureus* is considered likely (e.g., in patients with a chronic indwelling IV catheter or previous history of methicillin-resistant *Staphylococcus aureus* [MRSA] colonization), vancomycin can be given as initial empirical therapy, although this drug is considered to be less effective than a beta-lactam antibiotic for sensitive organisms. It should be noted that the combination of a beta-lactam and an aminoglycoside is highly effective in the setting of streptococcal and enterococcal IE and combination therapy is usually given for these patients.

In the case of early prosthetic valve endocarditis and endocarditis in patients with associated IV drug use, there is an increase in the incidence of beta-lactam-resistant organisms such as coagulase-negative staphylococci. In patients with these risk factors, vancomycin is often substituted for a beta-lactam pending culture and sensitivity results.

Once an organism is isolated, the results of routine antimicrobial resistance testing should be reviewed to further define the antimicrobial therapy. As far as the duration of antibiotic treatment, IE is generally treated with 4 to 6 weeks of IV antibiotics, depending on the causative organism, sensitivity data, and patient characteristics, such as the presence of a prosthetic valve.

Once initial therapy has been instituted, close monitoring of the patient should be maintained. Microbiologic data such as in vitro susceptibility testing and monitoring of bloodstream sterilization should be obtained. Close monitoring for complications that might require surgery (see earlier) is done with daily physical examination (to look for evidence of congestive heart failure [CHF] and embolic/immunologic phenomena), electrocardiograms (ECGs; monitoring for evidence of progressive heart block), and, if indicated, repeat echocardiograms.

Once therapy for IE has been completed, the patient should be monitored for late complications, generally related to **valvular dysfunction** such as development of CHF, the onset of atrial fibrillation, and so on. It is also important to prevent recurrences of IE (see later).

Prophylaxis of IE is recommended for patients with significant cardiac abnormalities that predispose to the development of IE who are undergoing certain procedures associated with high levels of bacteremia. The recent revision of these prophylaxis guidelines has greatly decreased the number of patients who require prophylaxis, mainly by decreasing the number of underlying conditions for which prophylaxis is recommended. The main conditions are a prosthetic cardiac valve or valve repair with prosthetic material, a history of IE, cardiac transplant patients with valvulopathy, unrepaired **cyanotic** congenital heart disease (CHD) or repaired CHD with residual structural defects. The complete recommendation for IE prophylaxis is published by American Heart Association (http://www.heart.org) and includes indications for prophylaxis along with suggested antibiotic regimens.

KEY POINTS

- Endocarditis is an infection of the endothelial lining of the heart by bacteria, fungi, and other microorganisms.

- The clinical diagnosis of endocarditis can be made by the presence of persistently positive blood cultures and echocardiographic evidence of infection (vegetations, abscesses, valve perforations).

- The major risk factor for the development of endocarditis is the presence of a structurally abnormal heart.

- Gram-positive organisms are the major cause of endocarditis, and empirical therapy is directed against these organisms, with subsequent adjustment based on the results of culture and susceptibility testing.

- Long courses of antimicrobial therapy are required to ensure sterilization of infected endovascular structures.

- Cardiac surgery, including valve replacement, may be required for severe valvular dysfunction.

- Prophylaxis of endocarditis is recommended for patients with abnormal hearts who undergo procedures that lead to bacteremia.

Meningitis classically presents with the triad of fever, headache, and signs of meningeal irritation. There are a number of etiologies. The important distinction is between acute bacterial meningitis (ABM) and meningitis due to other causes. The term **acute aseptic meningitis syndrome** refers to meningitis for which a cause is not apparent after initial examination and routine stains and culture of the CSF. Aseptic meningitis is most often viral (AVM) but can also be caused by noninfectious agents such as drugs. Whereas AVM and other aseptic meningitis syndromes are self-limited and uncomplicated, ABM is associated with a mortality rate of up to 30%, making its early diagnosis important.

EPIDEMIOLOGY

In the United States there are an estimated 20,000 to 25,000 cases of ABM a year. Previously, 70% of the cases of ABM occurred in children younger than 5 years. However, the institution of vaccination against *Haemophilus influenzae* type B decreased the incidence of this pathogen by 94%, and now the majority of cases of ABM occur in adults.

Among adults, bacterial meningitis can be divided into **community acquired** and **nosocomial**. Community-acquired meningitis generally occurs among patients older than 50 years. Nosocomial meningitis is most often, but not invariably, associated with recent neurosurgery, the presence of a neurosurgical device, or altered immune state (e.g., asplenia, immunosuppressive drugs, and immune globulin deficiencies).

Viral meningitis generally has increased prevalence in the summer months, whereas bacterial meningitis tends to have a winter predominance.

ABM caused by *Neisseria meningitidis* is unique in that it can occur in outbreaks, often among young, otherwise healthy adults who are in groups, such as college students and military recruits.

ETIOLOGY

The **etiologic agents of acute bacterial meningitis** vary depending on the age of the patient and whether the condition is community acquired or nosocomial (Table 34-1).

Among adult patients with community-acquired meningitis, well over half of all cases are caused by *Streptococcus pneumoniae*, whereas in nosocomial meningitis gram-negative bacilli are the most common pathogen.

The most common **etiologic agents of aseptic meningitis** are viruses, with non–polio enteroviruses accounting for more than 90% of cases for which an etiology can be identified. Other relatively common causes of aseptic meningitis include:

- Other viruses (mumps, lymphocytic choriomeningitis virus, arboviruses, Epstein-Barr virus [EBV], cytomegalovirus, varicella-zoster virus, herpes viruses, human immunodeficiency virus [HIV])
- *Mycobacterium tuberculosis*
- Fungi (*Candida* species, *Cryptococcus neoformans*)
- Rickettsia (Rocky Mountain spotted fever, *Coxiella burnetii*)
- Spirochetes (syphilis, leptospirosis, Lyme disease)
- Malignancy (metastatic leukemia, lymphoma, metastatic carcinomas)
- Medications (sulfamethoxazole, nonsteroidal anti-inflammatory agents, isoniazid)
- Vaccinations (mumps, measles)

■ **TABLE 34-1** Common Etiologies of Acute Bacterial Meningitis in Adults

Community Acquired	Nosocomial
Streptococcus pneumoniae	Gram-negative bacilli
Neisseria meningitidis	*Staphylococcus aureus*
Listeria monocytogenes	Streptococci Other staphylococci

CLINICAL MANIFESTATIONS

HISTORY

The classic history of acute meningitis is that of **severe headache**, **fever**, **altered mental status**, and symptoms of meningeal irritation such as **neck stiffness**. The severity of symptoms is such that patients generally seek medical care within 24 hours of symptom onset. Although one or more of these signs and symptoms may be absent in a given patient, if none of the three classic symptoms of fever, altered mental status, and neck stiffness is present, the diagnosis of meningitis is virtually ruled out. Other symptoms to inquire about include photophobia, seizures, and rash. An exposure history including travel, animal exposures, and ill contacts should be obtained.

Two elements of the history may help distinguish the likelihood of ABM versus AVM: (a) Patients with bacterial meningitis are more likely to be younger than 5 or older than 50 years, and (b) AVM has a peak incidence in the summer months.

PHYSICAL EXAMINATION

Eliciting signs of meningeal inflammation has been a classic aspect in working up suspected meningitis. **Nuchal rigidity**, or neck stiffness, is one typical finding. Other signs are the so-called **Kernig sign** and **Brudzinski sign**. Although these classic tests were first described over 100 years ago, a recent study showed that they have low sensitivity (~5%) in most patients.

Other elements of the physical examination include examination of the fundi (to look for papilledema indicative of increased intracranial pressure); skin examination for rashes (seen in meningococcal meningitis as well as viral meningitis); and neurologic examination (in particular cranial nerve examination, where deficits can be seen with herniation).

Given the lack of specific physical examination findings for meningitis, suspicion needs to be based on the complete clinical picture and then proceed with the diagnosis via CSF examination when appropriate (see later).

DIFFERENTIAL DIAGNOSIS

As mentioned at the outset, the key distinction is between ABM and other inflammatory processes. A number of other conditions can also present with fever, headache, and meningeal irritation, including:

- Brain abscess
- Cerebral and spinal epidural abscess
- Septic intracranial thrombophlebitis
- Infective endocarditis with cerebral embolization

DIAGNOSTIC EVALUATION

Analysis of **CSF** obtained by LP is the main diagnostic test used in the evaluation of possible meningitis. The fear of triggering brain herniation following LP has prompted some to recommend universal CT for patients prior to LP. However, this can lead to a delay in administration of antibiotic therapy, and therefore, the Infectious Diseases Society of America (IDSA) has published criteria outlining conditions/findings that identify **patients in whom CT should be performed prior to LP**:

- Immunocompromised state (HIV or immunosuppressive therapy)
- History of central nervous system (CNS) disease (mass, stroke, focal infection)
- New onset seizure (within 1 week)
- Papilledema
- Abnormal level of consciousness
- Focal neurologic deficit (dilated nonreactive pupil, abnormal ocular motility, visual field deficits, arm or leg drift)

When an **LP** is performed, the following **routine data** should be obtained:

- Opening pressure (normally between 70 and 180 mm Hg)
- Cell counts (often opening and closing) and white blood cell (WBC) differential
- Glucose and protein determination
- Gram stain and culture for bacterial organisms

Gram stain of CSF permits a rapid, accurate identification of the causative agent in approximately 60% to 90% of patients with bacterial meningitis, with nearly 100% specificity.

If other patient characteristics are present (e.g., HIV disease, immunocompromise, tuberculosis, STDs, CSF leak, or recent sinus surgery or neurosurgery), some or all of the following **additional CSF tests** can be sent:

- Acid-fast stains and mycobacterial culture
- Fungal stain and culture
- Polymerase chain reaction for herpes viruses
- India ink stain with or without cryptococcal antigen testing
- Serology for syphilis (Venereal Disease Research Laboratory [VDRL], rapid plasma reagin [RPR], microhemagglutination assay for *Treponema pallidum* [MHA-TP])
- Viral culture
- Anaerobic culture

Latex agglutination tests have been used extensively in the past, but because of studies that show problems with sensitivity and specificity of these tests, they are not recommended for general use in patients with suspected meningitis.

Blood cultures should be obtained because they can identify the infectious organism in a case of ABM. In patients who are to undergo cranial CT prior to LP, blood cultures should be drawn before proceeding to CT, if possible.

TREATMENT

Because of its life-threatening nature, potential bacterial meningitis should be considered a medical emergency. An LP should be performed immediately, followed by empirical antibiotics. If LP is to be delayed while a CT is obtained first to rule out signs of increased intracranial pressure, antibiotic therapy **should not be delayed**. Empirical antibiotics should be given prior to CT scan and then the LP performed. If the time delay between giving antibiotics and LP is less than 2 hours, culture yield will not be adversely affected by a large degree.

A number of factors, including patient characteristics and CSF examination, have been studied to see if they can reliably distinguish ABM from AVM prior to culture results becoming available (Table 34-2). However, although these clinical features are suggestive of ABM versus AVM, the relatively poor positive and negative predictive values preclude their use in deciding if empirical antibiotic therapy is necessary for a patient in whom definitive diagnosis of ABM is not made after initial examination of the CSF.

In adults, empirical antibiotic therapy for presumed community-acquired bacterial meningitis should target the most common organisms, that is, *S. pneumoniae*, *N. meningitidis*, and *Listeria monocytogenes*. The antibiotics need to readily pass the blood–brain barrier. Because of the increase in penicillin-resistant *S. pneumoniae*, vancomycin plus a third-generation cephalosporin such as ceftriaxone or cefotaxime will give good coverage of *S. pneumoniae* and *N. meningitidis*, including penicillin-resistant strains of *S. pneumoniae*. Ampicillin is generally added for coverage of *L. monocytogenes* in patients >50 years old and immunocompromised patients because of the increased incidence of this organism in these patient groups.

Corticosteroids reduce the incidence of complication in ABM in infants and children. Although traditionally not given to adults (because of the lack of controlled data supporting use) a study demonstrated that in patients with intermediate neurologic

■ **TABLE 34-2** Comparison of Clinical Features: Acute Bacterial Meningitis and Acute Viral Meningitis		
	Acute Bacterial Meningitis	**Acute Viral Meningitis**
CSF WBC count (cells/mm^3)	200 to 10,000; PMN predominance	25 to 100; lymphocyte predominance
CSF protein (mg/dL)	100 to 500	50 to 100
CSF glucose (mg/dL)	<40	>40
Opening pressure (mm H$_2$O)	>200	<180
Time of year	Winter	Summer
Age	Older adults and infants	Children and young adults

meningitis (judged by a Glasgow coma score of 8 to 11) caused by proven *S. pneumoniae*, there was a benefit to adjunctive dexamethasone. However, because attempted assessment of the Glasgow coma score could delay initiation of therapy, the IDSA recommends starting dexamethasone on all patients with suspected or pneumococcal pneumonia and continued only if Gram stain reveals gram-positive diplococci or if blood or CSF cultures are positive for *S. pneumoniae*. Because of the theoretic possibility of steroid therapy interfering with entry of vancomycin into the CSF and thus resulting in suboptimal treatment for penicillin-resistant organisms, some experts recommend the addition of rifampin in patients who are started on dexamethasone.

Once empirical antibiotics are started, the patient is monitored for clinical response. Defervescence, loss of meningeal signs, and improvement in mental status indicate response to treatment. Culture results allow narrowing the spectrum of antibiotic coverage. If the diagnosis of ABM is made, antibiotics are generally continued for 14 days, provided there is good clinical response.

In cases of probable AVM, once clinical improvement occurs and CSF cultures remain negative for bacteria for more than 48 hours, antibiotics can be discontinued early.

If a patient fails to improve on antibiotic therapy, this can be because of resistant organisms or the presence of other entities seen in the differential diagnosis of meningitis (see earlier). Radiographic (CT or MRI) imaging, along with repeat LP, may be indicated under such circumstances.

KEY POINTS

- Meningitis generally presents with fever, headache, and signs of meningeal irritation.

- The distinction needs to be made between ABM and so-called aseptic meningitis. Bacterial meningitis has a high mortality and must be diagnosed.

- LP is essential to the diagnosis, but empirical antibiotics should be administered immediately if LP is delayed.

HIV Part I: Primary Care of the HIV-Infected Patient

The recognition of the human immunodeficiency virus (HIV) epidemic and acquired immune deficiency syndrome (AIDS) in the early 1980s has resulted in a major change in the spectrum of infectious disease. Because HIV has spread to virtually every patient population, practitioners in all fields of medicine must know basic features of HIV-related conditions and how HIV infection affects the care they will give.

AIDS can be caused by HIV-1 and HIV-2. The majority of cases of AIDS in the United States are caused by HIV-1. HIV-2 is more closely related to a monkey virus called SIV and clinically produces a syndrome virtually identical to that caused by HIV-1. There is evidence that HIV-2–related AIDS progresses at a slower rate than AIDS because of HIV-1 infection. The remainder of this chapter focuses on HIV-1 (hereafter referred to as HIV) infection.

The **clinical syndrome of AIDS** is defined to include those HIV-infected individuals who either:

- Have a CD4 count (see later) that falls below 200 cells/mm^3 *or*
- Develop one of the so-called AIDS-defining illnesses (Fig. 35-1).

EPIDEMIOLOGY

There has been a shift in the epidemiology of HIV infection in the United States. HIV infection was initially recognized in young homosexual men, and male-to-male sexual contact remains the most frequently reported risk factor for HIV exposure among men. HIV infection has spread to other demographic groups. Rapidly rising rates of infection have been observed in racial and ethnic minorities, especially if there is concomitant intravenous drug use (IVDU). In the United States, transmission via heterosexual sex has been rising, but not to the extent seen in other areas of the world, especially sub-Saharan Africa and regions of the Far East (e.g., Thailand). Still, heterosexual contact now accounts for more than half of AIDS cases diagnosed among women and has surpassed IVDU as the predominant mode of HIV exposure for women.

In the United States, the peak incidence of symptomatic HIV infection occurs in those 30 to 39 years of age. Because of the association with male homosexual behavior, more males than females are infected, but as the infection continues to spread among heterosexuals, male preponderance is diminishing.

ETIOLOGY AND PATHOGENESIS

HIV-1 is an RNA virus belonging to the lentivirus subfamily of retroviruses. The life cycle of retroviruses is characteristic in that, following binding to their cell surface receptor (CD4 being the primary receptor in the case of HIV) and entry into the host cell, the viral RNA genome is first transcribed into a double-stranded DNA molecule via a viral enzyme called **reverse transcriptase** (RT). This DNA is then **integrated** into the genome of the host cell, where it

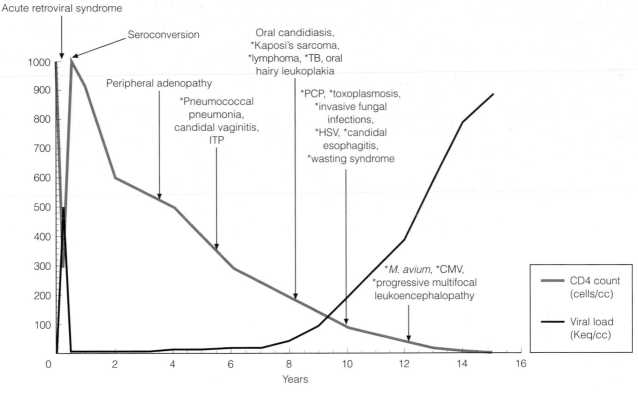

Figure 35-1 • Hypothetical natural course of an untreated HIV-infected individual. Asterisks indicate AIDS-defining illnesses.

is transcribed into RNA that codes for viral proteins as well as new RNA viral genomes. These products are then **processed and packaged** into new viral particles that bud from the surface of the host cell. These viral particles then travel to new cells to continue the life cycle. Several unique steps in the viral life cycle (Fig. 35-2) are the target of existing and proposed anti-HIV therapy.

HIV infects cells that carry the CD4 cell marker, generally T cells of the helper subclass, but also other CD4-positive (CD4) cells. Infection of CD4 lymphocytes results in their eventual death. Progression of HIV infection to frank AIDS is associated with a decline in circulating CD4 lymphocytes and may in part explain the decline in immune status.

HIV-1 is found in the highest concentrations in blood and semen but can be isolated from a number of other bodily fluids as well. **Transmission** commonly occurs via:

- Unprotected sexual contact (in the United States the highest risk is with anal receptive intercourse, but transmission also occurs with vaginal intercourse and oral–genital contact)
- IVDU

- Perinatal blood exchange (mother to child, either transplacentally, during childbirth, or by breastfeeding)
- Transfusion of blood and blood products (accounts for approximately 1% to 2% of the cases in the United States to date)

Transmission has not been firmly linked to casual (social) contact. Transmission appears to require unprotected sexual contact or exchange of blood or blood products.

CLINICAL PRESENTATION AND NATURAL HISTORY

Primary infection with HIV is linked with the **acute retroviral syndrome** in approximately 50% to 60% of cases. This manifests as a flulike illness with fever, myalgias, rash, and headache. The CD4 count may fall acutely during the acute retroviral syndrome, allowing for early appearance of opportunistic infections, but generally recovers to normal. High levels of viremia occur but then fall as the immune system appears to clear peripheral virus particles (Fig. 35-2).

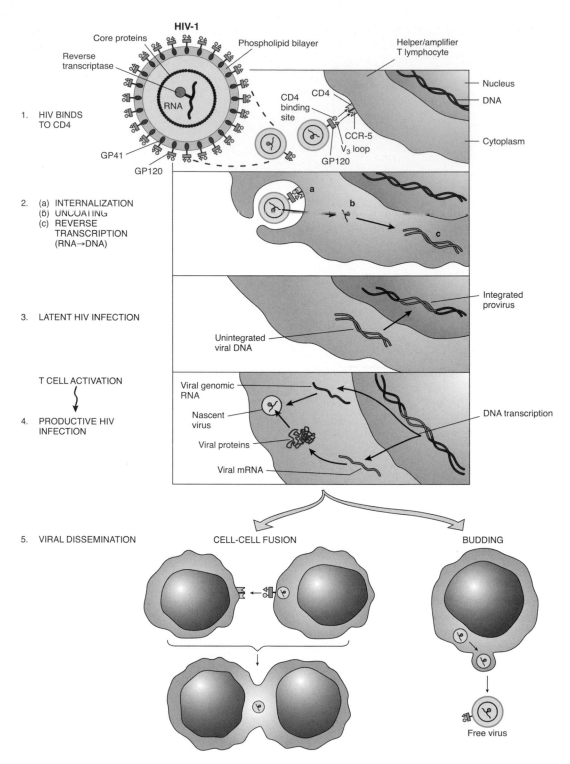

Figure 35-2 • The HIV replicative cycle and targets for antiviral therapy.
(From Rubin E, Gorstein F, Rubin R, et al. *Rubin's Pathology: Clinicopathologic Foundations of Medicine*, 4th ed. Baltimore: Lippincott Williams & Wilkins; 2005, with permission.)

Because of the nonspecific nature of the illness, few patients are diagnosed during this acute syndrome.

The natural history of HIV infection then enters a phase of **clinical latency**, where the patient is asymptomatic. Secondary markers of disease progression, such as peripheral CD4 count and peripheral viral titers, are relatively stable. What has become clear from recent studies is that despite clinical latency, there is no accompanying viral latency. Even during the asymptomatic phase, there are very high levels of viral replication, occurring mostly in the lymphoid tissues. This viral replication is felt to cause progressive damage to the immune system, eventually leading to an inability to control the infection and the reappearance of viremia.

As the peripheral CD4 count falls, the HIV-infected individual becomes more susceptible to a variety of opportunistic diseases and progression to the clinical syndrome of AIDS. The progression from HIV infection to AIDS has generally taken approximately 10 years in most untreated individuals. It is important to note that because of the advent of effect antiretroviral therapy, fewer patients follow this prototypical course, but a significant number patients are are still diagnosed with HIV infection at an advanced stage.

CLINICAL MANIFESTATIONS

HISTORY

The diagnosis of HIV infection is more frequently being made when patients are asymptomatic. Risk factors for HIV infection should be sought and patients with known risk factors screened (see later) for infection. Many times, screening is initiated by the patient. Physicians should inquire about HIV risk factors as part of every complete medical evaluation. Additionally, HIV infection needs to be considered in patients diagnosed with a sexually transmitted infection (see Chapter 29) or tuberculosis (Chapter 31). Additionally, as maternal–fetal transmission can be effectively prevented, assessment of HIV risk factors and screening should be offered to all pregnant women.

When the diagnosis of HIV infection is suspected, a **general review of systems** should be obtained, checking for:

- Constitutional symptoms: weight loss, fevers, night sweats, anorexia
- Visual disturbances, persistent headache, oral lesions

- Cough, shortness of breath, dyspnea on exertion
- Pain or difficulty in swallowing, nausea/vomiting, diarrhea, rectal pain
- Genital lesions, abnormal vaginal bleeding
- Rashes, pigmented lesions, nodules
- New or rapidly growing lymph nodes

The complete review of systems is also very important for each office visit of a known HIV-infected patient during follow-up. Progression of stable disease (whether or not the patient is currently taking antiviral medications) presents insidiously, and thus a thorough review of systems may be the only sign prior to laboratory evidence of decompensated HIV infection or an opportunistic disease.

PHYSICAL EXAMINATION

The baseline physical examination of a patient with newly diagnosed HIV infection should cover all organ systems, paying particular emphasis to those affected by the symptoms just listed. Women should have a complete pelvic examination, including Papanicolaou smear because of the increased risk of invasive cervical cancer among HIV-infected women.

Typical positive findings include:

- Generalized lymphadenopathy
- Oral candidiasis
- Angular cheilitis
- Pigmented lesions (Kaposi sarcoma, bacillary angiomatosis)
- Fungal nail infections

On initial presentation, particularly in those patients diagnosed on HIV screening performed secondary to known risk factors rather than symptoms, the physical examination may be entirely normal.

During follow-up of a known HIV-infected patient, a thorough physical exam needs to be repeated, paying particular attention to any areas of concern based on patient symptomatology or previous history.

DIAGNOSTIC EVALUATION

Testing for HIV infection is generally accomplished by a screening **ELISA** (enzyme-linked immunosorbent assay) that tests for the presence of antibodies directed against the virus. If the ELISA is positive, then a follow-up **Western blot** is performed to test for immunoreactivity against specific viral proteins and to confirm the diagnosis. The ELISA tests currently in use have a >99% specificity and a sensitivity of ~99.5%. When the test is used to screen the general population, even with this good test performance, there are a significant number of false-positive results. Thus, the Western blot is used for confirmation.

In addition to the ELISA and Western blot, a number of other tests can document as well as quantitate HIV infection. Assay for the **p24 antigen** of HIV is useful to detect virus prior to the appearance of antibody. Other direct tests for virus include **detection of viral RNA** by polymerase chain reaction (PCR) and other molecular biologic assays that are also used to follow progression of disease (see later).

When initially **evaluating a patient with newly diagnosed HIV infection**, the following **initial tests** are useful for establishing the stage of infection as well as the presence of possible opportunistic microorganisms:

- CD4 lymphocyte count
- HIV RNA quantitation (viral load)
- HIV resistance testing (genotyping)
- CBC
- Routine chemistries (electrolytes, creatinine, LFTs, lipid panel)
- Chest radiograph
- Titers of antibodies against cytomegalovirus, *Toxoplasma gondii*, hepatitis B, hepatitis C
- Purified protein derivative (PPD) to test for tuberculosis exposure along with anergy panel
- RPR or VDRL
- Screen for glucose-6-phosphate dehydrogenase (G6PD) deficiency (in patients with appropriate racial or ethnic background because of commonly used HIV drugs that predispose to hemolysis)
- Fasting lipid panel (because of metabolic disorders associated with antiviral therapy)
- Papanicolaou smear for women
- Testosterone level for men

TREATMENT

The management of the asymptomatic HIV-infected individual is twofold. The first goal is to **forestall the immunologic decline** caused by infection. This is done via the administration of **antiviral agents**. The second goal is to **prevent** and, if unsuccessful, to **initiate prompt treatment of opportunistic diseases** (Chapter 36). **Prophylaxis and routine surveillance** are the main tools used to accomplish this second goal. Various studies have shown that success in the management of HIV infection with antiviral agents is dependent on practitioner expertise and experience. Therefore, management of HIV antiviral treatment should be done in partnership with a specialist.

ANTIVIRAL AGENTS

The first class of antiviral agents developed were the **nucleoside reverse transcriptase inhibitors** (NRTIs), of which zidovudine was the first. An early study showed a modest survival benefit when zidovudine was given to patients with advanced-stage AIDS. A number of other nucleoside analogues that have been developed and various pairs of these drugs now form the core "backbone" of modern HIV treatment regimens. Many of these combinations are now available as coformulations of two drugs to aid in administration by decreasing pill burden. Resistance (because of mutations in reverse transcriptase) has arisen in viral isolates from patients on these agents. Genotyping of a patient's HIV isolates to look for resistance determinants can direct initial therapy and changes in existing therapy during virologic failure.

The **nonnucleoside reverse transcriptase inhibitors** (NNRTIs) have become important drugs to add to the NRTI backbone of therapy in treatment-naïve patients. Efavirenz or nevirapine are the approved drugs in the United States that are most commonly used for initial therapy. The deceased pill burden associated with efavirenz coupled with generally lower toxicity has made efavirenz the more commonly used drug. One notable exception is that efavirenz has high teratogenic potential (category D) and thus cannot be used in pregnant women and must be used with caution in women who may become pregnant.

The **protease inhibitors** (PIs) are the drugs that ushered in the modern age of potent combination antiretroviral therapy (commonly referred to as "highly active antiretroviral therapy" or HAART; see later). These agents inhibit the HIV protease, a virally encoded protein that is necessary for proper synthesis and assembly of viral particles, thus affecting a later stage in the viral infection than the RT inhibitors.

Additional drugs in various stages of development and use target other aspects of viral replication, including soluble CD4 to block viral entry, inhibitors of viral integration (which is mediated by a virally encoded protein), and blockers of HIV surface proteins. Enfuvirtide is a drug that inhibits HIV entry, and thus should demonstrate antiretroviral activity, even in patients with resistance to RT inhibitors and PIs. It is the first drug with this mechanism of action to receive approval from the Food and Drug Administration (FDA), although clinically its use is so reserved as part of a "salvage" regimen in the setting of treatment failure.

The use of potent combination antiretroviral therapy (i.e., HAART) has resulted in a revolution in the treatment of HIV infection. Most commonly consisting of either an NNRTI or PI (the base) added to a combination NRTI regimen (the backbone), institution of HAART is often followed by significant decreases in plasma HIV viral load, oftentimes below the detection limit of current PCR-based assays. Falling viral load is generally associated with an increase in CD4 counts and a decrease in the incidence of opportunistic infections.

The use of antiviral drugs is hindered by two main factors. The treatment regimens are often complex, often with multiple drugs taken multiple times, and the drugs have multiple side effects and drug–drug interactions. These factors can lead to poor patient compliance, which in turn can lead to the appearance of viral drug resistance and subsequent progression of disease. Even a cursory review of the various HAART regimens is beyond the scope of this chapter, but suffice it to say that the development of HAART has served to decrease the overall morbidity and mortality caused by HIV infection in developed countries. To provide up-to-date information on the recommendations for HIV antiretroviral therapy, the National Institutes of Health (NIH) has established a website that is constantly updated to provide the most current information: http://AIDSinfo.nih.gov. Further information on the antiviral drug classes and specific drugs in each class as well as recommendations on initial and follow-up treatment regimens can be found at this site.

The time to initiate antiretroviral therapy is somewhat controversial. Consensus exists to treat all patients with a history of an AIDS-defining illness or asymptomatic patients with a CD4 count of <200 cells per mm³. However, recommendation for treatment of other patients is less standardized. Many physicians who treat HIV-infected patients offer treatment to asymptomatic patients with CD4 cell counts between 201 and 350 cells per mm³. Asymptomatic patients with CD4 cell counts >350 cells per mm³ are not typically started on therapy unless they have plasma HIV RNA >100,000 copies per mL, in which case some clinicians consider starting antiretroviral therapy.

Most of the care of asymptomatic HIV-infected patients involves careful monitoring and patient education. Patients should be encouraged to ask whatever questions they may have. Modes of transmission should be reviewed, as well as the course of progression and treatment options. For asymptomatic patients, the psychosocial aspects of the disease are often the most difficult. Support groups and professional counseling are available and should be offered to the patient. As the disease progresses to the symptomatic stage, this support often becomes even more important.

The issue of partner notification is an ethical dilemma that needs to be faced. Patients need to be assured that the diagnosis will remain confidential but should also be encouraged to inform others who may have been infected by them. HIV is generally not a reportable disease; therefore, the physician may be placed in a position between maintaining patient confidentiality and protecting the health of others. Laws on partners vary from state to state, making it important for the physician to be aware of local regulations.

Patients who receive antiviral therapy need to be advised of the importance of strict adherence to therapy to prevent the emergence of drug-resistant virus. In addition they should be monitored for drug side effects and treatment response. As mentioned earlier, response is usually measured by monitoring CD4 counts and viral load. If CD4 counts fall or levels of viremia rise on therapy, consideration should be given to altering therapy, either by switching to different agents or adding other agents, particularly one of a different class. Development of opportunistic diseases can also be considered to be a sign of progression.

KEY POINTS

- HIV is the etiologic agent of AIDS, which is characterized by a progressive decline in immune function that leads to an increased susceptibility to a variety of opportunistic infections and conditions.

- HIV is transmitted by unprotected sexual contact, IVDU (with shared needles), perinatally, and by blood and blood products that have failed screening.

- After infection with HIV, there is generally a 5- to 10-year period of clinical latency during which there are relatively few signs or symptoms of infection despite high rates of viral replication within lymphoid tissues.

- The diagnosis of HIV infection is generally made by a screening ELISA test for presence of antiHIV antibodies, followed by a confirmatory Western blot if the ELISA is positive.

- The development of HAART, consisting of combinations of antiretroviral agents, represents a major advance in the treatment of HIV infection and has led to a decrease in the overall morbidity and mortality caused by HIV infection.

- The management of the asymptomatic HIV patient involves characterizing and following the progression of infection (via CD4 counts and viral load), preventing opportunistic diseases, and attempting to forestall immunologic decline by the administration of drugs that have activity against HIV itself.

HIV Part II: Prophylaxis and Treatment of Opportunistic Infections in HIV

The bulk of the morbidity and mortality associated with HIV infection is caused by conditions (most commonly secondary infections) that arise in the setting of the resultant immune defects. Early in the history of the HIV epidemic, most physicians waited for opportunistic diseases to arise and then attempted to treat them as best as possible. It was later demonstrated that **prophylaxis** was possible for a number of opportunistic infections—extending both the symptom-free periods and overall survival of HIV-infected individuals.

Given the dozens of HIV-associated opportunistic diseases, even a limited discussion of most of these is beyond the scope of this chapter. However, a few **common opportunistic diseases** are responsible for the bulk of the morbidity and mortality:

- *Pneumocystis* pneumonia (PCP, caused by *Pneumocystis jiroveci*, formerly known as *Pneumocystis carinii*)
- *Mycobacterium tuberculosis* infection
- Disseminated *Mycobacterium avium* complex (MAC) infection
- *Toxoplasma gondii* infection
- Recurrent *Streptococcus pneumoniae* infections
- Cytomegalovirus (CMV)
- Herpes simplex virus (HSV)
- Varicella-zoster virus (VZV)
- *Cryptococcus neoformans* infection

- *Histoplasma capsulatum* infection
- *Coccidioides immitis* infection
- *Candida albicans* infection
- Lymphoma
- Kaposi sarcoma (associated with infection by HHV-8)

In the United States, PCP remains the most common serious opportunistic infection (OI) among HIV-infected individuals. At least half of the cases of PCP occur in persons with previously undiagnosed HIV infection.

RISK FACTORS

Specific opportunistic diseases are encountered at particular degrees of immune suppression. If the CD4 count is used as a marker for immune status, certain conditions are rarely encountered until the CD4 count has fallen below a given level (see Fig. 35-1). For example, PCP is usually not encountered until the CD4 count is $<200/mm^3$, whereas CMV disease is not seen until the CD4 count is $<50/mm^3$. This has implications for both formulating a differential diagnosis for a symptomatic HIV-infected patient as well as influencing when prophylactic drugs are started.

Exposures (including remote infections) can influence the likelihood of a particular opportunistic condition. For example, CMV and central nervous system (CNS) toxoplasmosis are generally felt to be caused by reactivation of latent infection and therefore would be unlikely to occur in patients without serologic evidence of past infection. The endemic fungal infections are seen in particular geographic areas (histoplasmosis in the Mississippi River Valley and coccidioidomycosis in the Southwest). Animal exposures increase risk for certain infections (e.g., cryptococcosis with pigeons and *Bartonella* with cats).

CLINICAL MANIFESTATIONS

HISTORY

A given symptom complex in an HIV-infected patient can be important evidence for an opportunistic disease. The common HIV-specific differential diagnosis for various symptoms includes:

- **Constitutional symptoms (fever, weight loss, fatigue)**—mycobacterial infection (tuberculosis [TB] and MAC), HIV wasting syndrome, lymphoma, *Bartonella* infection
- **Visual changes, eye pain**—CMV retinitis, ophthalmic varicella-zoster
- **Headache, mental status changes**—toxoplasma encephalitis, CNS lymphoma, cryptococcal meningitis, progressive multifocal leukoencephalopathy
- **Cough, shortness of breath**—PCP, TB, recurrent bacterial pneumonia, influenza
- **Oral lesions**—thrush, oral hairy leukoplakia, aphthous ulcers, HSV
- **Odynophagia, dysphagia**—candidal esophagitis, CMV esophagitis, HSV esophagitis
- **Chronic diarrhea**—cryptosporidiosis, isosporiasis
- **GU symptoms**—recurrent HSV infection, syphilis, cervical cancer
- **Skin lesions**—Kaposi sarcoma, molluscum contagiosum, *Bartonella* infection (bacillary angiomatosis), scabies
- **Enlarged lymph nodes**—lymphoma, mycobacterial infection, HIV lymphadenopathy, *Bartonella*

PHYSICAL EXAMINATION

The physical examination of the symptomatic HIV-infected patient should be broad. In addition to examination of symptomatic regions, particular attention should be paid to:

- Mucosa (oral candidiasis, oral ulcers, genital lesions)
- Retina (retinopathy)
- Skin (pigmented lesions, rashes, ulcers)
- Lungs (consolidation, crackles)
- Lymph nodes (new or tender nodes, bulky adenopathy)
- Liver and spleen (hepatomegaly, splenomegaly)

TESTING

Once a differential diagnosis is formulated based on historical and clinical clues, focused testing (e.g., chest x-ray for suspected pneumonias/pulmonary symptoms or head computed tomography [CT]) for neurologic signs or symptoms (Fig. 36-1) should be initiated. Because of the range of opportunistic infections found in HIV-infected individuals, testing needs to be guided by the presenting clinical picture.

TREATMENT

The treatment of opportunistic diseases in HIV can be divided into the following categories:

- **Primary prophylaxis:** Lifestyle modifications and administration of drugs designed to prevent the appearance of an opportunistic disease
- **Treatment:** Specific therapy to cure or control an opportunistic disease
- **Secondary prophylaxis:** Continued drug therapy that is designed to prevent active recurrence of an opportunistic disease once initial treatment has been completed

In 2002, the U.S. Public Health Service and the Infectious Diseases Society of America (PHS/IDSA) revised their published guidelines on the prevention of opportunistic infections (see http://www.cdc.gov/mmwr/PDF/rr/rr5108.pdf). Table 36-1 summarizes some of the major recommendations.

Avoidance of exposure to opportunistic pathogens is desirable but not always possible. Some OIs are felt to be caused by reactivation of latent disease. Complete avoidance of certain exposures requires placing limitations on lifestyle.

In general, the following **lifestyle recommendations** can be considered:

- **Sexual exposure:** Use of latex condoms can reduce exposure to CMV, HSV, and other STDs. Latex

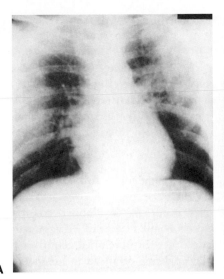
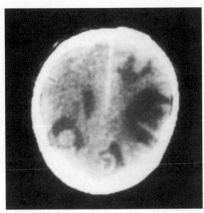

Figure 36-1 • **(A)** Chest radiograph showing features of PCP. **(B)** Brain CT scan showing focal lesions of toxoplasmosis.

■ **TABLE 36-1** Treatment and Prophylaxis of Major Opportunistic Infections in HIV-Infected Individuals

Pathogen	Treatment [Alternatives]	Indications for Prophylaxis	Primary Prophylaxis [Alternatives]	Secondary Prophylaxis [Alternatives]
Pneumocystis jiroveci	TMP-SMZ [dapsone aerosolized pentamidine, dapsone plus pyrimethamine]	CD4 count >200 μL or oral candidiasis	TMP-SMZ [dapsone, aerosolized pentamidine, dapsone plus pyrimethamine]	TMP-SMZ [dapsone, aerosolized pentamidine, dapsone plus pyrimethamine]
Mycobacterium tuberculosis	Isoniazid plus pyridoxine plus rifampin plus ethambutol (until sensitivity data are available)	Tuberculin test reaction >5 mm *or* history of positive test without treatment *or* contact with active case of TB	Isoniazid plus pyridoxine [rifampin]; rifampin or rifabutin (if suspected isoniazid resistance)	None
Toxoplasma gondii	Sulfadiazine plus pyrimethamine plus leucovorin [clindamycin as alternative to sulfa]	IgG antibody to *Toxoplasma* and CD4 <100 μL	TMP-SMZ [dapsone plus pyrimethamine plus leucovorin]	Sulfadiazine plus pyrimethamine plus leucovorin [clindamycin plus pyrimethamine plus leucovorin]
Mycobacterium avium complex	Clarithromycin or azithromycin plus one or more of rifabutin, ethambutol, clofazimine, ciprofloxican	CD4 <50 μL	Clarithromycin or azithromycin [rifabutin]	Clarithromycin or azithromycin plus one or more of rifabutin, ethambutol, clofazimine, ciprofloxican
Influenza virus	No recommendation [oseltamivir, zanamivir, rimantadine, amantadine]	All patients	Influenza vaccine [oseltamivir, zanamivir, rimantadine, amantadine]	None

continued

■ **TABLE 36-1** Treatment and Prophylaxis of Major Opportunistic Infections in HIV-Infected Individuals *(continued)*

Pathogen	Treatment [Alternatives]	Indications for Prophylaxis	Primary Prophylaxis [Alternatives]	Secondary Prophylaxis [Alternatives]
Hepatitis B virus	None [lamivudine for chronic active]	All susceptible (i.e., hepatitis B core antigen negative)	Hepatitis B vaccine	None
Hepatitis A virus	None	All susceptible (i.e., hepatitis A seronegative) and those at high risk (men who have sex with men, IV drug users) or with chronic liver disease	Hepatitis A vaccine	None
Streptococcus pneumoniae	Penicillin, cephalosporins	All patients	Pneumococcal vaccine	Pneumococcal vaccine
Cytomegalovirus	IV ganciclovir [foscarnet]	IgG antibody to CMV and CD4 <50 μL	Oral ganciclovir	IV ganciclovir [IV foscarnet, oral ganciclovir, cidofovir]
Herpes simplex virus	Acyclovir [famciclovir]	Not recommended	Not recommended	Acyclovir or famciclovir [valacylovir] for frequent and/or severe relapses
Herpes (varicella) zoster virus	Acyclovir [famciclovir]	Exposure to person with acute chicken pox or zoster	Varicella-zoster immune globulin (VZIG)	Acyclovir [famciclovir] for frequent and/or severe relapses
Candida species	Fluconazole [ketoconazole]	CD4 <50 μL	Fluconazole [ketoconazole]	Generally reserved for frequent or severe recurrences—fluconazole [ketoconazole, itraconazole, clotrimazole troches, nystatin]
Cryptococcus neoformans	Fluconazole [ketoconazole]	CD4 <50 μL	Fluconazole [ketoconazole]	Fluconazole [itraconazole, weekly IV amphotericin]
Histoplasma capsulatum	Itraconzole [fluconazole]	CD4 <100 μL and endemic area	Itraconzole [fluconazole]	Itraconazole [weekly IV amphotericin]
Coccidioides immitis	Fluconazole [ketoconazole]	CD4 <50 μL	Fluconazole [ketoconazole]	Fluconazole [itraconazole, weekly IV amphotericin]

condoms also prevent the transmission of HIV to others. Avoidance of sexual practices that can result in oral exposure to feces may reduce the risk of infections such as cryptosporidiosis, amebiasis, hepatitis, and giardiasis.

• **Environmental exposure:** Certain professions can result in increased risk of certain OIs: healthcare or work in shelters or correctional institutions (TB), child care (giardiasis, hepatitis, CMV), animal care (toxoplasmosis, campylobacteriosis, cryptosporidiosis), gardening (cryptosporidiosis, toxoplasmosis). Pet exposure should be monitored: cats (bartonellosis, toxoplasmosis), reptiles (salmonellosis), and fish (*Mycobacterium marinum*).

- **Food- and water-related exposures:** Avoid raw or undercooked eggs, meat, seafood, and dairy products. Avoid drinking untreated water, as well as swimming in lakes and rivers. Boiling of drinking water is advisable in areas with documented cryptosporidiosis.
- **Travel:** Exposures to any of the risks listed earlier may be increased in certain geographic areas. Particular attention needs to be paid to the risk of diarrheal illnesses (traveler's diarrhea). Killed vaccines (rabies, diphtheria-tetanus) can be given as recommended for all travelers, but live vaccines (polio, typhoid) should be avoided, with the exception of measles vaccine.

In general, the potential benefits of these lifestyle modifications need to be weighed against the hardships that may be imposed. For example, the companionship provided by a pet cat can be very beneficial. Provided certain preventive measures can be taken (washing hands after handling cat litter, keeping the cat indoors, and controlling fleas), pet ownership need not be prohibited. In addition, with the exception of condom use, the data supporting most of the preceding recommendations are limited.

Table 36-1 presents the treatments and primary and secondary prophylaxis for the most commonly encountered OIs. For most pathogens, alternative regimens exist, generally used in the setting of adverse drug reactions to the primary regimen.

There is currently no prophylaxis available to prevent secondary malignancies (lymphoma, Kaposi sarcoma, cervical cancer), although effective treatment of the underlying HIV infection appears to decrease the risk of developing a malignancy. The treatment of these diseases is generally undertaken in consultation with an experienced oncologist.

The development of highly active antiretroviral therapy (HAART) and the subsequent marked improvement in the clinical and surrogate markers of disease (CD4 count and viral load) in many patients has raised the question of whether prophylaxis can be discontinued if the patient's CD4 count increases above the threshold level considered to be an indication for the institution of prophylaxis. The revised PHS/IDSA recommendations (see earlier) outline guidelines for the discontinuation of primary and secondary prophylaxis for a number of infections, including PCP, MAC, toxoplasmosis, and cryptococcosis.

The standard of care for HIV-infected individuals is in a constant state of change. In general, it appears that a combination of antiviral therapy along with monitoring and prophylaxis for opportunistic diseases provides the best long-term outcome. The specific recommendations are changing; consultation with an infectious disease specialist can help ensure that the most recent recommendations are known.

KEY POINTS

- Opportunistic diseases cause the majority of the morbidity and mortality attributable to HIV infection.
- OIs are the most frequently encountered opportunistic diseases. Of these, PCP is the most common in the United States.
- A given opportunistic infection tends to occur at specific degrees of immune suppression. The CD4 count is used to quantify immune suppression.
- Prophylactic antibiotic regimens have been developed that decrease the risk of certain OIs.

Part 5

Gastrointestinal

Abdominal Pain

When a patient presents with abdominal pain, it is important to distinguish medical causes from surgical causes. This chapter discusses the evaluation of **acute abdominal pain** in the adult. Causes of chronic abdominal pain (e.g., peptic ulcer disease, irritable bowel syndrome) are discussed in subsequent chapters.

Abdominal pain can be caused by obstruction, perforation, ischemia, infection, or metabolic disturbances. Abdominal pain referred from the hollow **viscera** travels via the splanchnic (sympathetic) nerves. It is dull, vague, and poorly localized. Diseases involving the **parietal** peritoneum produce sharp, stabbing, well-localized pain.

DIFFERENTIAL DIAGNOSIS

The differential diagnosis of abdominal pain can be divided according to the predominant location of the pain. Although this can be a useful way to narrow the differential diagnosis, it should be made clear that these are only generalizations, and should not be relied on to definitively exclude any specific diagnosis.

Diffuse or Periumbilical
- Abdominal aortic aneurysm (AAA) (Chapter 10 [vascular disease])
- Ischemic bowel* (Chapter 10 [vascular disease])

Ischemic bowel may refer to chronic ischemia (intestinal angina) or acute ischemia. In this chapter, *ischemic bowel* refers to the latter syndrome. In general, ischemia of the bowel is secondary to underlying atherosclerotic disease or arterial embolism (from atrial fibrillation or valvular disease). However, ischemia may also be caused by vasculitis (Henoch-Schönlein purpura, polyarteritis nodosa; see Chapter 60) or by a crisis in sickle cell anemia.

- Bowel obstruction, especially small bowel
- Pancreatitis (Chapter 44 [pancreatitis])
- Gastroenteritis (Chapter 32 [gastroenteritis])
- Metabolic disturbances (see below)

Right Upper Quadrant
- Cholecystitis (Chapter 43 [cholestatic liver disease])
- Biliary colic (Chapter 43 [cholestatic liver disease])
- Hepatitis (Chapter 41 [hepatitis])
- Pyelonephritis (Chapter 30 [urinary tract infection])

Right Lower Quadrant
- Appendicitis
- Nephrolithiasis (Chapter 25 [nephrolithiasis])
- Crohn disease of terminal ileum (Chapter 40 [inflammatory bowel disease])

Left Upper Quadrant
- Splenic rupture
- Pyelonephritis (Chapter 30 [urinary tract infection])

Left Lower Quadrant
- Diverticulitis
- Nephrolithiasis (Chapter 25 [nephrolithiasis])
- Inflammatory bowel disease (Chapter 40 [inflammatory bowel disease])

Gynecologic sources of pain (pelvic inflammatory disease [Chapter 29], ovarian torsion, ectopic pregnancy) should be considered in all women with abdominal pain, especially lower quadrant pain.

Certain metabolic diseases may present with abdominal pain. Although these are uncommon causes, they should be considered in the differential diagnosis:

- Acute intermittent porphyria
- Diabetic ketoacidosis (DKA)

- Familial Mediterranean fever
- Narcotic withdrawal
- Lead toxicity

Acute intermittent porphyria is an autosomal dominant deficiency in hydroxymethylbilane synthase (formerly known as porphobilinogen deaminase), an enzyme in the heme synthesis pathway. **Familial Mediterranean fever** is an autosomal recessive disease, more common in people of Middle Eastern descent. It is characterized by recurring bouts of fever and inflammation of the peritoneum (serositis).

CLINICAL MANIFESTATIONS

HISTORY

Certain diseases may present with a "typical" pattern of pain. **Appendicitis** usually begins as vague, cramplike abdominal pain that moves to the right lower quadrant, becoming sharper in quality and more intense. **Biliary colic** can be characterized by severe, steady, aching pain in the right upper quadrant or epigastrium, lasting approximately 1 to 4 hours. Pain may be associated with a meal and often occurs at night. More persistent pain, associated with fever, is seen in **acute cholecystitis**, which may also be referred to the right scapula due to diaphragmatic irritation.

Pancreatitis often is epigastric/periumbilical in location and is a steady and boring pain, radiating to the back and relieved with sitting. A history of recent alcohol ingestion may be present. **Bowel ischemia** is often sudden and severe in onset. Patients often have history of atrial fibrillation, placing them at risk for arterial embolism. **Bowel obstruction** presents as crampy, midabdominal pain, occurring in paroxysms. Absence of recent bowel movement (constipation) or absence of flatus (obstipation) is another indicator. Most of these patients have a history of abdominal surgery because approximately 75% of bowel obstructions are caused by adhesions. **Nephrolithiasis** begins gradually and then escalates to a severe pain in 20 to 60 minutes, with flank pain radiating to the groin or testicle.

Nausea and vomiting are commonly associated symptoms in patients with acute abdominal pain. However, these two symptoms are very nonspecific, seen in a variety of disorders, including pancreatitis, cholecystitis, hepatitis, bowel obstruction, and appendicitis.

Patient age may suggest a particular cause. Appendicitis is more common in younger patients; elderly patients may have vascular causes (AAA, bowel ischemia) or diverticulitis.

PHYSICAL EXAMINATION

Fever occurs in infectious causes of abdominal pain but may also be present in inflammatory etiologies, such as acute pancreatitis. Jaundice is often seen in hepatitis and is usually absent in cholecystitis and biliary colic unless obstruction of the bile duct occurs. Evidence of vascular disease, such as diminished peripheral pulses, should increase the suspicion of bowel ischemia or AAA.

The abdominal examination should begin with assessing the **presence of bowel sounds** (often absent in pancreatitis and bowel ischemia; high pitched in bowel obstruction). **Rebound tenderness** indicates peritoneal irritation and requires immediate surgical evaluation. Although many conditions may demonstrate abdominal tenderness, **point tenderness** usually occurs in appendicitis, diverticulitis, and cholecystitis. Pain at McBurney's point is classic for appendicitis. This point is a third of the way between the right anterior superior iliac spine and the umbilicus. Murphy's sign (pain on palpation of right upper quadrant with inspiration) is associated with cholecystitis. **Palpable masses** may represent an aortic aneurysm and a large dilated loop of bowel. A rectal examination should be performed to examine for tenderness and the presence of occult blood. A pelvic exam should be performed in sexually active women to evaluate for cervical motion tenderness suggestive of PID or adnexal pain or mass suggestive of tubal ovarian abscess or ectopic pregnancy.

Conditions that are notable for **severe pain but relatively normal abdominal examinations** (pain out of proportion to findings) are ischemic bowel, pancreatitis, and acute intermittent porphyria.

DIAGNOSTIC EVALUATION

The extent of diagnostic testing depends on the history and physical examination. The well-appearing patient with the classic symptoms of gastroenteritis (diffuse abdominal pain, diarrhea, nausea) and a benign examination may only need observation. The acutely ill patient with peritoneal signs suggestive of a perforated viscus should go directly to the operating room for exploration. Physical examination and early testing should distinguish the surgical causes of abdominal pain from the nonsurgical causes.

The **abdominal plain film** may show free intraperitoneal air, seen under the diaphragm on an upright film, indicating perforation of a hollow viscus. Bowel obstruction reveals distended small bowel (>2.5 cm in diameter), large bowel (>9 to 10 cm), or both. Absence of air in the distal GI tract distinguishes bowel obstruction from adynamic ileus (Fig. 37-1). However, residual air may be present in early bowel obstruction. Edematous bowel loops or "thumbprinting" may be seen in bowel infarction. Most renal stones (>80%) and a smaller percentage of gallstones (15%) can be seen on a plain film.

Serum electrolytes may show an **anion gap acidosis** in bowel infarction, DKA, or severe pancreatitis.

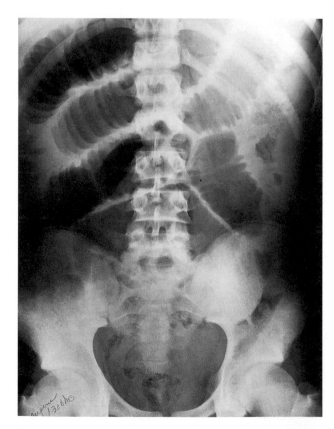

Figure 37-1 • Dilated small bowel with air-fluid levels in the small bowel obstruction. Note the paucity of air in the large intestine.

Hyperkalemia is seen in bowel infarction and represents tissue necrosis. Leukocytosis is a nonspecific finding and seen in many causes of abdominal pain. All women of reproductive age should have **human chorionic gonadotropin beta-subunit** sent to rule out pregnancy-related conditions. Serum **amylase** is markedly elevated in pancreatitis, although moderate elevation may be seen in biliary disease, bowel obstruction, DKA, and bowel ischemia. Liver function tests (**LFTs**) show marked elevations in transaminases in hepatitis and elevation in alkaline phosphatase in cholecystitis. LFTs may be normal in biliary colic.

A urine sample should be sent to evaluate for hematuria (nephrolithiasis). Mild amounts of pyuria may be seen in diverticulitis and appendicitis. Ketones are detected in the urine in most patients who have not been eating because of the abdominal pain; however, large amounts of ketones raise the suspicion of DKA.

Ultrasonography may be used to evaluate the liver and biliary tree in patients with upper quadrant pain. However, the presence of stones in the gallbladder does not confirm cholecystitis because many patients have asymptomatic stones. Approximately 5% to 10% of patients with cholecystitis have **acalculous** cholecystitis; no stones are visualized in these patients. **Sonographic findings of cholecystitis** include:

- Gallbladder wall thickening
- Sonographic Murphy's sign (tenderness with pressure applied by probe over gallbladder)
- Pericholecystic fluid

Abdominal ultrasound can also show an aortic aneurysm or reveal a dilated ureter in nephrolithiasis.

Standard computed tomography (CT) is not needed in most evaluations of abdominal pain. However, it is very sensitive in detecting inflammation in the pancreas (pancreatitis) and large bowel (diverticulitis). Splenic rupture or laceration may be seen with abdominal CT. Bowel wall edema, as seen in bowel ischemia, can also be detected. More recently, the use of helical CT has been shown to have good sensitivity and specificity in diagnosing acute appendicitis in patients. Importantly, this test has good negative predictive value (up to 99% in some studies) and thus can be used to rule out appendicitis in equivocal cases.

The **Watson-Schwartz test** is used to detect elevated levels of porphobilinogen seen in attacks of acute intermittent porphyria. This test can be performed in patients with a suspicious history or findings of a neuropathy in addition to the abdominal pain.

TREATMENT

Surgical evaluation and probably surgery should be performed immediately in patients with suspected appendicitis, bowel infarction, ruptured AAA, or splenic rupture. Surgery is usually delayed 24 to 72 hours in the stable patient with cholecystitis while antibiotics are given. Treatment of medical causes of abdominal pain is discussed in the specific chapters related to each element of the differential diagnosis as noted above.

KEY POINTS

- Pregnancy or ectopic pregnancy should be considered in all women of reproductive age with abdominal pain.

- Vascular causes of abdominal pain (bowel ischemia, AAA) should be considered in elderly patients.

- Point tenderness is suggestive of appendicitis, diverticulitis, and cholecystitis.

- Abdominal films should be obtained in patients with suspected obstruction or perforation.

- DKA can produce abdominal pain, vomiting, ketonuria, and an anion gap acidosis.

Adults normally produce approximately 150 g of stool per day. Diarrhea can be simply defined as an increase in the volume of stool. Although not part of this functional definition, this increase in volume is often accompanied by increased stool fluid content and frequency. There are four basic **pathophysiologic causes of diarrhea**:

1. **Increased secretion** of electrolytes and water into the bowel lumen
2. **Increased osmotic load** within the intestine, leading to water retention in the bowel lumen
3. **Inflammation** leading to exudation of protein and fluid from the intestinal mucosa
4. **Altered intestinal motility**, leading to rapid transit times

In addition to classification based on pathophysiology, diarrhea can also be divided into **acute**, which usually has a sudden onset and often has a benign self-limited course, and **chronic**, which may persist for weeks to years, sometimes with a waxing and waning course.

DIFFERENTIAL DIAGNOSIS

Causes of diarrhea can be grouped according to the underlying pathogenic mechanism.

Increased Secretion
- Enterotoxin producing bacteria (e.g., ADP-ribosylating toxin like cholera toxin, guanylate cyclase activators like *E. coli* heat stable toxin)
- Noninvasive microbial gastroenteritis (e.g., viral gastroenteritis, *Giardia*)
- Carcinoid syndrome
- Vasoactive intestinal peptide-secreting tumor (VIPoma)
- Villous adenoma

Increased Osmotic Load
- Sorbitol ingestion (sugar-free candy diarrhea)
- Bile salt malabsorption
- Pancreatic insufficiency (due to lipid malabsorption)
- Lactase deficiency (lactose intolerance)
- Other malabsorption syndromes (e.g., celiac disease/ gluten intolerance)
- Postantrectomy rapid gastric emptying (dumping syndrome)
- Magnesium-containing laxatives

Inflammation
- Ulcerative colitis (see Chapter 40)
- Crohn disease (see Chapter 40)
- Radiation-induced enteritis
- Invasive microbial gastroenteritis (e.g., *Shigella*, *Entamoeba*)
- Cytotoxic bacterial infection (e.g., *Clostridium difficile*, enterohemorrhagic *E. coli* infection)

Altered Intestinal Motility
- Thyrotoxicosis
- Irritable bowel syndrome (IBS)
- Neurologic disease (e.g., diabetes-associated enteropathy)

CLINICAL MANIFESTATIONS

HISTORY

History helps determine whether the illness is acute or chronic and provides hints as to the underlying etiology. For example, infectious diarrhea may occur in outbreaks associated with particular foods or environmental exposures, such as swimming or drinking of stream water. The physical **nature of the stool** can give important clues to etiology:

- Watery (secretory)
- Bulky, greasy (osmotic)
- Bloody, with or without leukocytes (inflammatory)

A **medication history** is important because many drugs, including antibiotics, antihypertensives, anti-inflammatory agents, and diuretics, can cause diarrhea. **Laxative abuse** is a very common cause of chronic secretory diarrhea.

Other important historical features to obtain include the presence of fever, abdominal pain, flatulence, and extraintestinal symptoms such as arthritis, rashes, weight loss, or edema. An association with meals or fasting should be sought because this can help identify a malabsorption syndrome.

PHYSICAL EXAMINATION

Important elements of the physical examination are the degree of hydration, the presence of abdominal tenderness, rectal mass or blood, and characterization of bowel sounds. Along with providing etiologic clues, these elements indicate the severity of the illness.

DIAGNOSTIC EVALUATION

The approach to diagnostic testing is based on whether the diarrhea is acute or chronic. Because acute diarrhea (if not associated with drugs) is often infectious (see Chapter 32), the principal tests used are examination of the stool coupled with culture. Not every patient who presents with diarrhea needs to be evaluated with these expensive and time-consuming tests. If the patient is clinically well, watchful waiting and symptomatic therapy with oral fluids are all that may be necessary. However, certain **clinical features** should **trigger a stool examination**:

- High fever
- Evidence of dehydration
- Systemic toxicity
- Bloody stool
- Immunocompromise
- Overseas or outdoor (e.g., hiking) travel

- Male homosexuality
- Recent antibiotic use

The presence of blood and/or leukocytes in the stool suggests an invasive microbial (e.g., *Shigella*, *Campylobacter*, or *Entamoeba*) rather than a viral or toxin-mediated cause. It is important to also consider the possibility of ulcerative colitis, Crohn disease, and other inflammatory diarrheas when blood and/or leukocytes are found in the stool. **Culture** for bacterial pathogens and **examination for parasites** can identify etiologic organisms.

Chronic diarrhea is usually not inflammatory. Exceptions include inflammatory bowel disease and radiation enteritis, but the history usually suggests these causes of chronic diarrhea. Evaluation of chronic diarrhea often centers on the differentiation between an osmotic diarrhea and a secretory diarrhea. A simple and useful diagnostic test is to assess the clinical change resulting from fasting. Osmotic diarrhea (which is generally caused by some sort of malabsorption syndrome) improves with fasting, whereas secretory diarrhea persists during fasting.

Another rapid way to distinguish between secretory and osmotic diarrhea is to calculate the stool osmotic gap using the following formula:

$$\text{Osmotic Gap} = \text{Osmolality} - 2(\text{Stool Na} + \text{Stool K})$$

Stool osmolality is usually estimated using the measured plasma osmolality. An osmotic gap >50 mOsm per kg H_2O suggests an osmotic diarrhea.

Further diagnostic testing is generally only necessary in the workup of chronic diarrheas. **Endoscopy**, either sigmoidoscopy or full colonoscopy with biopsy, can reveal a number of findings that are suggestive or diagnostic of a particular etiology:

- Inflammation with pathology indicative of inflammatory bowel disease
- Melanosis coli in laxative abuse
- Villous adenoma
- Pseudomembranous colitis (C. *difficile*)
- Flask-shaped ulcers in amebiasis

If initial workup reveals an osmotic diarrhea, various **studies** can be used to check for the presence of a number of **malabsorption syndromes**:

- D-Xylose test (measures absorptive capacity of the proximal small bowel)
- Schilling's test (evaluates the terminal ileum)
- Bile salt breath test (evaluates the terminal ileum)

- Measurement of pancreatic secretions (to test formal digestion from pancreatic insufficiency)
- Lactose challenge (to test for lactase deficiency)
- Antiendomysial antibody titers (to rule out celiac disease)

When further diagnostic tests fail to reveal an organic cause for chronic diarrhea, the diagnosis of **irritable bowel syndrome** (IBS) should be entertained. IBS is defined as a syndrome characterized by chronic abdominal pain and altered bowel habits (can be either diarrhea or constipation). In the United States, IBS is the most commonly diagnosed GI condition, with a prevalence estimated to be 10% to 20% of the general population. Although only a minority of patients with actually seek medical care, those that do are responsible for a significant healthcare cost, estimated to be as high as $1.3 billion. Although IBS is defined by the lack of an organic cause, the symptoms of IBS have a physiologic basis. The current opinion is that IBS results from the interaction of three key factors: altered gut reactivity in response to luminal or environmental stimuli, a hypersensitive gut with enhanced visceral perception and pain, and dysregulation of the brain–gut neurologic axis.

The AGA recommends diagnosis based on symptom-based criteria, the so-called **Rome criteria** (Table 38-1), most recently updated in 2006. With regard to treatment, the strategy is based on the nature and severity of symptoms. Patients with mild symptoms can generally be treated with education, reassurance, and simple treatments including diet (avoidance of "trigger foods," caffeine), addition of fiber and bulk agents (psyllium), drugs (antispasmodics), and psychological management (stress reduction). Patients with more severe symptoms and a greater degree of impairment may require a combination of psychological treatments and pharmacologic treatments directed at altered gut physiology. The use of newly developed agents that act at the level of the 5-HT (serotonin) receptor provided significant promise. However, the use of these agents has been hampered by the development of rare, but severe complications including ischemic cardiac events and ischemic colitis. These problems, along with the severe impact of IBS on health related quality of life are prompting many researchers to try and find safe and efficacious treatment regimens.

■ **TABLE 38-1** Rome III Diagnostic Criteria for Irritable Bowel Syndrome

Abdominal pain or discomfort of at least 3 days a month for the past 3 months (with symptom onset at least 6 months before diagnosis) that is associated with two or more of the following characteristics:
1. Relieved with defecation; and/or
2. Onset associated with a change in frequency of stool; and/or
3. Onset associated with a change in form (appearance) of stool
The diagnosis of a functional bowel disorder always presumes the absence of a structural or biochemical explanation for the symptoms.

Note: Evaluation also includes a complete physical examination, sigmoidoscopy, and additional testing when indicated. Other studies may include examination of the stool (ova and parasites, occult blood, laxatives), complete blood count (CBC), sedimentation rate, and serum chemistries. In certain cases, imaging studies (e.g., upper GI series, colonoscopy with rectal biopsy) are needed.

KEY POINTS

- Diarrhea is the increase in stool volume (usually with increased fluid content and frequency).
- The four major pathogenic mechanisms for diarrhea are increased secretion, osmotic load, inflammation, and altered intestinal motility.
- Osmotic and secretory diarrhea can be distinguished by the calculation of the stool osmolar gap or the response to fasting.
- Irritable bowel disease is a very common GI complaint that results in significant morbidity and associated healthcare costs.

Dyspepsia

Dyspepsia, or epigastric discomfort, is a common complaint. The variety of disorders that can result in dyspepsia is broad. Peptic ulcer disease (PUD), gastroesophageal reflux disease (GERD), and gastritis are important causes of dyspepsia and will be discussed in this chapter. It should be noted, however, that a majority of patients in some series do not have a biochemical or structural cause for their dyspepsia, so-called functional dyspepsia.

EPIDEMIOLOGY

Most people experience transient episodic epigastric pain. As noted above, the causes of dyspepsia are varied. Furthermore, the incidence and prevalence of each of these underlying causes have been changing.

The lifetime incidence of PUD in the United States and other industrialized countries is 5% to 10%. The epidemiology of PUD varies widely worldwide with hygiene and socioeconomic status, which are important factors for **infection with *Helicobacter pylori*** (see later).

Gastritis, the **inflammation of the gastric mucosa**, occurs in a variety of settings and as such is not a single disease. The epidemiology is thus quite varied and reflects the prevalence of the underlying conditions that lead to the condition (see later). GERD is a condition that results from the reflux of gastric contents that leads to symptoms and/or esophageal complications. The condition is common, but since many patients never seek medical attention, the true prevalence of the condition is difficult to measure. It is estimated that at least a quarter of the population experiences reflux symptoms, and in about a third of these the symptoms are clinical significant.

ETIOLOGY AND PATHOPHYSIOLOGY

In gastritis, inflammation is limited to the gastric mucosa. It can be an acute or chronic disease, each with a particular pathogenesis. In **acute gastritis**, there is erosion and damage to the gastric mucosa, and a brisk inflammatory infiltrate. This damage can be diffuse or patchy in distribution. Acute gastritis can occurs in the setting of a serious systemic illness, such as trauma, burns, sepsis, liver and renal failure, and shock, but is more **commonly due to direct mucosal injury** due to agents such as nonsteroidal anti-inflammatory drugs (NSAIDs), ethanol, steroids (high doses), and strong alkali and acid agents.

Chronic gastritis is characterized by mononuclear cell infiltrates and lack of mucosal erosions. Chronic infection with *H. pylori* is associated with at least three types of chronic gastritis: **chronic active gastritis**, **atrophic gastritis**, and so-called **type B gastritis**. Atrophic gastritis is believed to be a precursor to some gastric cancers.

In contrast to gastritis, **ulcers** are focal areas of **deep erosion** through the mucosa and, in some cases, through the submucosa. They commonly occur in the stomach and the duodenum. There are differences between the pathogenesis of gastric and duodenal ulcers. In **duodenal ulcers, excess gastric acid** is necessary for ulcer formation (hence the dictum, "no acid, no ulcer"). In contrast, patients with **gastric** ulcers tend to have **normal or even reduced gastric acid** secretion.

H. pylori infection appears to be associated with >90% of duodenal ulcers and 70% to 80% of gastric ulcers. The precise pathogenesis of *H. pylori* infection resulting in peptic ulcer is not clear but appears to involve both bacterial and host factors. Only approximately one in six individuals who are infected with *H. pylori* develops ulcers.

H. pylori infection is also associated with the development of gastric cancer and low-grade non-Hodgkin gastric lymphoma. Only a small (1% to 2%) number of *H. pylori*–infected individuals develop gastric cancer, and it appears that those who have gastric ulcers are more prone to develop cancer than those who have duodenal ulcers.

The pathogenesis of GERD centers on the movement of gastric contents into the esophagus. This implies a failure of the antireflux mechanisms that function at the gastroesophageal junctions. This can occur via physiologic pathology (e.g., decreased pressure of the lower esophageal sphincter [LES]) or anatomic pathology (e.g., the presence of a hiatal hernia. The role of *H. pylori* infection in the pathogenesis of GERD is controversial, although there has been some evidence suggesting that *H. pylori* infection may play a causative role in GERD, there is also a suggestion that chronic *H. pylori* infection may actually protect against the development of GERD. According to this hypothesis, the rising incidence of GERD, particularly in industrialized areas, may actually be a reflection of decreasing rates of infection with *H. pylori*.

Although the term functional dyspepsia implies that there is not a structural reason for the dyspepsia, there is a great deal of evidence that there is a physiologic basis, parallel to that hypothesized to be acting in irritable bowel syndrome (Chapter 38). This includes abnormalities in upper gastrointestinal motor function, visceral sensitivity, and a variety of psychosocial factors.

RISK FACTORS

Besides *H. pylori* infection, other risk factors for the development of **peptic ulcer** include male gender, stress, NSAID use, steroid use, and cigarette smoking. These non-*H. pylori* risk factors are also shared for acute gastritis.

The risk factors for **GERD** include obesity, cigarette smoking, foods that can reduce lower esophageal sphincter pressure (caffeine, chocolate, alcohol), and the presence of a hiatal hernia.

CLINICAL MANIFESTATIONS

HISTORY

Patients with dyspepsia present with **epigastric pain**. Some features of the pain may be suggestive of a particular etiology, but are rarely diagnostic. Patients with ulcer disease often report a **gnawing**, **burning**, or **aching** discomfort. In patients with duodenal ulcer, the pain typically occurs within 2 to 3 hours of a meal (presumably reflecting increased acid and pancreatic enzyme load in the duodenum). The pain awakens the patient in the middle of the night, but pain occurring before breakfast is rare. Food and antacids generally provide prompt relief. The relationship between food and pain in the setting of gastric ulcer is more variable; food may actually aggravate gastric ulcer pain.

Other symptoms that can be seen in PUD are nausea, vomiting, early satiety, and emesis of undigested food (in the setting of obstruction), melena, hematemesis, and back or shoulder pain (often in the setting of posterior penetration of a duodenal ulcer). The nonspecificity of these symptoms is highlighted by the fact that both functional dyspepsia and GERD can have identical presentations. Symptoms that are more suggestive of GERD include retrosternal pain and a sensation of reflux of gastric contents into the mouth or hypopharynx (often perceived as an "acid taste").

In patients with gastritis, pain is often less prominent. Occult or frank GI bleeding (with melena or hematemesis) is often the only finding.

PHYSICAL EXAMINATION

On physical examination, patients with PUD may exhibit epigastric tenderness. Other findings that are usually seen in the setting of complications of ulcer disease include:

- "Succussion splash," a sound produced by air and fluid in a distended stomach several hours postprandially because of gastric outlet obstruction
- Peritoneal signs (rigid abdomen, diminished bowel sounds, rebound tenderness) in the setting of perforation
- Occult blood on rectal examination

Similar to symptomatology, however, physical examination is poor at distinguishing the various causes of dyspepsia.

DIFFERENTIAL DIAGNOSIS

Besides the conditions discussed here, the differential diagnosis of epigastric pain, variably associated with food ingestion, includes:

- Pancreatitis
- Myocardial ischemia
- Cholecystitis

DIAGNOSTIC EVALUATION

Since history and physical exam often are unrevealing in patients with dyspepsia, a number of diagnostic schemes have been proposed to search for underlying etiologies. These can involve a variety of invasive and noninvasive tests as well as empiric pharmacologic treatment with antisecretory agents. The choice as to which strategy to follow in a given patient depends on a number of considerations. For example, in a patient younger than 55 years old who doesn't have any symptoms that could be suggestive of a gastric malignancy (e.g., unexplained weight loss, odynophagia or progressive dysphagia, hematemesis, jaundice, or a palpable mass), many providers will try a trial of antisecretory agents. Some immediately test for *H. pylori* infection (see below) whereas others will rapidly proceed to endoscopy. The relative merits of each strategy are still being debated (e.g., in terms of cost, long-term outcome etc.) but no definitive data from randomized trials exist to provide the best approach.

The main techniques by which peptic ulcers can be documented are **radiographic studies** (barium swallow; Fig. 39-1) and **endoscopy**. The presence of gastritis can generally be documented only by endoscopy. **GERD** can be documented by esophageal manometry and pH monitoring. In long-standing GERD, esophageal ulcers and mucosal changes (including Barrett's esophagus) can be documented by endoscopy.

The diagnosis of possible *H. pylori* infection can be accomplished by a number of means, all of which have a sensitivity of >90%:

- Culture of biopsy specimen (the gold standard but rarely performed outside of research protocols)
- Serology (high sensitivity, lower specificity)
- Direct urease test (requires endoscopic biopsy)
- Urease breath test

TREATMENT

Treatment of dyspepsia will depend on the underlying cause for the condition. The medical treatment of peptic ulcers and gastritis is designed to relieve symptoms and to accelerate the healing. If possible, removal of the inciting insult is included. In general, an avoidance of NSAIDs and aspirin is recommended. Cessation of smoking is another important intervention. Treatment of GERD can be symptomatic with antisecretory agents and can also target the underlying cause (e.g., repair of a hiatal hernia). Treatment

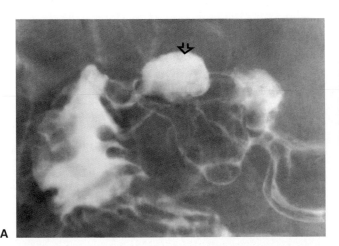
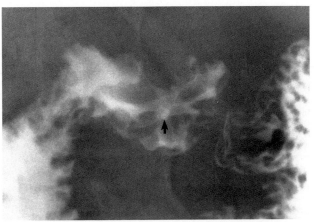

A **B**

Figure 39-1 • Duodenal ulcer (two patients). **(A)** Ulcer seen as a large collection of barium in the duodenal cap (*arrow*). **(B)** Mucosal fold radiating to a central ulcer crater (*arrow*).

of functional dyspepsia is tailored to specific patients based on symptomatology and patient characteristics (see later).

As noted above, in some cases, empiric treatment is initiated prior to obtaining a definitive diagnosis, particularly in younger patients (e.g., <50 years) without symptoms worrisome for malignancy or severe complications of PUD or GERD.

Traditional pharmacologic treatment is designed to inhibit or neutralize gastric acid or protect the mucosa. The major classes of drugs used are:

- **H_2 receptor antagonists** (cimetidine, ranitidine, famotidine, nizatidine)—limit both basal and stimulated acid secretion
- **Antacids** (aluminum hydroxide, magnesium hydroxide, calcium carbonate, and others)—neutralize gastric acid and provide relatively prompt relief of symptoms once started
- **Proton pump inhibitors** (lansoprazole, omeprazole)—most potent antisecretory agents, which limit the terminal step in acid secretion
- **Sucralfate**—mucosal protectant without significant antacid effect

Empiric dyspepsia treatment typically involved 4 to 6 weeks of an H_2-receptor antagonist or omeprazole along with antacid use as needed for symptoms. Treatment can be extended if there is incomplete response.

The realization that *H. pylori* infection is the underlying etiology in most ulcers has changed the nature of treatment. Treatment of concomitant *H. pylori* infection is believed by many to be a necessary component of therapy for patients with ulcer disease. A number of effective antibiotic regimens have been developed.* One of the first shown to be efficacious is the combination of tetracycline, metronidazole, and bismuth, given for 2 weeks. Other regimens using proton pump inhibitors (omeprazole) and antibiotics such as clarithromycin and amoxicillin have subsequently been developed. Cost, patient compliance, and side effects are considerations when choosing among the various regimens with proven efficacy. Since the role of *H. pylori* infection in GERD and functional dyspepsia is not clear, most experts do not feel there is an indication for treatment of *H. pylori* infection in these patients.

If patients with PUD unable to obtain relief from medical therapy, and endoscopy fails to yield another complication such as a malignancy, surgery may be an option. Surgery is also performed in an emergency setting of perforation, obstruction, and uncontrolled bleeding. Generally, a vagotomy (partial or selective) is combined with a pyloroplasty or antrectomy for untraceable duodenal ulcer disease. Vagotomy with or without a partial gastrectomy was previously a common procedure for unresponsive gastric ulcer disease. With the recognition of the role of *H. pylori* infection in PUD, surgery is performed much less often than in the past for this condition.

Patients with functional dyspepsia may respond to antisecretory therapy. In others, therapeutic trials of prokinetic agents or antidepressants may be efficacious. These patients often represent diagnostic and treatment dilemmas for the clinician, most likely reflecting the fact that this patient population is heterogeneous in terms of underlying pathophysiology. There is currently a significant amount of research into the causes and treatment of functional dyspepsia to try and improve the management of these patients.

---

*More details are available at http://www.cdc.gov/ulcer.

KEY POINTS

- PUD (gastric and duodenal ulcers) generally manifests as chronic epigastric pain.
- Gastritis is superficial mucosal inflammation, as opposed to the deeper damage seen in ulcer disease.
- Infection with *H. pylori* increases the risk of developing PUD.
- Treatment of underlying *H. pylori* infection is a key component of the therapy of peptic ulcers in addition to antacid therapy with or without mucosal protective agents to increase the rate of healing.

40 Inflammatory Bowel Disease

The inflammatory bowel diseases (IBDs)—ulcerative colitis and Crohn's disease—are both idiopathic, chronic, inflammatory conditions of the bowel, but their clinical and pathologic features are quite different.

Ulcerative Colitis

- Involves only the colon (large intestine), with 95% of cases involving the rectum.
- Disease is limited to the mucosa.
- There is uniform and continuous involvement of affected areas.

Crohn's Disease

- May involve any part of the GI tract from mouth to anus.
- Approximately 30% of cases affect small intestine only, 30% affect large intestine only, and 40% affect both.
- Only approximately 50% of cases of Crohn's disease involve the rectum.
- Disease may involve the entire bowel wall (transmural).
- Diseased bowel may be separated by healthy bowel (skip lesions).

EPIDEMIOLOGY

Both types of IBD occur more often in whites than in blacks. These diseases most often present between 15 and 30 years of age, but there is a second peak in patients 60 to 70 years of age.

ETIOLOGY

The underlying pathophysiology of IBD remains unknown. The increased relative risk of disease (4- to 20-fold) in first-degree relatives of IBD patients suggests a genetic predisposition. A crucial development has been the identification of specific genetic abnormalities in a subset of familial cases of Crohn's disease (see later). No infectious agents have been universally implicated in the etiopathogenesis of IBD, but the effectiveness of antibiotics in the treatment of a fraction of patients suggests at least a partial role for the indigenous intestinal microbiota. Finally, the pathology of the disease, with inflammation and, in some cases, granuloma formation, supports the concept of a dysregulated immune response as a key factor in the development of IBD. This inappropriate and chronic inflammatory immune response is hypothesized to be caused by an intrinsic (genetic) defect in immune regulation and driven by elements of the intestinal microbiota.

The relationship between the host immune system and the indigenous intestinal microbiota in the pathophysiology of IBD has been highlighted by the discovery that mutations in the *NOD2* locus underlie the development of Crohn's disease in a subset of patients with familial disease. *NOD2* belongs to the class of "pattern recognition receptors," molecules that can detect so-called microbial-associated molecular patterns and then either drive or regulate host inflammatory responses. Thus, the finding that a subset of patients with Crohn's disease have abnormalities in the system that is responsible for detecting and regulating inflammatory responses following microbial stimulation provides further support for the theory that IBD represents a breakdown in the normal interaction between indigenous microbes and the host immune system. Additional disease susceptibility loci have been found, and in many cases also encode for proteins that are involved in host/microbe interactions.

CLINICAL MANIFESTATIONS

HISTORY

The patient with ulcerative colitis often presents with **bloody diarrhea** and **abdominal pain**. There may also be a complaint of tenesmus, or painful urgency to move the bowels. A travel history (dysentery) and recent antibiotic use (*Clostridium difficile*) should be obtained to evaluate other possible etiologies.

Crohn's disease presents with similar symptoms, but the pain may be more cramplike, with accompanying **fever** and **weight loss**. Acute ileitis (inflammation of ileum) may mimic appendicitis with right lower quadrant pain.

Patients with **irritable bowel syndrome** (Chapter 38) may have many similar symptoms, including abdominal pain, bloating, and diarrhea. However, with irritable bowel syndrome, symptoms have often been prolonged, and there is an absence of bleeding and weight loss. Bowel movements often relieve symptoms in irritable bowel syndrome.

PHYSICAL EXAMINATION

Vital sign abnormalities are present in the severely ill patient with IBD, such as tachycardia, orthostatic hypotension, and fever. On abdominal examination, abdominal tenderness is often present, but rebound tenderness necessitates consideration of appendicitis, perforation, or other causes of a surgical abdomen (see Chapter 37). Patients with Crohn's disease may have fullness or palpable masses, representing adherent loops of bowel. Rectal fistulas in Crohn's disease may present as a perirectal abscess.

Skin examination may show the characteristic **pyoderma gangrenosum**, an ulcerating lesion usually located on the trunk, or **erythema nodosum**, violaceous subcutaneous nodules located most often on the lower legs. Aphthous ulcers of the oral cavity occur in 5% to 10% of patients with Crohn's disease. Finally, uveitis, arthritis, and other extraintestinal inflammatory conditions may be associated with IBD.

DIFFERENTIAL DIAGNOSIS

In the patient with **lower GI bleeding**, consider diverticulosis, colon cancer or polyps, arteriovenous malformations, or hemorrhoids. In the patient with **bloody diarrhea**, consider infectious etiologies such as *Yersinia*, *Campylobacter*, *Shigella*, *Salmonella*, amebiasis, or *C. difficile*. In the **elderly patient** with a presentation suggesting IBD, consider the preceding diagnoses along with diverticulitis or ischemic bowel.

DIAGNOSTIC EVALUATION

Helpful initial studies include a complete blood count (CBC), serum albumin, and alkaline phosphatase. These studies may reveal signs of inflammation (leukocytosis, increased ESR) or malabsorption (decreased albumin). Anemia is often multifactorial, and causes include iron, folate, and B_{12} deficiencies or chronic disease.

Increased alkaline phosphatase level may represent underlying liver disease, which occurs at a higher frequency in patients with IBD. **Hepatobiliary diseases** associated with IBD include:

- Sclerosing cholangitis (mostly ulcerative colitis)
- Cholelithiasis (mostly Crohn's disease)
- Fatty liver
- Autoimmune hepatitis
- Cholangiocarcinoma

Two interesting laboratory findings are the presence of perinuclear antineutrophil cytoplasmic antibodies (P-ANCAs) in the majority of patients with ulcerative colitis and the presence of anti–*Saccharomyces cerevisiae* antibodies in the majority of patients with Crohn's disease. Genetic tests for various disease susceptibility loci are available, but are not generally used as screening test.

Definite diagnosis in IBD is made by direct visualization of the GI tract and biopsy. **Sigmoidoscopy** or **colonoscopy** reveals erythematous, friable mucosa with longitudinal ulcerations (**cobblestone** appearance) in Crohn's disease, or regeneration of the mucosa around a diseased colon that gives the appearance of **pseudopolyps** in ulcerative colitis.

Histopathologic examination of biopsy specimens in Crohn's disease shows involvement of the entire bowel wall, with **granuloma formation** or lymphoid aggregates. The histopathology in ulcerative colitis is generally limited to the mucosa, but **crypt abscesses** may be present.

TREATMENT

The natural history of IBD varies with the type of disease and severity of the initial presentation. In ulcerative colitis, disease limited to the rectum has a relatively benign course. In fact, 20% of patients with ulcerative colitis are relapse free a decade after the initial presentation. Crohn's disease, however, tends to be more severe, with frequent relapses. Initial treatment for IBD consists of medical therapy to keep disease in remission. Surgery is reserved for:

- Intractable disease
- Obstruction
- Perforation
- Prophylactic resection to prevent colon cancer (in ulcerative colitis)

Removal of the entire colon cures ulcerative colitis but leaves the patient with a colostomy. However, new surgical techniques strip the mucosa off the rectum while leaving the sphincter intact. An ileoanal anastomosis is then performed (often with formation of an ileal loop pouch to provide continence) to avoid colostomy. Surgery in Crohn's disease is never curative. The disease will often recur around the surgical resection.

Sulfasalazine and other 5-aminosalicylate derivatives remain the first-line treatment for mild to moderate ulcerative colitis. Sulfasalazine consists of a sulfapyridine moiety and 5-aminosalicylic acid (5-ASA), also known as mesalamine. The active drug is the 5-ASA, which is liberated in the colon by bacterial enzymatic cleavage. Sulfasalazine (4 to 6 g per day in divided doses) is effective in treatment of mild to moderate ulcerative colitis and in maintaining remissions in these patients. It is less effective in the treatment of Crohn's disease because the drug is not active in the small intestine. **Side effects** of sulfasalazine include:

- Nausea
- Headache
- Allergic reactions
- Hepatitis
- Bone marrow suppression

Recognition that the last three side effects are caused by the inactive sulfa moiety has led to the development of **5-ASA dimers** (olsalazine) and **coated 5-ASA** that are not degraded in the proximal bowel and **mesalamine enemas** for distal disease. The coated 5-ASA drugs have active drug released in the ileum and seem to be useful in maintaining remissions in Crohn's disease and ulcerative colitis.

Prednisone is commonly used for controlling moderate to severe IBD, often in doses of 40 to 60 mg per day. However, because side effects (bone loss, hyperglycemia, cataracts) are common with chronic use and steroids are not effective at maintaining remission, they should be tapered off when possible. Topical steroids (in the form of enemas and foam) can be used as alternatives for 5-ASA–based drugs for distal disease.

Patients who become steroid dependent may benefit from **immunomodulators**. Examples (with side effects) include:

- Azathioprine, 6-mercaptopurine (bone marrow suppression, pancreatitis)
- Methotrexate (diarrhea, stomatitis, bone marrow suppression, hepatic fibrosis)
- Cyclosporin A (hypertension, renal dysfunction, seizures)

These drugs are effective at maintaining remissions and decreasing steroid use in IBD patients. Cyclosporin A has a role in preventing colectomy in patients with severe ulcerative colitis refractory to IV steroids.

A treatment unique to a subset of patients with Crohn's disease is the use of antibiotics, such as **metronidazole**. This drug can control mild to moderate Crohn's disease and increase healing of perianal disease. Ciprofloxacin has been used in these situations. There is minimal evidence that antibiotics are effective in ulcerative colitis, although it can be successful in patients with ileal-anal pouch anastomoses who develop so-call pouchitis.

New biologic agents have been developed to target specific inflammatory mediators in IBD. A number of agents have been developed, including **specific monoclonal antibodies**, that target the elements of the immune system such as infliximab and adalimumab that block cytokine tumor necrosis factor. These agents are effective at inducing remissions in Crohn's disease. Other treatments have been developed to target leukocyte adhesion molecules and interleukins. Although sometimes touted as "steroid-sparing" therapeutics, it is important to note that life-threatening infections have developed in patients taking various biologic agents. Other drug toxicities have included hypersensitivity, autoimmunity, and a serum sickness–type reaction.

Patients with IBD may develop several different complications, which should be suspected in patients with acute deterioration. **Enteric fistulas** or **bowel obstruction** may occur in 20% to 30% of patients with Crohn's disease. Fistulas may be intraintestinal, enterovaginal, or enterovesical. **Toxic megacolon** in ulcerative colitis may present with fever, pain, and a

■ TABLE 40-1 Diagnosis and Treatment of Inflammatory Bowel Disease

	Crohn's Disease	**Ulcerative Colitis**
Location	Entire GI tract; mostly small intestine and colon	Limited to colon
Rectal involvement	Often spared	Almost always involved
History	Abdominal pain, weight loss	Bloody diarrhea
Colonoscopy	Skip lesions, "cobblestone" mucosa	Continuous involvement, pseudopolyps
Treatment	Metronidazole, immunomodulators	Sulfasalazine or 5-ASA drugs, immunomodulators
Complications	Bowel obstruction, fistulas	Toxic megacolon, colon carcinoma

distended colon (>6 cm on abdominal radiograph). There may be air in the bowel wall. Treatment is conservative at first, with bowel rest, parenteral nutrition, steroids, empirical antibiotics, and surgery only if needed.

Finally, patients with diffuse ulcerative colitis are at extremely high risk for **colon carcinoma** after 10 years of active disease. Patients should be screened with colonoscopy every 1 to 2 years depending on the clinical course. Colectomy is recommended if colonoscopy reveals high-grade dysplasia or any dysplasia associated with a mass. Although patients with Crohn's disease are at increased cancer risk as well (not as high as with ulcerative colitis), optimal treatment and best approach to surveillance remain to be defined.

Table 40-1 summarizes the key features of diagnosis and treatment of IBD.

KEY POINTS

- Crohn's disease involves the entire GI tract, mostly the small intestine and colon, whereas ulcerative colitis is limited to the colon.

- The rectum is often spared in Crohn's disease but is almost always involved in ulcerative colitis.

- Abdominal pain and weight loss are often seen in Crohn's disease, whereas ulcerative colitis often presents with bloody diarrhea.

- Colonoscopy reveals skip lesions and cobblestone mucosa in Crohn's disease and continuous involvement and pseudopolyps in ulcerative colitis.

- The medical treatment of IBD involves the tailored use of anti-inflammatories, immunomodulators, and antibiotics.

- Complications of Crohn's disease include bowel obstruction, abscesses, and fistulas; complications of ulcerative colitis include toxic megacolon and colon carcinoma.

Hepatitis

Hepatitis refers to inflammation of the liver parenchyma that can be caused by a variety of infectious and noninfectious etiologies. This inflammation can be acute or chronic. By convention, **chronic hepatitis** is defined as hepatitis that persists for >6 months.

ETIOLOGY AND PATHOPHYSIOLOGY

A number of **viruses** can cause hepatitis. Overall, viral hepatitis (both acute and chronic) is the most common type of hepatitis encountered in the United States and worldwide. The hepatitis viruses differ regarding the nature of their genome, transmission, ability to cause chronic infection, and severity of disease (Table 41-1). Hepatitis D virus (HDV) is unique in that it is a defective virus and requires coexisting hepatitis B virus (HBV) infection to establish a productive infection.

Hepatic injury caused by hepatitis virus infection is believed to be a result of the **host immune response against infected hepatocytes**. The viruses (with the possible exception of hepatitis C virus [HCV]) are not believed to be directly cytotoxic themselves. In chronic viral hepatitis caused by HBV, HCV, and HDV, the host immune response is insufficient to clear the infection, and there is **ongoing viral replication**. Despite the inability of the immune system to clear the infection, there is continued immune-mediated hepatic injury. A number of host and viral factors influence the development of chronic hepatitis, including age of infection (the younger the age at which infection is acquired, the higher the chance of developing chronic disease), hepatitis virus type (HCV most commonly becomes chronic), and immunosuppression (increased risk of chronic disease).

In addition to the hepatitis viruses, other viral infections can cause hepatic damage, including **cytomegalovirus**, **herpes simplex virus**, and **Coxsackie viruses**. Other candidate hepatitis viruses include hepatitis G virus (HGV, also known as hepatitis GV virus C) and transfusion-transmitted virus (TTV), but their precise significance as causes of hepatitis is as yet unknown. Various **drugs** can cause acute and chronic hepatitis:

- Oxyphenisatin (a laxative, no longer used in the United States; one of the first drugs proven to cause chronic hepatitis)
- Acetaminophen (important because it is unknowingly consumed by patients as a component of a variety of prescription and over-the-counter medications)
- Halothane (causes a rare, idiosyncratic, severe acute hepatitis)
- Isoniazid (approximately 10% of adults on isoniazid have transient liver function test (LFT) elevations because of a toxic metabolite; in <1%, an acute hepatitis can result, which can be fatal)
- Methyldopa (associated with chronic hepatitis)
- Azole antifungals (ketoconazole and fluconazole have been associated with acute hepatitis)

Alcohol can cause a severe, even fatal, acute hepatitis. Chronic alcohol use can lead to a condition known as **alcoholic fatty liver** and eventually **cirrhosis**

■ **TABLE 41-1** Features of Viral Hepatitis

	Viral Genome	Epidemiology	Acute Mortality (%)	Chronic Disease (%)	Laboratory Markers
HAV	ssRNA	Fecal-oral	0.2	None	HAV antigen, anti-HAV, HAV RNA
HBV	dsDNA	Parenteral, sexual, perinatal	0.2 to 1.0	2 to 7	HBsA, HBeAg, anti-HBaAg, anti-HBeAg, HBV DNA
HCV	ssRNA	Parenteral, sexual	0.2	50 to 70	HCV antigen, anti-HCV
HDV	ssRNA	Parenteral, sexual	2 to 20	?50	HDV antigen, anti-HDV
HEV	ssRNA	Fecal-oral	0.2	None	HEV Ag, anti-HEV

(see Chapter 42). In addition, acute anoxic liver injury can result in a syndrome that resembles acute viral hepatitis.

There is a rare idiopathic form of chronic hepatitis known as **autoimmune chronic active hepatitis** (ACAH). As suggested by the name, this disease is characterized by chronic hepatic inflammation and the production of a number of autoantibodies. Three fourths of patients with this disease are women of childbearing age. Patients with ACAH have a higher than normal incidence of other autoimmune disorders. ACAH is also associated with other immune diseases including celiac disease.

A chronic form of hepatitis is associated with the **hereditary disorders** Wilson disease, hemochromatosis, and α_1-antitrypsin deficiency. When unrecognized, these diseases can progress to cirrhosis (see Chapter 42).

CLINICAL MANIFESTATIONS

HISTORY

Patients who present with **acute hepatitis** generally report the following:

- Jaundice
- Dark-colored urine (from bilirubin in urine)
- Abdominal pain or discomfort (often in the right upper quadrant)
- Fever
- Nausea/vomiting

Other associated symptoms can include fatigue, malaise, headache, myalgias, and arthralgias. Patients who present with severe **fulminant acute hepatitis** can present with signs of **liver failure**, such as encephalopathy, coagulopathy, ascites, and renal failure. Patients with mild cases of acute hepatitis can be **minimally symptomatic** or entirely **asymptomatic**.

The clinical presentation of **chronic hepatitis** is commonly insidious. A few patients with chronic viral hepatitis may recall an acute episode of jaundice (especially with hepatitis B). In many other cases, nonspecific symptoms such as **fatigue**, **malaise**, **anorexia**, and **arthralgias** are the only presenting complaints. Many times the diagnosis is only entertained when screening LFTs (see later) reveal chronic elevated transaminases. Other patients with chronic hepatitis are only diagnosed when they present with cirrhosis and end-stage liver disease.

PHYSICAL EXAMINATION

Findings in **acute hepatitis** generally include:

- Jaundice (see Color Plate 13)
- Hepatomegaly (often tender)
- Splenomegaly
- Adenopathy

More severe cases can present with complications from **hepatic failure** such as ascites, edema, encephalopathy (e.g., asterixis), or gastrointestinal (GI) bleeding.

In **chronic hepatitis**, the physical examination is often unrevealing unless significant hepatic impairment is present, at which time findings of chronic liver failure are present (see Chapter 42).

DIFFERENTIAL DIAGNOSIS

For **acute hepatitis**, the major differential diagnosis is between the etiologies listed previously and other conditions that can cause direct (toxic) hepatic injury and/or result in cholestasis:

- Biliary tract disease (acute cholecystitis, cholangitis, obstructing common duct stone)
- Drug-induced cholestasis (see Chapter 43)
- Direct hepatotoxins (acetaminophen overdose, *Amanita* mushroom poisoning, carbon tetrachloride)
- Right-sided heart failure (caused by hepatic congestion)
- Anoxic liver injury

The differential diagnosis for **chronic hepatitis** includes:

- Chronic biliary tract disease (primary biliary cirrhosis, primary sclerosing cholangitis)
- Nonalcoholic steatohepatitis (a condition characterized by fatty deposits and inflammation throughout the hepatic lobule, seen in obese women with hyperlipidemia)

DIAGNOSTIC EVALUATION

Hepatitis leads to **hepatocyte necrosis** and release of hepatic enzymes. Clinically, increases in the serum levels of the **aminotransferases** aspartate transaminase (AST) and alanine transaminase (ALT) have proven to be useful in detecting hepatocellular necrosis. Excretion and, to a lesser extent, conjugation of bilirubin are also impaired by hepatocyte injury, leading to elevation of the **serum bilirubin** level.

The **pattern of aminotransferase elevation** may give clues to the underlying etiology. In general, acute viral hepatitis causes a greater absolute elevation than alcoholic hepatitis. Furthermore, in alcoholic hepatitis, the serum AST is usually elevated out of proportion to the ALT, leading to an AST-to-ALT ratio greater than 2. A single measurement of aminotransferase level, however, is a poor indicator of the absolute degree of hepatic damage.

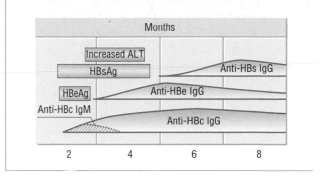

Figure 41-1 • The evolution of hepatitis B: occurrence of hepatitis B virus markers and antibodies in the blood of infected patients.
(Courtesy Communicable Disease Surveillance Centre.)

The diagnosis of **viral hepatitis** is aided by the availability of specific **serologic tests** that detect specific viral proteins and/or host antibodies directed against these viral proteins (see Table 41-1 and Fig. 41-1). Multiple serologic tests are available, but for the most commonly encountered situations, the following recommendations for their use can be made.

For the diagnosis of presumed **acute viral hepatitis**:

- IgM antihepatitis A virus (antiHAV)
- IgM antihepatitis B core antigen (antiHBcAg)
- Hepatitis B surface antigen (HBsAg)
- Anti-HCV (variably present in acute disease, may need serial serology)

If HBsAg is present, testing for coexisting HDV by anti-HDV is appropriate, particularly if there are risk factors (IV drug use or exposure to blood or blood products).

For the diagnosis of presumed **chronic viral hepatitis**:

- HBsAg
- Anti-HCV

Again, testing for HDV is appropriate if HBsAg is present.

The presence of anti-HBsAg (IgG) indicates **distant resolved infection** with HBV or successful immunization against HBV. Patients with chronic HBV infection do not develop anti-HBsAg, which is protective and also develops in response to successful immunization against HBV (see later). In contrast, the development of anti-HCV simply indicates infection with HCV; the development of anti-HCV is seen in patients with chronic HCV infection, and these antibodies are not protective.

In chronic viral hepatitis, the degree of viral replication can be determined by the measurement of HBV DNA or HCV RNA (using an assay based on the polymerase chain reaction).

In patients in whom a diagnosis of **autoimmune chronic active hepatitis** (ACAH) is suspected (e.g., a woman with chronically elevated aminotransferases and without serologic evidence of chronic viral hepatitis), measurement of **autoantibody** titers can be useful:

- Antinuclear antibody, primarily in a homogeneous pattern
- Anti–smooth muscle antibody
- Anti–liver-kidney microsomal antibodies
- Anti–cytokeratin antibodies

When present in high titers, these autoantibodies can be useful in making the diagnosis of ACAH, but they are not invariably present. Another common laboratory abnormality seen in ACAH is **hyperglobulinemia**.

Percutaneous liver biopsy can be performed in cases in which the diagnosis remains uncertain. Done in consultation with a gastroenterologist, the procedure is relatively safe and yields important diagnostic information because specific causes of hepatitis have characteristic histologic appearances.

An assessment of the degree of hepatocellular impairment can be determined by measurement of:

- PT
- Serum albumin level
- Serum ammonia level

TREATMENT

For **acute viral hepatitis**, there are **no well-accepted specific therapies**. In many cases, close outpatient follow-up with laboratory monitoring to document resolution of hepatic injury is sufficient. Hospitalization for closer monitoring may be required in more severe cases. For drug- or alcohol-related hepatitis, therapy involves removal of the offending agent followed by supportive care. Note that documented viral hepatitis should be reported to local or state health departments.

The recognition that an insufficient immune response appears to be a factor in continued productive viral infection has revolutionized the treatment of **chronic viral hepatitis** (HBV and HCV). The administration of interferon alpha to bolster the immune response and allow clearance of the virus has proven to be successful in approximately 50% of patients with chronic stable HBV or HCV. In the case of chronic HCV, the antiviral agent ribavirin is generally added to the treatment regimen. For chronic HBV the antiviral agents lamivudine, adefovir dipivoxil, or entecavir have been used to supplement interferon therapy. Although the combination of interferon and antiviral agents represent an important advance in the treatment of chronic HBV and HCV infection, the high cost and the relatively high rate of recurrent disease/treatment failure have prompted a search for even more potent agents/ regimens.

Interferon treatment is complicated by the development of significant side effects including a chronic influenzalike syndrome with fatigue, nausea, and low-grade fevers (because of the augmented inflammatory response). Anemia and leukopenia can also arise and need to be monitored for. In patients who have HCV and are also receiving ribavirin, adequate contraception is necessary because this agent is highly teratogenic. Interferon therapy should not be administered to patients with chronic HBV or HCV who have evidence of decompensated liver disease because interferon therapy actually results in increased hepatic inflammation, which can be extremely harmful in this case.

In cases of severe alcoholic hepatitis (as judged by marked hyperbilirubinemia and prothrombin time prolongation), there is the suggestion that administration of glucocorticoids may increase survival, but the use of steroids in such patients is by no means universal.

For patients with autoimmune chronic active hepatitis, administration of glucocorticoids (alone or in combination with azathioprine) is the treatment of choice. Up to 80% of patients respond with symptomatic, biochemical, and histologic improvement and with an increase in survival. It is unclear if the development of cirrhosis is prevented by steroid therapy. Additionally, patients who fail to respond with early (within 2 weeks of initiating therapy) improvements in laboratory indicators of liver dysfunction have a poorer overall prognosis.

Patients who are diagnosed with acute HBV or HCV infection should be followed for the development of chronic hepatitis. For HBV, resolution of infection is marked by the appearance of anti-HBsAg and normalization of transaminase levels. For HCV, recovery is marked by normalization of transaminases alone because there is no serologic marker of recovery.

For patients with fulminant acute hepatitis or chronic hepatitis that progresses to end-stage liver failure, orthotopic liver transplantation is a limited, but potentially lifesaving, option. It is interesting to note that a significant subset of patients who undergo liver transplantation for autoimmune hepatitis have a recurrence of disease affecting the orthotopic organ.

Prophylaxis against some forms of viral hepatitis is available: HAV immune globulin (all preparations of immune globulin have some anti-HAV activity), HAV vaccine, HBV recombinant HBV vaccine, and hepatitis B immune globulin (recommended for postexposure prophylaxis, e.g., after needle stick, in a nonimmunized individual). There is currently no available postexposure prophylaxis for HCV. Such an individual should be monitored for the development of infection, with consideration for interferon and ribavirin treatment if infection does develop.

KEY POINTS

- Hepatitis, acute or chronic inflammation of the liver, can be caused by infectious and noninfectious causes.
- Hepatitis viruses are responsible for most cases of acute and chronic hepatitis seen worldwide.
- Noninfectious causes of hepatitis include drugs, hereditary disorders such as Wilson disease, and an idiopathic disorder called autoimmune chronic active hepatitis (ACAH).
- Chronic hepatitis (both infectious and noninfectious) can lead to cirrhosis and end-stage liver failure.
- Treatment of acute hepatitis is mainly supportive. Some cases of chronic viral hepatitis respond to interferon therapy. Corticosteroids are the treatment of choice for ACAH.
- Immunoprophylaxis is available for hepatitis A and hepatitis B virus infection.

Cirrhosis

Cirrhosis is defined as irreversible hepatic injury, characterized histopathologically by fibrosis that distorts the normal hepatic architecture and the presence of regenerative nodules. The normal **function of the liver** includes:

- Production of protein
- Filtering of mesenteric blood flow
- Metabolism of endogenous (e.g., bilirubin) and exogenous (e.g., drugs) substances

Loss of these functions in cirrhosis leads to the common complications of ascites, portal hypertension, jaundice, and encephalopathy.

ETIOLOGY

The underlying **causes of cirrhosis** include:

- Alcohol
- Chronic hepatitis B or C
- Biliary disease (including primary biliary cirrhosis)
- Cardiac disease
- Autoimmune hepatitis
- Inherited diseases (hemochromatosis, Wilson disease, α_1-antitrypsin deficiency)
- Nonalcoholic fatty liver disease (a condition characterized by lobular inflammation and some degree of pericellular fibrosis, often in patients with diabetes mellitus or metabolic syndrome).

In the United States, alcoholism and chronic hepatitis C infection are the most common causes of cirrhosis; viral hepatitis (mostly hepatitis B) is the leading cause worldwide. Biliary disease is discussed in Chapter 43.

INHERITED DISORDERS

Hemochromatosis is an autosomal recessive disorder of **increased iron absorption** and results in excess deposition of iron in certain organs. It is characterized by liver, heart, and gonadal failure. Pancreatic failure, leading to glucose intolerance, combined with increased skin pigmentation, has resulted in hemochromatosis being described as "bronze diabetes." Secondary hemochromatosis (in contrast to hereditary) may occur in patients who are transfusion dependent, such as in thalassemia major.

Wilson disease is an autosomal recessive disorder of **copper excretion**, resulting in increased accumulation of copper in the liver and brain. Patients may present with fulminant or chronic hepatitis, cirrhosis, psychiatric involvement, or neurologic disease (tremor, rigidity).

α_1-Antitrypsin deficiency is an autosomal recessive disorder characterized by abnormal alleles of serum α_1-antitrypsin. This disease often presents as early emphysema and asymptomatic cirrhosis.

PATHOPHYSIOLOGY

Mortality and morbidity in cirrhosis are usually caused by its complications. **Ascites** is the accumulation of fluid within the peritoneal cavity. It is the result of multiple factors, including increased capillary hydrostatic pressure (portal hypertension), decreased plasma oncotic pressure (hypoalbuminemia), and increased sodium reabsorption by the kidney.

Esophageal varices develop from portal vein hypertension that is transmitted to systemic collateral veins in the gastroesophageal junction. Rupture of these veins and the resultant bleeding depend on the size of the varices and the extent of portal hypertension. Bleeding from esophageal varices usually presents as painless massive hematemesis and/or melena. Because other etiologies of UGI bleeding are also common in cirrhotic patients (gastritis, peptic ulcer disease), variceal bleeding should be confirmed with endoscopy (even in the patient with known varices).

Hepatic encephalopathy is characterized by confusion, personality changes, and asterixis and may progress to obtundation and coma. The etiology is unknown; increased ammonia levels have been implicated in the pathogenesis, but the theory remains unproved. Recent evidence suggests that increased levels of γ-aminobutyric acid may have an etiologic role.

CLINICAL MANIFESTATIONS

HISTORY

The patient with end-stage liver disease may present without specific complaints other than fatigue and malaise. However, failure of liver function may result in leg edema, easy bruisability, and increased abdominal girth (from ascites). Bleeding from esophageal varices can present dramatically.

Evaluation for possible causes of cirrhosis should include a detailed alcohol history (which the patient may deny), past episodes of hepatitis, or risk factors for hepatitis (IV drug use, high-risk sexual behavior, blood transfusions). Family history may suggest an inherited liver disease; however, because most such diseases are autosomal recessive, the patient's parents are usually unaffected.

PHYSICAL EXAMINATION

The abdominal examination in cirrhosis liver that is enlarged, normal or small, depending on the stage of disease, although when palpable, it is generally firm. Flanks may be bulging because of ascites, and shifting dullness may be present. Portal hypertension will lead to **splenomegaly**, **internal hemorrhoids**, and **caput medusae** (prominent periumbilical veins). Men may present with gynecomastia and testicular atrophy.

Skin findings in cirrhosis include **jaundice** and **spider telangiectases**. Examination of the hand may reveal:

- Clubbing
- Palmar erythema
- Dupuytren's contracture (permanent flexion of the third or fourth metacarpal phalangeal joint)

A sign of hepatic encephalopathy is **asterixis**, a coarse unintentional flapping of the wrist when the wrists are held in complete extension (as if stopping traffic).

DIFFERENTIAL DIAGNOSIS

In the patient presenting with **ascites**, consider:

- Abdominal malignancy (pancreatic, ovarian)
- Nephrotic syndrome
- Cardiac failure
- Peritoneal tuberculosis
- Peritoneal mesothelioma

See Chapter 43 for the differential diagnosis of the patient presenting with jaundice.

DIAGNOSTIC EVALUATION

The following **laboratory findings** are seen in cirrhosis:

- Hyponatremia because of increased antidiuretic hormone secretion (effective renal blood flow is reduced)
- Decreased BUN level because of malnutrition and decreased protein production
- Decreased albumin level
- Increased bilirubin level (mostly direct)

Hematologic abnormalities include:

- Increased PT because of decreased production of vitamin K–dependent clotting factors
- Macrocytic anemia (mean cell volume >100) because of increased RBC membrane in liver disease, which may also be caused by concomitant alcohol use or folate deficiency
- Thrombocytopenia secondary to splenomegaly and decreased production of thrombopoietin

If an **inherited disease** is suspected from history and physical finding, the following tests can be useful:

- Hemochromatosis: increased ferritin and increased iron to total iron-binding capacity ratio (>55%)
- Wilson disease: decreased ceruloplasmin (<20 mg per dL)
- $<\alpha_1$-Antitrypsin deficiency: absence of α-globulin spike on immunoelectrophoresis and decreased serum α_1-antitrypsin

■ TABLE 42-1 Serum Ascites-Albumin Gradient Test for Cause of Ascites	
SAAG <1.1 mg/dL	**SAAG ≥1.1 mg/dL**
Malignancy	Cirrhosis (portal hypertension)
Tuberculosis	Hepatic metastases
Pancreatitis	Budd-Chiari syndrome
Nephrotic syndrome	Cardiac disease Myxedema

These hereditary diseases are then confirmed by liver biopsy. Identification of the causative genes is available for hemochromatosis and α_1-antitrypsin deficiency.

Patients with new-onset ascites should undergo **paracentesis** to determine the etiology of ascites and rule out infection. Two useful tests on ascitic fluid are a cell count and an albumin level. The difference between the serum albumin and ascites albumin level, the so-called **serum ascites-albumin gradient** (SAAG), is the most specific test to differentiate between causes of ascites (Table 42-1).

An absolute polymorphonuclear count of >250 cells per mL is consistent with **spontaneous bacterial peritonitis** (SBP) and should be treated (see later). Ascitic fluid should be inoculated into blood culture bottles at the bedside to improve sensitivity of bacterial culture.

TREATMENT

The most important intervention in the patient with cirrhosis is complete **abstinence from alcohol**. Patients who continue to drink after diagnosis of alcoholic cirrhosis have an extremely poor prognosis.

The patient should be monitored for the **complications of cirrhosis**, which include:

- Bleeding esophageal varices
- Ascites
- Hepatic encephalopathy

Prognosis in cirrhosis is influenced by the development of these complications and has been summarized by the Child's criteria (Table 42-2).

Liver transplantation is usually indicated when the patient has refractory ascites, recurrent encephalopathy, recurrent variceal bleeding, or progressive malnutrition. Absolute **contraindications to transplantation** include:

- Infection outside of the hepatobiliary system (including AIDS)
- Metastatic liver disease
- Uncorrectable coagulopathy

The 5-year survival rate for liver transplantation is approximately 70%.

THERAPEUTICS

Treatment of Ascites

- Sodium restriction (<2 g NaCl per day).
- Diuretic therapy: **Potassium-sparing** diuretics (spironolactone, amiloride, triamterene) are the drugs of choice to counteract the high aldosterone state in cirrhosis. Urinary sodium should exceed urinary potassium during therapy. Many patients require the addition of furosemide.
- **Large-volume paracentesis:** Removal of 6 to 8 L of peritoneal fluid is an effective and prompt method to decrease ascites. Concerns about precipitating hypotension and renal failure have led to the practice of transfusing albumin during the procedure, although randomized trials have not demonstrated much benefit.

■ TABLE 42-2 Child's Criteria for Prognosis in Cirrhosis			
	A	**B**	**C**
Bilirubin (mg/dL)	<2.3	2.3 to 2.9	>2.9
Albumin (g/dL)	>3.5	3.0 to 3.5	<3.0
Ascites	None	Easily controlled	Poorly controlled
Encephalopathy	None	Mild	Advanced
Nutrition	Excellent	Good	Fair

- **Peritoneovenous (LeVeen) shunt:** This plastic shunt connects the peritoneum to the vena cava. Although effective in decreasing ascites, complications include thrombosis or infection of the shunt and DIC.

Patients with ascites may develop **spontaneous bacterial peritonitis** because of a low amount of albumin and bacteriostatic proteins in the ascitic fluid. Symptoms may include fever, abdominal pain, and worsening mental status, but often symptoms are minimal (such as malaise, anorexia). If paracentesis confirms the diagnosis, empirical treatment directed at gram-negative enteric organisms (*Escherichia coli*, *Klebsiella*) and *Streptococcus pneumoniae* should be started, commonly with a third-generation cephalosporin such as cefotaxime. Patients who fail to improve or appear seriously ill warrant treatment for *Enterococcus* and anaerobic organisms (<10% of all cases) with a drug such as ampicillin/sulbactam. Aminoglycosides should be avoided in patients with cirrhosis because of the increased risk of nephrotoxicity. Newer quinolones such as levofloxacin and third-generation cephalosporins are alternatives. Severely ill patients with SBP may benefit from the addition of IV albumin.

Treatment of Esophageal Varices

- Replacement of blood products and coagulation factors if needed.
- IV **vasopressin analogues** (somatostatin, octreotide, terlipressin): Constricts portal blood flow and controls bleeding in approximately 80% of cases. Vasopressin itself is no longer used because of a poor side-effect profile (including cardiac ischemia).
- Endoscopic **sclerotherapy** (injection) or **band ligation** of varices: Immediate treatment reduces rebleeding rates, and follow-up treatments are required to obliterate varices. Both are very effective, although band ligation has gained recent preference because of lower rebleeding and complication rates.

As "salvage treatment" in patients who fail endoscopic hemostasis, emergency TIPS (see later) placement can be effective but is a technically demanding procedure without universal availability. Balloon tamponade is rarely used, even as a treatment of last resort.

Nonselective β-blockers (such as propanolol) reduce the hepatic venous pressure gradient and are used in the prevention of initial bleeding from large varices. Band ligation may be as or more effective than balloon tamponade.

Treatment of Hepatic Encephalopathy

- Correction of precipitating factors, including infection, GI bleeding, excess dietary protein, hypokalemia, hypovolemia, alkalosis, and drugs (especially narcotics and benzodiazepines).
- Lactulose (30 mL two to four times daily): A nonabsorbable disaccharide that decreases ammonia absorption; dose is adjusted until diarrhea occurs.
- Neomycin (500 mg every 6 hours): A broad-spectrum antibiotic that decreases ammonia production from bacteria in the GI tract. Although systemic absorption is minimal, its use may still be limited by nephrotoxicity.

CONTINUED CARE

Portosystemic Shunts

Shunt procedures are reserved for patients who are refractory to standard treatments or have recurrent variceal bleeding or diuretic-refractory ascites. **TIPS** is a relatively noninvasive method to treat the complications of portal hypertension. A radiologist places a stent from the inferior vena cava through the liver parenchyma into the portal system, decompressing the portal system. Complications include increased hepatic encephalopathy (20% to 30% of patients) and shunt thrombosis or stenosis. A more permanent solution is **distal splenorenal shunt**, which connects the splenic vein to the distal left renal vein. However, in addition to perioperative mortality and morbidity, this surgery may increase the risk of hepatic encephalopathy (although the risk is lower than with earlier portocaval shunts).

Hepatocellular Cancer

Cirrhosis is the most important predisposing risk factor for hepatocellular cancer (HCC), and HCC should be suspected in the stable cirrhotic patient with new clinical deterioration. α-Fetoprotein may be elevated in HCC, but its use as a screening test is limited because of its relatively low sensitivity and specificity. Treatment is surgical resection for localized disease in patients who are eligible for surgery. Hepatic artery embolization and chemoembolization are options for other patients.

KEY POINTS

- Alcohol consumption is the primary cause of cirrhosis in the United States.
- The patient with ascites caused by cirrhosis generally has a serum ascites-albumin gradient of >1.1 g per dL.
- Causes of a low gradient (<1.1 g per dL) include malignancy, pancreatitis, and tuberculosis.
- The patient with spontaneous bacterial peritonitis should be treated empirically with an antibiotic such as cefotaxime that covers enteric gram-negative rods and streptococci.
- In the patient with new-onset hepatic encephalopathy, an underlying precipitant should be suspected, including infection, GI bleeding, hypokalemia, and drugs.

Cholestatic Liver Disease

Bile is formed in the hepatic lobules and secreted into bile canaliculi; it then flows into bile ducts. These ducts drain into the common hepatic duct, which is joined by the cystic duct of the gallbladder to form the common bile duct. Obstruction of normal bile flow from the liver at any of these sites results in **cholestasis**.

Diseases that cause cholestasis are classified as **intrahepatic** or **extrahepatic** obstructions. This distinction must be made early in the evaluation because treatment strategies differ greatly. Cholecystitis (inflammation of the gallbladder) and cholelithiasis (gallstones) do not cause obstruction of biliary flow (except in the case in which gallstones enter the common bile duct) and are not discussed in this chapter.

EPIDEMIOLOGY

Some etiologies of cholestasis involve particular populations. **Primary biliary cirrhosis** (PBC) affects predominantly middle-aged women, whereas **primary sclerosing cholangitis** (PSC) affects mostly men. For diseases where the obstruction is a result of another disease (e.g., cholelithiasis, pancreatic tumor), the epidemiology will obviously follow that of the underlying etiology.

ETIOLOGY AND RISK FACTORS

Both PBC and PSC seem to have an **autoimmune etiology**. PSC is associated with inflammatory bowel disease (especially ulcerative colitis) in up to 90% of cases (see Chapter 40).

Many **drugs** are known to cause cholestatic liver disease and, along with PBC and PSC, are the major causes of intrahepatic obstruction. Space does not allow for a complete listing, but some of the more well-known agents include:

- Erythromycin
- Oral contraceptives and estrogen
- Anabolic steroids
- Sulfonamides
- Chlorpromazine

Extrahepatic obstruction is generally **mechanical** in nature (e.g., bile duct strictures, tumor, common bile duct stones).

CLINICAL EVALUATION

HISTORY

Symptoms of **cholestatic liver disease** include:

- Pruritus
- Fatigue
- Steatorrhea
- Jaundice

Malabsorption of fat-soluble vitamins (A, D, E, K) may lead to symptoms as well (see Chapter 53). Patients with pancreatic carcinoma may present with the classic triad of jaundice, weight loss, and back or abdominal pain. Patients with extrahepatic bile duct obstruction may also present with signs of **ascending cholangitis**:

- Fever and chills
- Right upper quadrant pain
- Jaundice
- Nausea and vomiting

PHYSICAL EXAMINATION

In early cholestatic disease, the physical examination may be completely normal. Later, jaundice and scleral icterus appear. Splenomegaly, ascites, telangiectasia, and lower extremity edema are signs of cirrhosis that may be seen in advanced cases of PBC or PSC.

DIFFERENTIAL DIAGNOSIS

Cholestasis must be differentiated from other causes of **jaundice**, such as:

- Hepatocellular injury
- Hemolysis
- Acute and chronic pancreatitis
- Gilbert disease

The differential diagnosis of cholestasis may be divided into **extrahepatic bile duct obstruction**:

- Pancreatic carcinoma
- Cholangiocarcinoma
- Parasitic infections (e.g., *Ascaris*, liver flukes)
- Bile duct strictures
- Choledocholithiasis

and **intrahepatic duct obstruction**:

- Primary biliary cirrhosis (can also cause extrahepatic obstruction)
- Primary sclerosing cholangitis
- Drug reactions
- Viral hepatitis
- Nonalcoholic steatohepatitis

DIAGNOSTIC EVALUATION

Elevation of alkaline phosphatase is almost always seen in cholestatic liver disease. Because bone disease also increases alkaline phosphatase, the hepatic source of the elevation is confirmed by an elevated **5-nucleotidase** or **gamma glutamyl transpeptidase** (GGT). **Bilirubin**, predominantly direct (conjugated), may also be increased and indicates more advanced obstruction. Serum transaminases (aspartate aminotransferase and alanine aminotransferase) are usually mildly elevated (except in the case of cholestasis due to acute viral hepatitis). This pattern of liver function tests is in contrast to hemolysis (in-

direct hyperbilirubinemia) and hepatocellular dysfunction (transaminases elevated more than alkaline phosphatase).

After determining that the patient has evidence of cholestasis, the next step is to classify the problem as intrahepatic or extrahepatic. **Ultrasound** is the initial test. Bile duct dilation indicates obstruction at or below the common bile duct (extrahepatic obstruction). Gallstones may be visualized in the common bile duct. However, obstruction may not produce duct dilation during the first 24 hours.

In the patient with extrahepatic obstruction, a cholangiogram must then be performed to localize the obstruction. **Endoscopic retrograde cholangiopancreatography** (ERCP) is one technique used to visualize the bile ducts. If a common bile duct stone proves to be the cause of obstruction, removal may be achieved through a papillotomy (opening of the pancreatic ampulla). Biopsy or brushings may be performed during ERCP to diagnose pancreatic or biliary malignancy. Percutaneous hepatic cholangiogram is another diagnostic alternative but has a higher incidence of complications.

Abdominal computed tomography may be useful to:

- Visualize bile ducts if ultrasound is inadequate
- Look for pancreatic masses as a cause of obstruction
- Identify common bile duct stones
- Stage pancreatic carcinoma or cholangiocarcinoma (hepatic metastasis)

In the patient without bile duct dilation, diagnosis depends on blood tests and possibly liver biopsy. **Antimitochondrial antibody** (AMA) is positive in 95% of patients with PBC. AMA is not present in PSC, although 60% of PSC cases have the peripheral pattern of **perinuclear antineutrophil cytoplasmic antibody** (P-ANCA). PSC may also be diagnosed by the narrow-beaded appearance of both intra- and extrahepatic ducts on ERCP. If the diagnosis remains in doubt, **liver biopsy** is used to confirm the diagnosis and assess prognosis.

TREATMENT

Treatment is determined by the nature of the obstruction. Extrahepatic obstruction will require an intervention to relieve the obstruction, whereas intrahepatic obstructions are treated medically.

INTRAHEPATIC OBSTRUCTION

For drug-induced cholestasis, removal of all possible offending agents is indicated. Liver enzymes usually return to normal, although continued worsening may occur. In PBC, medical treatment may slow the progression of disease. **Ursodiol** (ursodeoxycholic acid), 13 to 15 mg/kg/day, has been shown to decrease liver function test abnormalities and decrease pruritus in PBC. It presumably decreases the accumulation of toxic bile salts. Long-term results also suggest that treatment with ursodiol delays need for liver transplantation. In fact, several studies indicate that appropriate treatment of early stage disease will result in normal life expectancy. Medical treatment is less successful for PSC. Balloon dilation of a predominant stricture is sometimes used for PSC, but this does not change the natural history of the disease.

EXTRAHEPATIC OBSTRUCTION

Discovery of a common duct stone necessitates early removal to prevent continued obstruction and possible cholangitis. ERCP has become the preferred method of stone extraction, although surgery is occasionally necessary. In patients with pancreatic carcinoma or cholangiocarcinoma, surgical resection may be considered, but the malignancy has almost always spread by the time of diagnosis. In cases of advanced malignancy, endoscopically placed stents will relieve symptomatic obstruction but do little to change the course of disease.

Cholestyramine, a bile acid resin, is often used to control symptoms of pruritus in patients with long-standing cholestasis. Patients should also be followed for development of **deficiencies of fat-soluble vitamins**:

- Vitamin D (osteoporosis, hypocalcemia)
- Vitamin A (night blindness)
- Vitamin K (increased prothrombin time)
- Vitamin E (ataxia, neuropathy)

Given the young age at which PSC often occurs and coupled with the fact that the disease is generally progressive and leads to cirrhosis, patients with end-stage liver disease should be considered for **liver transplantation**. As noted above, with modern treatment (ursodoxycholic acid) end stage cirrhosis is encountered much less often in the setting of PBC. Transplantation is usually indicated when the patient has refractory ascites, recurrent encephalopathy, recurrent variceal bleeding, or progressive malnutrition and, as such, is similar to the criteria for transplantation for other patients with end-stage liver disease. Additionally, criteria specific for timing of transplantation have been developed using prognostic criteria based on clinical and laboratory data. In general, referral for transplantation is made when the criteria predict a six-month survival of less than 80%. Both PBC and PSC have been known to recur in transplanted livers.

KEY POINTS

- Laboratory findings in cholestatic liver disease generally include increased alkaline phosphatase with normal to slightly elevated transaminases (alanine and aspartate).

- A hepatic source of an elevated alkaline phosphatase is confirmed by an elevated 5-nucleotidase or GGT.

- The initial test in evaluating cholestatic liver disease is the right upper quadrant ultrasound to determine whether the obstruction is intrahepatic or extrahepatic.

- Primary biliary cirrhosis occurs mostly in middle-aged women and often presents with pruritus or asymptomatic elevations in alkaline phosphatase; antimitochondrial antibody is present in most cases.

- Primary sclerosing cholangitis is usually seen in association with inflammatory bowel disease; patients may present with ascending cholangitis (fever, right upper quadrant pain, jaundice).

44 Pancreatitis

Pancreatitis is the consequence of inappropriate activation of enzymatic precursors (zymogens) in the pancreas. Activation leads to autodigestion of the organ, triggering further enzyme activation and release of systemic toxins. Despite extensive research, the precise initiating factors remain unknown.

ETIOLOGY

Alcohol and **gallstones** are the underlying etiology in 80% of cases. The most common cause depends on the specific patient population being discussed. Less common causes (10% of cases) include **direct injury** (postoperative, traumatic, post-endoscopic retrograde cholangiopancreatography [ERCP]), **viral infections** (mumps, Coxsackie virus, hepatitis, cytomegalovirus), vascular injury (cholesterol embolism, vasculitis), and **metabolic abnormalities** (hypertriglyceridemia, hypercalcemia). Pancreatic cancer uncommonly presents as pancreatitis (2% of all cancers). Numerous drugs have been implicated in pancreatitis; Table 44-1 lists the most common offenders.

Pancreas divisum is a common congenital abnormality (7% on autopsy series) in which the embryonic dorsal and ventral buds of the pancreas fail to fuse. Therefore, the main pancreatic duct drains through the dorsal remnant, the minor papilla. Although pancreas divisum can be found in patients with pancreatitis, its etiologic role continues to be debated. Idiopathic pancreatitis makes up the remaining 10% of cases. However, careful investigation of these cases has revealed microlithiasis (also known as biliary sludge) or spasm of the sphincter of Oddi as possible underlying causes.

CLINICAL MANIFESTATIONS

HISTORY

The predominant symptom in pancreatitis is severe **abdominal pain**. It is characteristically epigastric in location, steady and boring in nature, radiating to the back, and relieved with sitting. **Nausea** and **vomiting** are usually present.

PHYSICAL EXAMINATION

The abdominal examination is often less impressive than the presenting pain, although tenderness and rebound may certainly be present. Vital sign abnormalities, such as hypotension and tachycardia, indicate volume depletion and a potentially unstable patient. Low-grade temperature is often seen, but higher temperatures may indicate an underlying infection.

Other physical findings that may be suggestive of severe disease include:

- Erythematous skin nodules (because of fat necrosis)
- Dullness to percussion and decreased breath sounds (indicating pleural effusion, most often on the left)
- Blue periumbilical discoloration (Cullen sign) and bruising on the abdominal flanks (Grey-Turner sign), both suggesting severe necrotizing disease

DIFFERENTIAL DIAGNOSIS

Pancreatitis must be distinguished from other causes of abdominal pain, especially those with

■ **TABLE 44-1** Drugs Associated with Pancreatitis
Azathioprine/6-mercaptopurine
Valproic acid
Estrogens
Furosemide
Metronidazole
Sulfonamides
Tetracyclines
Cytarabine
Dideoxyinosine
Pentamidine
Salicylates

elevated serum amylase levels (marked with an asterisk):

- Perforated viscus*
- Cholecystitis*
- Small bowel obstruction*
- Mesenteric ischemia/thrombosis*
- Dissecting aneurysm
- Renal colic
- Diabetic ketoacidosis
- Ruptured ectopic pregnancy*

DIAGNOSTIC EVALUATION

The most sensitive test is the **serum amylase**, which is elevated within 6 to 12 hours of symptoms. Because other diseases may also present with abdominal pain and increased amylase, some experts recommend measurement of the **serum lipase** to increase the accuracy of the diagnosis. Lipase remains elevated several days longer than amylase and may be useful for patients presenting after a prolonged episode. Although amylase levels do not predict severity, higher levels are more specific for the diagnosis of pancreatitis. Similarly, these enzyme levels should not be used to monitor disease, and thus daily measurement in patients with pancreatitis is unnecessary. Other laboratory findings include the following:

- Increased hematocrit (hemoconcentration)
- Increased white blood cell (WBC) count (nonspecific, usually in the 10,000 to 25,000 range)

- Hypocalcemia (because of fat necrosis and saponification)
- Increased liver function tests (LFTs) (alanine aminotransferase greater than three times normal is highly suggestive of a biliary etiology)
- Hyperbilirubinemia (with biliary obstruction)
- Hypoxemia (pleural effusion or impending acute respiratory distress syndrome [ARDS])
- Hypertriglyceridemia (seen only in 20% of patients; likely represents preexisting lipid disorder or alcohol binge)

High triglycerides may make the amylase level falsely normal in acute pancreatitis. A **plain film of the abdomen** should be obtained to rule out other causes, such as perforation or obstruction. Nonspecific signs include ileus and a "sentinel loop" of bowel (dilated segment in the region of the pancreas). Calcification in the pancreas is pathognomonic for chronic pancreatitis, although acute pancreatitis may certainly coexist.

Abdominal US is useful to identify cholelithiasis as a possible etiology and to rule out biliary obstruction. It is not a good method to identify pancreatic disease. **Abdominal CT** has a high sensitivity for severe disease (e.g., necrotizing pancreatitis), although the pancreas may appear normal in mild cases. Obtaining a CT is advocated when the diagnosis is uncertain, the pancreatitis is clinically severe, the patient appears septic, or the patient fails to improve.

TREATMENT

Pancreatitis spans the spectrum from mild self-limited disease to fulminant multiorgan system failure and death. Mild pancreatitis resolves in 3 to 7 days in most patients (85%). Prediction of the severity of pancreatitis is thus important in identifying patients who may benefit from aggressive, targeted intervention, and this has led to the development of a number of scoring systems for acute pancreatitis. One commonly used system is the Ranson criteria (Table 44-2). Patients with fewer than three criteria have very low mortality (1%), whereas those with six or seven criteria approach 100% mortality. However, as these criteria take 48 hours to complete and can only be used once, other experts recommend the use of APACHE (Acute Physiology and Chronic Health Evaluation) score in combination with CT scanning to help determine disease severity.

■ TABLE 44-2 Ranson Criteria for Pancreatitis

On Admission	Within 48 Hours
Age >55 yr	Hct decrease >10% points
WBC >16,000/mL	BUN increase (mg/dL) >5
LDH (IU/mL) >350	PaO_2 (mm Hg) <60
SGOT (IU/mL) >250	Calcium (mg/dL) <8
Glucose (mg/dL) >200	Base deficit (mEq/dL) >4 Fluid deficit (L) >6

(From Ranson JHC, Rifkind KM, Rose DF, et al. Prognostic signs and the role of operative management in acute pancreatitis. *Surg Gyn Obstet* 1974;139:69 81.)

After establishing the diagnosis, the following treatment plan should be undertaken:

1. **Correction of underlying causes/factors:** Discontinuation of any suspected causative toxins/drugs is important. If obstruction from gallstones is suspected, early ERCP may be indicated.
2. **Intravenous fluids:** Patients with severe disease often require large volumes of fluid (think of pancreatitis as a retroperitoneal burn) and should be treated aggressively. Urine output and vital signs need to be closely followed.
3. **Analgesics:** Morphine has been traditionally avoided because it constricts the sphincter of Oddi and theoretically worsens pancreatitis, although objective clinical data are lacking. Meperidine is typically given (one should be careful of accumulation of its metabolite, especially in renal failure) with fentanyl as an option for patients with large analgesic requirements.
4. **Bowel rest:** Patients should not eat for several days. If stable and improving, they may advance diet on day 3. Patient hunger is a good marker to advance diet.

The development of pancreatic infection is a leading cause of morbidity and mortality in patients with severe pancreatitis; the use of prophylactic antibiotics remains controversial, however, with some experts recommending empirical agents such as imipenem for patients with severe, acute necrotizing pancreatitis. The development of pancreatic infection should be suspected with persistent fevers and treated if necessary. Diagnosis of infection may require percutaneous sampling of peripancreatic fluid. Attempts to decrease pancreatic secretion with glucagon, H2-receptor antagonists, and octreotide are ineffective and not routine.

There is a trend toward early institution of enteral feeding (often via a jejunal feeding tube to avoid stimulation of pancreatic secretion) even in cases of severe pancreatitis. One of the benefits proposed for early enteral feeding is maintenance of the intestinal barrier function, thus limiting bacterial translocation.

ERCP should be performed early (within 24 to 48 hours) in patients with evidence of biliary obstruction (dilated bile ducts, elevated bilirubin). Use of ERCP in suspected biliary pancreatitis without obstruction is currently not routine. ERCP is suggested in traumatic cases when ductal disruption or fistula is suspected (before definitive surgery).

Mortality because of pancreatitis is most often attributable to infection or multiorgan system failure. ARDS presents with worsening hypoxemia and bilateral pulmonary infiltrates. Other consequences of pancreatitis are:

- **Pancreatic abscess/infected necrosis:** Should be suspected when fever continues and patient remains ill. Diagnosed by CT, followed by CT-guided percutaneous needle aspiration. Surgery is required to treat early abscess/infected necrosis.
- **Pancreatic pseudocyst:** Suspected if mass palpated, or hyperamylasemia or abdominal pain persists. Diagnosed by CT. Often resolves on its own within 6 weeks; surgery is required if expanding or remains symptomatic. Percutaneous or endoscopic drainage may be used depending on the location and nature of the pseudocyst.
- **Chronic pancreatitis:** Seen most often as a consequence of alcohol-induced or idiopathic pancreatitis. Symptoms include recurrent pain and malabsorption. Diagnosis confirmed by ERCP, showing beaded dilated pancreatic duct ("chain of lakes"). Treatment is mainly symptomatic, with pancreatic enzyme replacement if needed. In severe cases, diabetes may develop as well. Ductal stenting has relieved pain in some patients.

KEY POINTS

- Alcohol and biliary tract disease are the underlying etiologies in most cases of pancreatitis; metabolic causes and drugs should be ruled out.

- Diagnosis is based on the typical picture of abdominal pain associated with increased amylase and lipase levels. Imaging studies, such as radiograph and US, may be used to rule out other abdominal pathology.

- Treatment is mainly supportive with IV fluids and analgesia.

- The development of infection is a major cause of morbidity and mortality and requires appropriate diagnosis and therapy. Empirical antibiotic use in cases of documented severe necrosis is advocated by some, but not all experts. Abscess formation requires drainage (by surgery or, in selected cases, percutaneous drain placement).

- Complications, such as pseudocyst or abscess, are detected by CT.

Colorectal Cancer

Colorectal cancer ranks third in cancer incidence and second in cancer-associated mortality in the United States, making primary prevention, screening, diagnosis, and therapy of concern to most physicians who care for adults.

EPIDEMIOLOGY

In the United States, an estimated 150,000 new cases of colorectal cancer are diagnosed each year, with approximately 55,000 deaths related to the disease. The overall lifetime risk is approximately 5% for the general population. Men have a slightly higher age-adjusted death rate than women. The incidence of colorectal cancer increases with age, beginning to rise after 40 years of age and then significantly after 55 years of age.

Worldwide, colorectal cancer rates vary depending on geographic location. The United States (with a rate of 14 per 100,000 population) is near the upper end of a broad range. Rates in Australia and several European countries are higher (up to 30 per 100,000 in the Czech Republic) whereas rates in most Asian and South American countries are much lower (3 per 100,000 in Ecuador). Environmental factors are suggested to play a role because persons from an area of low incidence assume a significantly higher risk when they migrate to areas of high incidence.

ETIOLOGY

The current hypothesis is that most colorectal cancers arise from preexisting benign adenomatous polyps that undergo sequential malignant transformation. **Adenomas** are neoplastic lesions that display abnormal cellular differentiation and are of varying architecture, size, and shape. Histologically, adenomas can be classified as:

- Tubular (80% to 85% of all adenomas)
- Tubulovillous (8% to 16%)
- Villous (3% to 15%)

Although adenomatous polyps are considered to be premalignant lesions, only approximately 5% are estimated to develop into cancer.

Factors associated with malignant transformation are:

- Increasing size (<1% of polyps <1 cm diameter develop into frank malignancies, whereas approximately 10% of those larger than 2 cm will)
- Villous histology

At the molecular level, neoplastic and malignant transformations are believed to be caused by an **accumulation of damage to the DNA** of the mucosal cells of the colon. Two key events are believed to be the activation of the ras oncogene and the inactivation of one or more of the so-called tumor-suppressor genes (e.g., APC, dcc, and p53). The DNA damage can be caused by **endogenous agents** (e.g., oxidizing and alkylating products of cellular metabolism) or **exogenous agents** (e.g., carcinogens, viruses, and radiation).

Cancers can initially be confined to the mucosa (carcinoma in situ) and then progress to the submucosa, muscularis propria, and adjacent tissues. Once the cancer invades past the mucosa, it can metastasize to regional lymph nodes and distant sites. Invasive cancer involving the rectum differs from other colon cancers in that local recurrences after resection are more common.

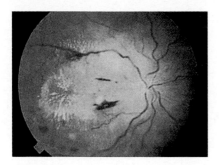

Plate 1 • Papilledema, exudates, and retinal hemorrhages in hypertensive retinopathy.

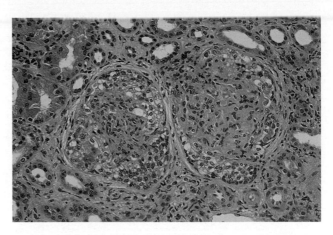

Plate 2 • Rapidly progressive (crescentic) glomerulonephritis. Appearance of cellular crescents on light microscopy.

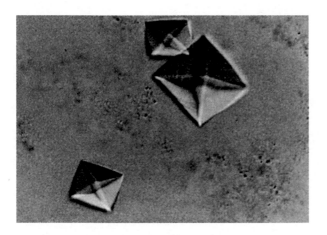

Plate 3 • Calcium oxalate dihydrate crystals commonly seen in nephrolithiasis. *N Engl J Med* 1992;326:1142. Used with permission.

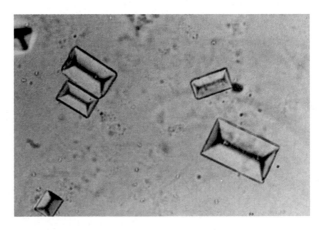

Plate 4 • Coffin-lid shaped struvite crystals commonly seen in nephrolithiasis. *N Engl J Med* 1992;326:1142. Used with permission.

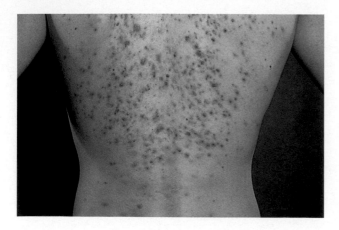

Plate 5 • Maculopapular rash on the back of a patient with acne vulgaris.

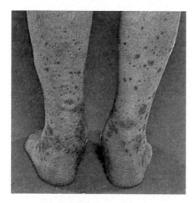

Plate 6 • Petechiae and purpura on the legs of a patient with allergic vasculitis.

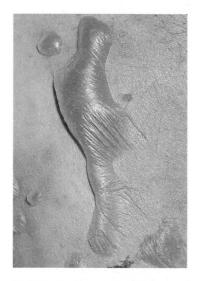

Plate 7 • Vesicles and bulla on a patient with bullous pemphigoid.

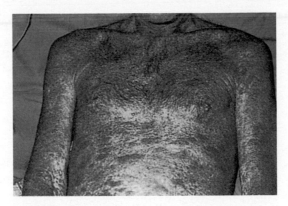

Plate 8 • Diffuse erythema on an AIDS patient with acute drug eruption.

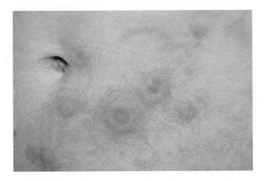

Plate 9 • Urticaria on a patient with acute allergic reaction.

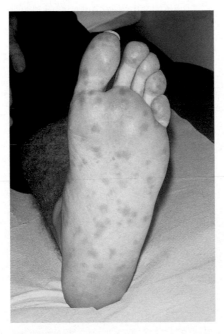

Plate 10 • Macular rash on the soles of the feet of a patient with secondary syphilis.

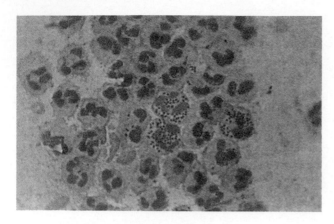

Plate 11 • Gram stain appearance of urethral discharge showing Gram-negative intracellular diplococci.

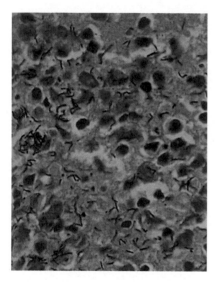

Plate 12 • Multiple acid-fast bacteria in a caseating mediastinal lymph node. Sputum samples from a patient with active primary pulmonary tuberculousis usually do not reveal such large numbers of organisms except in cases of military or cavitary disease.

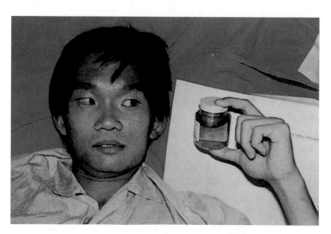

Plate 13 • Hepatitis A: Typical appearance of jaundice and dark urine in viral hepatitis; the patient is no longer suffering from fever or malaise.

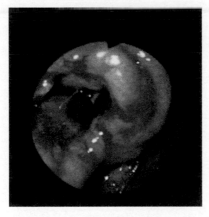

Plate 14 • Colonoscopic view of cecum showing annular ulcerated bleeding carcinoma.

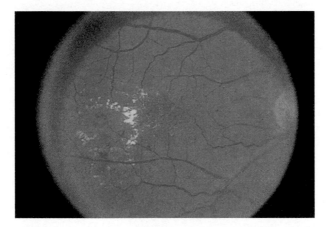

Plate 15 • Diabetic retinopathy fundoscopic examination shows microaneurysms (*red dots*) and hard exudates (*yellow patches*).

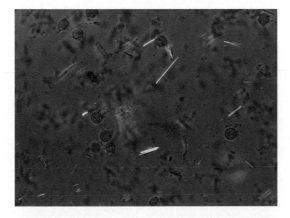

Plate 16 • Urate crystal (gout). Needle-shaped crystals that are yellow (negative birefringence) when parallel to the polarized light axis.

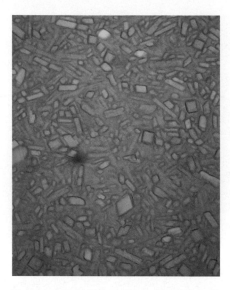

Plate 17 • Calcium pyrophosphate (pseudogout). Rhomboid-shaped crystals that are blue (positive birefringence) when parallel to the axis.

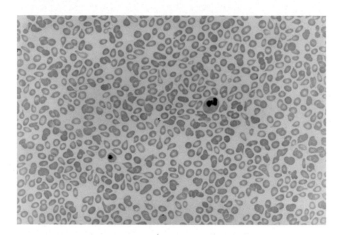

Plate 18 • Peripheral blood smear in myelofibrosis. Numerous teardrop cells are present.

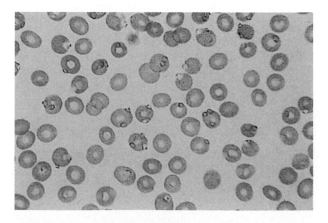

Plate 19 • Parasitic ring forms in malaria.

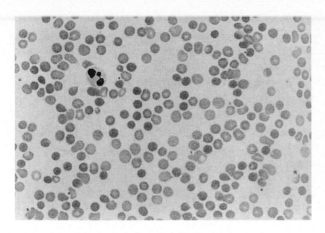

Plate 20 • Peripheral smear for question #1.

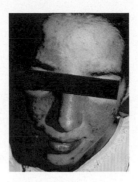

Plate 21 • Malar rash seen in systemic lupus erythematosus
(From Goodheart HP. *Goodheart's Photoguide of Common Skin Disorders,*
2nd ed. Philadelphia: Lippincott Williams & Wilkins, 2003.)

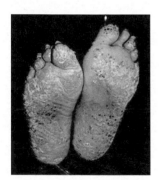

Plate 22 • Keratoderma blennorrhagica in reactive arthritis
(From Goodheart HP. *Goodheart's Photoguide of Common Skin Disorders,*
2nd ed. Philadelphia: Lippincott Williams & Wilkins, 2003.)

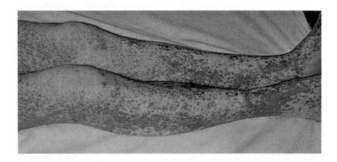

Plate 23 • Petechiae of the lower limbs due to severe thrombocytopenia associated with AML.

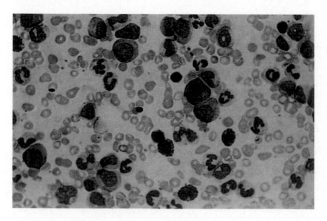

Plate 24 • Myeloblasts in peripheral smear in CML.

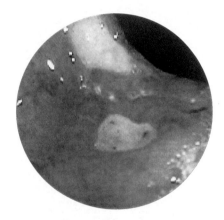

Plate 25 • Color plate for question 20
(From Rubin E, Gorstein F, Rubin R, et al. *Rubin's Pathology: Clinicopathologic Foundations of Medicine*, 4th ed. Baltimore: Lippincott Williams & Wilkins, 2005.)

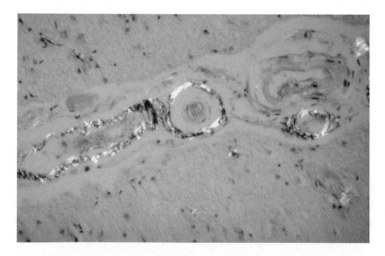

Plate 26 • Cerebrovascular amyloid in a case of Alzheimer disease. The section was stained with Congo red and examined under polarized light.

RISK FACTORS

A number of **risk factors** are associated with the development of colorectal cancer:

- History of adenomatous polyps
- Inflammatory bowel disease (greater in ulcerative colitis than Crohn disease)
- Familial disorders (familial adenomatous polyposis, hereditary nonpolyposis colorectal cancer)
- Personal history of another malignancy (ovarian, endometrial, breast)
- Family history of colon cancer in first-degree relatives

A number of studies have looked at dietary and lifestyle risk factors, with conflicting and inconclusive results. The strongest positive associations are as follows:

- High animal fat consumption (red meat)
- Low fiber consumption (lack of fruits and vegetables)
- Obesity
- Ethanol
- Refined sugar
- Cigarette smoking

There is the suggestion that regular use of aspirin may **lower** the incidence of colorectal cancer. Additionally, because high animal fat consumption and low fiber consumption is associated with increased risk, a number of studies have attempted to determine if certain dietary habits can be protective. Strong evidence indicates that increased dietary fiber may significantly reduce colon cancer risk, although prospective data are lacking.

CLINICAL MANIFESTATIONS

HISTORY

Most neoplastic colorectal lesions present without symptoms. Symptoms generally occur in more advanced (e.g., metastatic) disease. For this reason, screening (see later) is advocated for the detection of neoplasms in asymptomatic patients. When present, the most common **symptoms** of colorectal cancer are:

- Gastrointestinal (GI) bleeding (may be occult and variably associated with iron-deficiency anemia)

- Change in bowel habits (narrowed caliber of stool, chronic diarrhea, constipation)
- Abdominal pain
- Anorexia/weight loss (generally late, with advanced metastatic cancers)

PHYSICAL EXAMINATION

In a manner similar to the history, patients with colorectal cancer generally have few specific physical examination findings. A mass may be found on external palpation of the abdomen or on digital rectal examination, but this is uncommon.

DIAGNOSTIC EVALUATION

The main studies used for screening and diagnosis of colorectal cancer are as follows (Table 45-1):

- Fecal occult blood test
- Barium enema (Fig. 45-1)
- Sigmoidoscopy
- Colonoscopy (Color Plate 14)

While various combinations of modalities can be used for screening (see below), workup of patients with symptoms of colorectal cancer is generally done by colonoscopy, given the ability to directly visualize tumors and to obtain material to make a histopathologic diagnosis. In these patients, computed tomography can also be used as part of a staging workup, revealing local tumor extension, lymph node involvement and distant metastasis.

TREATMENT

The overall management of colorectal cancer involves both primary prevention, by reducing the potential risk factors listed earlier, and secondary prevention, by screening to detect and treat asymptomatic cancers and premalignant precursors. Multiple guidelines exist for the surveillance of colorectal cancer using the methods just listed (Table 45-2).

Polyps and carcinoma in situ are detected and then subsequently cured by excisional biopsy with sigmoidoscopy or colonoscopy. If invasive cancer is detected, the next step is to determine the local extent of the tumor and the presence of metastatic disease. Abdominal CT is generally of use for this staging.

■ TABLE 45-1 Tests for Colorectal Neoplasms*

Test	Characteristics	Advantages	Disadvantages
Fecal occult blood testing	Screening test with sensitivity and specificity approximately 50%; certain foods (rare red meat, radishes, broccoli) can give false-positive results; false negatives because of intermittent nature of blood loss	Inexpensive; easy to do	Poor sensitivity and specificity; does not localize source of blood loss (upper GI vs. lower GI)
Sigmoidoscopy	Screening examination; 60-cm flexible scope (formerly a 20- to 25-cm rigid scope was used)	Allows direct visualization and biopsy/removal of lesions; safer than colonoscopy; can be performed in the office without need for sedation/anesthesia	Inability to demonstrate lesions in the proximal colon, therefore lower sensitivity compared with barium enema and colonoscopy
Barium enema	Sensitivity of 80% to 90% for lesions >1 cm; sensitivity of 50% to 75% for lesions <1 cm	Allows visualization of proximal and distal colon; minimal discomfort to patient	Lower sensitivity for potentially clinically important but smaller lesions; no ability to biopsy/remove lesions
Colonoscopy	"Gold standard" for diagnosis; sensitivity of approximately 95%, near 100% sensitivity	Allows visualization of proximal and distal colon; allows direct visualization and biopsy/removal of lesions	High cost; increased risk to patient (sedation, possibility of perforation); uncomfortable for patient and requires extensive bowel preparation

*See http://cancer.gov/cancerinfo/pdq/screening/colorectal/healthprofessional/.

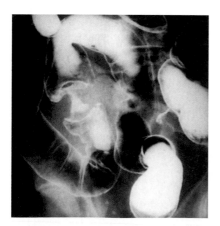

Figure 45-1 • Barium enema showing annular colonic carcinoma in the sigmoid colon. Note the shouldered margin giving the characteristic "apple core" appearance.

Colectomy is the treatment modality of choice for invasive colon cancer. Adjuvant therapy with chemotherapy and/or radiation therapy is added if the clinical situation warrants—generally, if there are nodal metastases. Colon cancer with nodal metastases is generally treated with postoperative 5-fluorouracil (5-FU) and levamisole. Because of the higher risk of local recurrences, rectal cancers characterized by invasion through the muscularis, with or without nodal disease, and all tumors with nodal involvement are treated with surgery plus postoperative 5-FU and high-dose pelvic irradiation.

Once colorectal neoplasms are discovered and treated, monitoring for recurrence must be maintained because the patient is now at higher than average risk for future neoplasms. This includes patients who are discovered to have benign polyps as well as those with malignant disease.

■ TABLE 45-2 Guidelines for Colorectal Cancer Screening

Risk Factor	Recommendation
None	Starting at age 50: annual fecal occult blood test, digital rectal examination, flexible sigmoidoscopy every 3 to 5 years *or* colonoscopy every 10 years
Ulcerative colitis	Colonoscopy after 8 to 10 years of disease, then surveillance colonoscopy every 1 to 2 years
Adenomatous polyps	Surveillance colonoscopy every 3 to 5 years after excision—every 1 to 3 years if multiple, large (>1 cm), villous, malignant (noninvasive)
Familial polyposis disorder (suspected)	Genetic counseling ± screening, flexible sigmoidoscopy by age 20
Familial nonpolyposis disorder (suspected)	Genetic counseling ± screening, colonoscopy or barium enema by age 35 to 40 (or 10 years younger than youngest relative diagnosed with colon cancer), then surveillance every 3 to 5 years
Positive family history	Screening as for average risk; consider barium enema or colonoscopy

Note: This table is a synthesis of a number of guidelines. Individual guidelines can be found at the National Guideline Clearinghouse: http://www.guideline.gov.

 KEY POINTS

- Colorectal cancers are believed to arise from malignant transformation of benign adenomatous polyps.
- Environmental and dietary factors are believed to play a role in the development of colorectal neoplasms, and primary prevention may be possible.
- Fecal occult blood testing, sigmoidoscopy, barium enema, and colonoscopy are the commonly available screening and diagnostic tests.
- Early detection via screening, the intensity of which is tailored to relative risk, may result in significant decreases in mortality.
- Surgery, followed by chemotherapy and/or radiation for more extensive disease, is the therapy of choice for invasive disease.

Part 6

Endocrine

46 Weight Loss

Maintenance of weight is determined by the balance of caloric intake and metabolic consumption of calories. Whereas obesity is usually caused by benign excess caloric intake and insufficient exercise, **involuntary weight loss** is usually a sign of underlying serious systemic disease and associated with up to 25% mortality within 18 months. Involuntary weight loss often leads a patient to seek medical care, in particular because of concern regarding underlying malignancy. However, the underlying causes of weight loss are actually quite numerous, and the differential diagnosis can be outlined according to the pathophysiology. Involuntary weight loss of 5% or more of body weight in <12 months should prompt medical evaluation.

PATHOGENESIS

The **mechanisms of pathologic weight loss** include alterations of the balance of dietary intake and metabolic output. Dietary intake is linked to appetite, which is controlled by the hypothalamus and related neurohormonal processes. Leptin works through this process, suppressing release of a hypothalamic appetite stimulant. Gastrointestinal (GI) peptides (glucagons, somatostatin, ghrelin, cholecystokinin) also signal satiety. Chronic inflammatory cytokines (e.g., tumor necrosis factor-α [TNF-α] and interferon gamma) can induce cachexia by reducing appetite while also increasing metabolic demand. Metabolic output is largely related to basal metabolic needs. For the average person, approximately half of ingested food energy is used for basal processes such as maintaining normal body temperature; approximately 40% is used for exercise, and 10% is used for digestion and metabolism itself.

ETIOLOGY

The causes of involuntary weight loss can be categorized based on their primary effects on caloric intake or caloric output.

- **Decreased intake:** Elderly patients are at risk for a number of conditions that limit intake of calories, including the five Ds: depression, dementia, poor dentition, dysgeusia (altered taste), and side effects of drugs. Malignancy, chronic heart or lung disease, advanced human immunodeficiency virus (HIV) infection, adrenal insufficiency, or hypercalcemia may also lead to anorexia. Conditions that lead to abdominal pain with eating (cholelithiasis, chronic mesenteric ischemia, gastric ulcer) cause the patient to decrease food intake. In anorexia nervosa, patients limit intake but are not concerned with the weight loss (in fact, they show a preoccupation with being too heavy).

- **Decreased absorption:** Malabsorption limits the uptake of nutrients. Major causes include amyloidosis (Chapter 62), pancreatic insufficiency, celiac sprue, inflammatory bowel disease (Chapter 40), intestinal parasites, and cholestasic liver disease (Chapter 43).

- **Accelerated metabolism:** Many illnesses increase basal metabolic energy expenditure. Hyperthyroidism, chronic infection (e.g., tuberculosis, subacute bacterial endocarditis), and malignancy lead to increased metabolic demand. In malignancy, a combination of accelerated metabolism mediated by cytokines and anorexia is the usual mechanism. The cytokine TNF, produced in response to certain malignancies, was originally called *cachectin* because of its effect on body mass. Cancers directly involving a segment of the GI system can also interfere with the digestion and/or absorption of food. An **increased adrenergic state** (such as in pheochromocytoma or amphetamine abuse) also increases metabolic demand.

- **Accelerated caloric loss:** Excessive caloric loss through nonmetabolic paths includes persistent vomiting, chronic diarrhea, fistulous drainage, and diabetic glucosuria.

CLINICAL MANIFESTATIONS

Evidence for an underlying etiology can usually be found with a careful history and physical examination. **Loss of appetite** and a **dietary history** are important factors in all patients. Patients with weight loss from excess metabolic demand often describe increased appetite and food consumption. However, elderly patients may have apathetic hyperthyroidism (see Chapter 47). Medications should be reviewed to look for those medicines that affect appetite. Because GI and lung cancers are the most common malignancies associated with involuntary weight loss, history should address risk factors and symptoms of those diseases (see Chapters 45 and 19). **Fever** and **night sweats** are associated with tuberculosis and lymphoma. Patients with **malabsorption** can report increased flatulence, steatorrhea, and abdominal pain after meals. **Symptoms of depression** should be assessed, particularly in the elderly patient. In addition to loss of appetite, a depressed patient can have difficulty with sleep (too much or too little), loss of interest in activities or work, feelings of worthlessness or guilt, and decreased concentration. In the elderly, depression is about as frequent a cause of unexplained weight loss as an occult malignancy. A thorough review of systems can sometimes localize a particular etiology, such as malignancy. A travel history can reveal risks for intestinal parasites.

On physical examination, the patient's weight should be documented and compared with previous values. Oral thrush indicates immune deficiency. The thyroid should be assessed for enlargement or nodularity. Cardiopulmonary examination may reveal chronic disease. Examination for possible malignancy should include lymph node exam, rectal exam, and breast exam. A detailed exam of the abdomen and pelvis is necessary to assess for abdominal masses or malignant hepatomegaly. Skin may show pallor or jaundice.

DIAGNOSTIC EVALUATION

Provided a specific cause is not readily apparent after a thorough history and physical examination, it is reasonable to send the following **initial screening tests:**

- Complete blood count (CBC) (with differential)
- ESR (usually significantly elevated with malignancies, chronic infections, and chronic inflammatory conditions)
- Albumin level (can provide an assessment of the degree of malnutrition)
- Liver function tests (LFTs)
- Serum calcium level
- Screening thyroid-stimulating hormone (TSH) (see Chapter 47)
- Fasting glucose level
- Urinalysis angina (UA)
- Chest radiograph (especially in smokers)

These tests are relatively inexpensive and can detect a variety of conditions that may cause weight loss. **HIV antibody testing** can be performed in a patient with any risk factors. Additional diagnostic tests should be performed only to confirm a diagnosis suggested by the preliminary workup. The patient with a history suggestive of malabsorption can be assessed with qualitative examination for fecal fat, stool exam for ova and parasites, and serum B_{12} levels.

When the initial evaluation is suggestive of an abdominal process, **abdominal CT** may be considered, given the high frequency of GI etiologies. Upper and/or lower GI **endoscopy** may be considered for malignancy screening as well as diagnostic biopsy when malabsorption is a prominent feature.

In general, extensive workup searching for occult malignancy is not warranted if the initial evaluation is unrevealing. Routine age-based and gender-based cancer screening examinations should be encouraged as usual. The patient should be closely followed for new symptoms and continued weight loss. Some conditions that can escape detection on initial evaluation include pancreatic cancer, amyloidosis, and depression.

TREATMENT

If a specific cause is found, correction of this etiology, if possible, is of obvious importance. **Calorie supplementation** to promote the restoration of body mass may also be appropriate while correcting the underlying abnormality. This can be accomplished by enteral or parenteral means. In the absence of complicating conditions (e.g., aspiration risk, obstructing lesions), the enteral route is generally preferred. Parenteral therapy requires the placement of an indwelling catheter with its attendant risks. In patients with anorexia, a number of pharmacologic agents can be used to improve appetite, including cannabinoid derivatives (dronabinol) and certain progestational agents (megestrol acetate).

 KEY POINTS

- Involuntary weight loss occurs through one or more of the following mechanisms: decreased intake, decreased absorption, accelerated metabolism, or accelerated caloric loss.
- Malignancy, depression, and benign (nonmalignant) GI causes are the most common etiologies detected in patients with weight loss.
- Risk factors for malignancies, especially lung and GI malignancies, should be taken into account when evaluating a patient with weight loss.
- Elderly patients can have atypical presentations for both hyperthyroidism and depression. Symptoms of depression and TSH should be assessed for all patients with involuntary weight loss.

Hyperthyroidism

Hyperthyroidism is characterized by oversecretion of thyroid hormone. In the normal physiologic state, elevated levels of free thyroxine (FT_4) or triiodothyronine (T_3) give feedback to the pituitary gland, resulting in suppression of thyroid-stimulating hormone (TSH). Hyperthyroidism results from autonomous thyroid nodules, diffuse thyroid hormone overproduction (Grave's disease), damage to the thyroid (subacute thyroiditis), or rarely TSH overproduction (pituitary disease).

EPIDEMIOLOGY

Hyperthyroidism occurs more often in women. Grave's disease is the primary cause of hyperthyroidism in younger individuals, generally occurring between 20 and 50 years of age, but it can also occur in the elderly. There does appear to be a genetic predisposition to Grave's disease based on twin concordance studies. Multinodular goiter is more common in the elderly. Smoking is a risk factor for both Grave's disease and multinodular goiter. Subacute thyroiditis tends to occur in middle age (30 to 50 years of age). Pituitary diseases resulting in excess TSH secretion are rare.

ETIOLOGY AND PATHOGENESIS

Grave's disease is an autoimmune thyroid disease caused by production of antibodies to the thyroid gland's TSH receptor. These antibodies stimulate the receptor and are therefore called thyroid-stimulating immunoglobulins (TSIs). Receptor stimulation then leads to increased thyroid gland hormone production. In the hyperthyroidism from thyroid nodules in **multinodular goiter**, autonomously secreting nodules produce thyroid hormone without need for TSH receptor stimulation.

Subacute thyroiditis includes granulomatous and lymphocytic thyroiditis. Granulomatous thyroiditis, also known as de Quervain or painful thyroiditis, is most likely viral in origin, often following a flulike syndrome. The initial inflammatory process causes thyroid follicle destruction with release of thyroid hormones. As the initial hyperthyroidism abates, there can follow a period of hypothyroidism during glandular recovery and restoration of euthyroid secretion. Lymphocytic thyroiditis (painless or silent thyroiditis) appears to be an autoimmune process, also causing a brief thyrotoxic state followed by hypothyroidism then resolution. It is often seen in postpartum women. Hashimoto thyroiditis, a chronic autoimmune thyroiditis that causes chronic hypothyroidism, may initially present with hyperthyroidism.

Ectopic thyroid hormone production is a rare cause of hyperthyroidism. Ovarian teratomas (struma ovarii) or functional metastatic thyroid cancer are two such rare etiologies.

CLINICAL FINDINGS

HISTORY

Symptoms of hyperthyroidism are:

- Heat intolerance
- Palpitations
- Weight loss
- Nervousness
- Fatigue and weakness
- Oligomenorrhea
- Frequent or loose bowel movements

The elderly are more likely to present with **apathetic hyperthyroidism**, characterized by weight loss, anorexia, and fatigue.

Neck pain mimicking pharyngitis is a prominent feature in de Quervain thyroiditis and can be associated with a fever. An abrupt onset of symptoms may follow an upper respiratory illness. As you might expect, silent thyroiditis can present subtly; clinicians must remember to address suggestive symptoms in postpartum patients.

The history should also investigate the possibility of **ingestion of excess exogenous thyroid hormone**. The most obvious mechanism is iatrogenic overreplacement with levothyroxine for other thyroid diseases. However, patients may also ingest excess bovine thyroid hormone by eating ground beef prepared from neck muscles. Finally, some patients inadvertently or surreptitiously abuse levothyroxine, usually as a method of weight loss. Healthcare professionals with medical knowledge and access to drugs may be more likely to do this than other patients.

A **recent iodine exposure** (such as a diagnostic study with IV contrast material) may precipitate hyperthyroidism in the patient with a multinodular gland. This is known as the Jod-Basedow effect. **Amiodarone** is an antiarrhythmic medication that can contribute to hyperthyroidism in a small percentage of patients. The excess iodine in amiodarone can lead to increased production (in patients with autonomous nodules), or amiodarone can directly cause a thyroiditis (by inflammation or direct injury).

PHYSICAL EXAMINATION

Tachycardia is present in most patients, and an irregular pulse may be a sign of atrial fibrillation. Fever can be present in subacute thyroiditis.

Signs of the high metabolism seen in hyperthyroidism include:

- Warm, moist skin
- Lid lag (upper eyelid does not cover sclera above iris with downward gaze)
- Tremor

Thyroid examination reveals an enlarged, painless thyroid in Grave's disease. With TSH-producing pituitary macroadenomas, the thyroid is also diffusely enlarged and nontender. In granulocytic (de Quervain's) thyroiditis, the gland is exquisitely tender. Nodules may be palpated in thyroid adenoma (single) or multinodular goiter (multiple). Patients taking excessive exogenous hormone have nonpalpable glands.

Two findings are seen exclusively in Grave's disease. **Proptosis** is visible protrusion of the eye and believed to be secondary to an autoimmune reaction in the retro-orbital space. **Pretibial myxedema** is a brawny thickening of skin in the lower extremities. Although the name *myxedema* suggests it is seen in hypothyroidism, it is a feature of hyperthyroidism.

DIFFERENTIAL DIAGNOSIS

The differential diagnosis of **hyperthyroidism** can be divided physiologically by iodine uptake on thyroid scan (see later).

High Uptake
- Grave's disease
- Toxic multinodular goiter
- Solitary adenoma
- TSH-secreting pituitary tumor (rare)

Low Uptake
- Thyroiditis
- Exogenous thyroid use
- Ovarian teratoma (struma ovarii)
- Metastatic functional thyroid cancer

DIAGNOSTIC EVALUATION

The initial step in diagnosing hyperthyroidism is the presence of an increased FT_4. When associated with a **decreased TSH** (<0.05 μU per L), the hyperthyroidism is considered primary. When associated with an increased TSH (>5.0), the hyperthyroidism is considered secondary (rare). Free T_4 is preferred to total T_4, which is influenced by increases in thyroid-binding globulin (TBG). If FT_4 is normal (but TSH is low), the patient may have T_3 thyrotoxicosis (elevated T_3 levels) or subclinical hyperthyroidism. A low TSH can also be seen in patients recovering from illness, but the FT_4 and T_3 are normal (Fig. 47-1).

A **thyroid scan** is used to evaluate uptake of radioactive iodine (RAI) in the thyroid gland. The RAI used is ^{123}I, which is different from the ^{131}I used to ablate the thyroid gland (see Treatment). Normal uptake is 30%. Low uptake ($<5\%$) in the setting of hyperthyroidism indicates either damage to the gland or an ectopic source of T_4 (see Differential Diagnosis).

Antithyroid peroxidase antibody (formerly known as antimicrosomal antibody) is present in autoimmune thyroid diseases (Grave's disease, lymphocytic thyroiditis). Antithyroglobulin antibody is less commonly seen in Grave's disease. These antibodies do

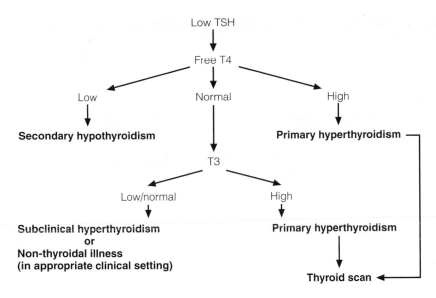

Figure 47-1 • Diagnostic approach to the patient with low TSH.

not add much additional information to the clinical presentation and thyroid scan. In multinodular goiter, nodule biopsy is not necessary unless there is a clearly dominant or enlarging nodule. An electrocardiogram (**ECG**) may show atrial fibrillation or sinus tachycardia with any etiology of hyperthyroidism.

TREATMENT

Patients with **thyroiditis** improve on their own in a few weeks. Management consists of treating the hyperthyroid symptoms (tachycardia, nervousness) with β-blockers (see later) until hyperthyroidism resolves. In de Quervain (painful) thyroiditis, a short course of nonsteroidal anti-inflammatory drugs (NSAIDs) or glucocorticoids (prednisone, 20 to 40 mg daily) results in prompt resolution of the pain and inflammation. Patients recovering from hyperthyroidism caused by thyroiditis should be monitored for a recurrence of symptoms or progression to hypothyroidism. The resultant hypothyroidism may require thyroid hormone replacement therapy, although patients usually recover normal thyroid function after weeks to months.

In diseases characterized by **overproduction of thyroid hormone** (e.g., Grave's disease, autonomous nodules), treatment is aimed at **reducing T₄ production** by:

- Radioactive iodine
- Antithyroid drugs (methimazole, propylthiouracil)
- Surgery

RAI has the advantage of being highly effective but usually requires lifelong replacement therapy because of destruction of the thyroid gland in Grave's disease. Overactive thyroid adenomas may preferentially take up iodine, destroying the adenoma and leaving the normal gland intact. The dose given to the patient depends on the size and iodine uptake of the gland. RAI should *not* be used in pregnant women because of the risk of fetal hypothyroidism. Despite earlier concerns, there appears to be no long-term risk of increased cancer in patients treated with RAI. It has become a popular treatment for Grave's disease given the simplicity of the regimen (one dose) and the success rate. The risk of hypothyroidism, however, following RAI approaches 90% and is permanent.

Antithyroid drugs interfere with the production of T₄. In Grave's disease, these drugs are associated with a remission rate of 30% to 50%. Table 47-1 lists the features of the two antithyroid drugs used (methimazole and propylthiouracil). Methimazole has the advantage of once-daily dosing, although it is a second-line agent in pregnancy because of early reports of an increased incidence of scalp defects (aplasia cutis) in newborns.

Major side effects of antithyroid drugs include:

- Agranulocytosis
- Hepatitis

Fever or sore throat may be the first sign of agranulocytosis in patients taking these medications. Patients should be instructed to seek medical attention if these symptoms occur.

Surgery is usually reserved for a patient who fails medication and RAI or who has an extremely large

■ TABLE 47-1 Antithyroid Drugs

	Usual Initial Dose	Half-Life	Use in Pregnancy
Propylthiouracil	100 mg 3 times per day	1 to 3 hr	Yes
Methimazole	30 mg once daily	6 to 8 hr	Maybe

goiter causing difficulty swallowing or airway compromise. A subtotal thyroidectomy is performed in Grave's disease or multinodular goiter, whereas solitary nodules are removed with preservation of the gland. Complications of thyroid surgery include recurrent laryngeal nerve paralysis and hypoparathyroidism (leading to hypocalcemia).

Before antithyroid medications or RAI takes effect, relief of symptoms (palpitations, tremor) with a beta adrenergic blocker is important. **Propranolol** (20 to 40 mg 2 to 4 times daily) has the added benefit of preventing conversion of T_4 to the more active T_3. However, the convenience of once daily dosing makes atenolol a common choice.

In subclinical (asymptomatic) hyperthyroidism, some advocate treating elderly patients because they are at increased risk for atrial fibrillation and osteoporosis with long-standing subclinical hyperthyroidism.

KEY POINTS

- Hyperthyroidism is diagnosed by the presence of increased FT_4. TSH is suppressed in primary hyperthyroidism (common) and increased in secondary hypothyroidism (pituitary, rare). An exception is T_3 thyrotoxicosis (T_3 high and FT_4 normal).

- The most common causes of hyperthyroidism are Grave's disease and mutlinodular goiter.

- A thyroid scan is useful to differentiate the etiologies into high-uptake and low-uptake causes. Important causes of a low-uptake scan and hyperthyroidism include thyroiditis and surreptitious use of thyroid hormone.

- Hyperthyroidism may be treated by radioactive iodine or antithyroid drugs. Most patients treated with RAI eventually become hypothyroid.

Hypothyroidism

Hypothyroidism is characterized by underproduction of thyroid hormone. In primary hypothyroidism, low levels of thyroid hormone result in an increased production of thyroid-stimulating hormone (TSH) by the pituitary (high TSH, low free T_4). When TSH production is increased to maintain normal thyroid hormone levels (high TSH, normal free T_4), this is called subclinical hypothyroidism. In secondary hypothyroidism, thyroid hormone production is reduced because of inappropriately low pituitary TSH production (low TSH, low free T_4).

Although hypothyroidism is often suspected in patients with common complaints such as fatigue and weight gain, many patients with hypothyroidism are completely asymptomatic. Conversely, profound hypothyroidism may present with **myxedema coma**.

EPIDEMIOLOGY AND PATHOGENESIS

The incidence of hypothyroidism (both overt and subclinical) is between 2% and 10%. The most common cause of hypothyroidism worldwide is **iodine deficiency**. Iodine deficiency is rare in the United States and Europe, but it is still prevalent in parts of Africa and Asia. In the United States, dietary iodine is sufficient and hypothyroidism is usually caused by an autoimmune disease (e.g., Hashimoto thyroiditis) or iatrogenesis (following radiation treatment).

Hashimoto thyroiditis occurs more often in **women**, typically presenting between 30 and 50 years of age, but is also common at older ages. The thyroid gland suffers lymphocytic infiltration with follicular atrophy and cytotoxic thyroid cell destruction.

RISK FACTORS

Patients with a history of other so-called autoimmune diseases are at increased risk for autoimmune hypothyroidism. These diseases include diabetes mellitus, Addison disease, pernicious anemia, and vitiligo. A family history of thyroid disease also increases a patient's risk. Patients with a history of head and neck **irradiation** are at risk for hypothyroidism because of either primary thyroid failure (neck radiation) or panhypopituitarism (cranial irradiation).

CLINICAL FINDINGS

HISTORY

Symptoms of hypothyroidism include:

- Cold intolerance
- Weight gain
- Fatigue
- Constipation
- Hoarseness
- Memory loss
- Menstrual changes
- Decreased libido
- Dry skin

In the elderly, symptoms of hypothyroidism are often incorrectly ascribed to aging. Patients may also present for evaluation of a condition associated with hypothyroidism, such as **carpal tunnel syndrome**, or **anemia**. History should note any prior radioactive iodine therapy or head and neck irradiation. Medication survey should include amiodarone and lithium use. Amiodarone contains a high iodine load, with resultant inhibitory effects on the deiodinase that converts T_4 to T_3. **Lithium ingestion** impairs secretion of thyroid hormone and may cause hypothyroidism in certain individuals.

PHYSICAL EXAMINATION

Diastolic blood pressure (BP) is often mildly elevated in hypothyroidism. In severe cases, bradycardia and hypothermia are present. Some patients have dry skin, coarse hair, retarded nail growth, and thinning of the lateral third of the eyebrows.

A **goiter**, or enlarged thyroid, is often present in patients with Hashimoto thyroiditis. The gland is firm and sometimes lobulated. The gland may not be palpable after radiation or ablative therapy.

Neurologic examination may be notable for a **delayed relaxation of deep tendon reflexes**. Carpal tunnel syndrome may be evident, with median nerve compromise. Patients with **myxedema** have a characteristic edematous face with periorbital edema and nonpitting pretibial edema. Myxedema coma is a late and severe manifestation, with depression of all organ systems including the cardiac, respiratory, and central nervous systems.

DIFFERENTIAL DIAGNOSIS

The causes of **hypothyroidism** include:

Primary Hypothyroidism
- Hashimoto (chronic lymphocytic) thyroiditis
- Iodine deficiency
- Recovery from subacute thyroiditis (transient)
- Lithium or amiodarone use
- Postradiation or postablative therapy
- Infiltrative disorders (amyloidosis, sarcoidosis, scleroderma)

Secondary Hypothyroidism
- Panhypopituitarism
- Hypothalamic disease

DIAGNOSTIC EVALUATION

The characteristic laboratory values for primary hypothyroidism are a **low or low-normal free thyroxine (T_4)**, in association with an **elevated TSH** (>5 µU/ml). In secondary/central hypothyroidism, as seen in panhypopituitarism, TSH is low to normal (see Chapter 53). Patients with an elevated TSH but normal free T_4 are said to have subclinical (or compensated) hypothyroidism.

Nonthyroid studies that can be abnormal in hypothyroidism include:

- Hypercholesterolemia and hypertriglyceridemia
- Elevated creatine phosphokinase
- Anemia
- Abnormal electrocardiogram (ECG) (decreased voltage, T-wave flattening)

Thyroid autoantibodies (**TPO antibody** and **thyroglobulin antibody**) are found in Hashimoto thyroiditis and are useful in confirming the autoimmune diagnosis. They are negative, however, in a small percentage of patients with autoimmune thyroid disease. Fine-needle aspiration biopsy is very rarely needed for the diagnosis of autoimmune thyroiditis.

TREATMENT

MANAGEMENT STRATEGY

Treatment in hypothyroidism is based on the severity of symptoms and the degree of hypothyroidism. Patients with subclinical hypothyroidism may be followed without treatment. Approximately 5% of these patients each year progress to symptomatic hypothyroidism. When treatment is instituted, therapy consists of exogenous thyroid hormone because the underlying cause of hypothyroidism is usually not correctable (with the exception of iodine deficiency). **Levothyroxine** is the treatment of choice because of its long half-life (1 week) and once-daily dosing. The typical dose is 1.7 µg per kg body weight, with most patients controlled with between 100 and 150 µg daily. The **speed of the replacement** depends on the patient's age and medical condition. In the elderly and in patients with known coronary artery disease, replacement should be started on a low dose (25 µg) that is increased in 25-µg increments every few weeks advanced slowly over months. Patients with myxedema coma are rapidly treated with intravenous levothyroxine (300 to 500 µg bolus, followed by 50 to 100 µg daily).

An important caveat is needed for patients with suspected **panhypopituitarism** or **myxedema coma**. Because these patients often have concomitant adrenal insufficiency, thyroid replacement may increase the metabolism of the small amount of the body's remaining cortisol, thereby precipitating an **adrenal** crisis. Therefore, patients with known or highly suspected panhypopituitarism and patients with myxedema coma should always begin hydrocortisone treatment prior to thyroid replacement therapy.

CONTINUED CARE

Levothyroxine therapy should be monitored by following **serum TSH**. Initially, TSH should be measured every 4 to 6 weeks (reflecting the time required to achieve a steady state with a medication that has a one-week half-life). Patients often feel least symptomatic when TSH is on the low end of normal. However, overreplacement increases the risk of atrial fibrillation and excessive bone loss. Once a stable replacement dose is achieved, TSH can be monitored every 6 months. It is important to inform the patient of medication interactions with levothyroxine; calcium, ferrous sulfate, and antacids with aluminum hydroxide can interfere with thyroid hormone absorption.

Patients with a history of radiation exposure are at increased risk for **thyroid cancer**, and physical examination should concentrate on the presence of new nodules that may represent cancer. Patients with Hashimoto thyroiditis have an increased incidence of **thyroid lymphoma**, which usually presents as an enlarging thyroid mass. Therapeutic radioactive iodine does *not* apparently increase the risk of thyroid malignancy.

KEY POINTS

- Hashimoto thyroiditis is an autoimmune disease that is the most common cause of hypothyroidism in the United States. Most patients have anti-TPO antibodies.

- Patients with a low T_4 and low-to-normal TSH may have central (pituitary) hypothyroidism.

- Many signs and symptoms of hypothyroidism (fatigue, weight gain, constipation, hypercholesterolemia) are common and nonspecific. TSH is therefore commonly tested for many complaints.

- Replacement of thyroid hormone in patients with central hypopituitarism or myxedema coma may cause adrenal crisis by increasing the metabolism of cortisol.

- Levothyroxine therapy is monitored by following TSH levels. TSH takes weeks to months to respond to a new dose of levothyroxine. Replacement should be instituted slowly in the elderly and in patients with coronary artery disease.

Diabetes Mellitus

Diabetes mellitus (DM) is a chronic metabolic disorder characterized by abnormal regulation of glucose, resulting in hyperglycemia. It is a serious cause of morbidity and mortality. In the United States, it is the leading cause of adult blindness and end-stage renal disease.

DM is subdivided on the basis of its etiology. Type 1 DM is caused by autoimmune destruction of the pancreas leading to insulin deficiency; type 2 DM is caused by peripheral resistance to insulin, and hyperglycemia develops despite above-average levels of insulin. The old term "non–insulin-dependent" DM to describe type 2 DM was misleading because many patients with type 2 DM eventually require insulin for control of hyperglycemia. Similarly, age-related terms such as "adult onset" or "juvenile" are no longer in use because type 1 and type 2 DM can occur in widely overlapping age ranges.

EPIDEMIOLOGY

Type 2 DM is a major public health problem in the United States, affecting approximately 8% of the population. Risk factors include family history, older age, and obesity. Because of the rising problem of childhood obesity, type 2 DM continues to grow as a national problem. According to the Centers for Disease Control and Prevention, the lifetime risk of type 2 DM for individuals born in 2000 is approximately 35%. Prevalence of type 2 DM is highest in Native Americans and Pima Indians. Blacks and Hispanics have intermediate risk, and whites have lowest risk (still approximately 7%). Type 2 DM often presents in persons in their fourth or fifth decade, but it is increasingly being seen in the obese young.

Type 1 DM is less prevalent, affecting only approximately 0.5% of the world population. It presents in childhood and adolescence, with a peak at approximately 14 years of age. Family history of type 1 DM is a risk factor.

PATHOPHYSIOLOGY

Type 1 DM begins with **autoimmune destruction** of the pancreatic islet beta cells. However, an environmental trigger (perhaps a viral infection or early childhood dietary antigen exposure) is necessary to promote autoimmunity because genetic predisposition alone does not seem to be sufficient. Without insulin, these patients are prone to develop **ketoacidosis**, which is caused by the lack of insulin and the increased release of glucagon. This leads to increased gluconeogenesis, release of fatty acids, and oxidation of fatty acids to form ketone bodies. Glucagon accelerates the oxidation of fatty acids by increasing their carnitine-mediated transport into the mitochondria, where the oxidation occurs.

Type 2 DM is characterized by **peripheral insulin resistance**, impaired regulation of hepatic gluconeogenesis, and a relative impairment of beta-cell function. Insulin resistance, characterized by hyperinsulinemia without frank hyperglycemia, is the earliest detectable abnormality and may precede the diagnosis of DM by years. Eventually, beta cells are unable to compensate, and insulin levels are inadequate to maintain normoglycemia. In addition, rising glucose levels may further inhibit beta-cell function (glucotoxicity). The abnormalities in type 2 DM leading to insulin resistance are the result of genetic predisposition and weight gain. Weight loss, exercise, and decreased caloric intake improve sensitivity to insulin.

Hyperglycemia contributes to the long-term **microvascular** complications of diabetes: retinopathy, nephropathy, and neuropathy. The incidence of complications increases with worsening glucose control and longer duration of disease. In addition, patients with DM are at increased risk for **macrovascular** complications, including coronary artery disease, peripheral vascular disease, and stroke.

CLINICAL MANIFESTATIONS

HISTORY

Patients with type 1 DM who present with diabetic ketoacidosis appear quite ill and complain of nausea, vomiting, and polyuria. In contrast, patients with type 2 DM are often asymptomatic or minimally symptomatic, and the condition is discovered by routine testing. A positive family history of DM and a personal history of obesity are often present in type 2 diabetics. Symptomatic patients often present with polyuria, polydipsia, polyphagia, fatigue, or blurred vision. Patients with poor wound healing or recurrent candidal vaginitis should also be tested for DM. A minority of patients initially present with a manifestation of microvascular or macrovascular complications, such as peripheral numbness (neuropathy), loss of vision (retinopathy), angina (coronary artery disease), or claudication or impotence (peripheral vascular disease).

PHYSICAL EXAMINATION

The physical examination in patients with DM focuses on end-organ complications. Funduscopic examination should be performed to look for **retinopathy** (see Color Plate 15). Nonproliferative retinopathy consists of microaneurysms, hard exudates (vascular leakage), soft exudates (ischemic injury), and macular edema. Proliferative retinopathy is a result of overcompensation for an ischemic retina and produces neovascularization of the retina or optic disc. Because direct funduscopic examination is not sensitive for many of these changes, a dilated pupil examination with a slit lamp should be performed at least annually on these patients.

Patients with **peripheral neuropathy** have decreased sensation to vibration and light touch, initially in the feet and then in the hands (stocking-and-glove pattern). If sensation is severely impaired, foot ulcers may appear over areas of increased pressure such as metatarsophalangeal joints. Another complication is autonomic neuropathy, often presenting as orthostatic hypotension. Examination should also look for evidence of coronary artery disease (increased jugular venous pressure [JVP], fourth heart sound, displaced point of maximal impulse) and peripheral vascular disease (decreased peripheral pulses, bruits).

Patients presenting in diabetic ketoacidosis should be assessed for dehydration and should be fully examined for possible precipitating illnesses such as infection and myocardial infarction.

DIFFERENTIAL DIAGNOSIS

Not all patients with hyperglycemia have type 1 or type 2 diabetes; the following may also increase blood glucose levels:

- Drugs (e.g., corticosteroids, thiazide diuretics, protease inhibitors)
- Administration of dextrose-containing IV fluids
- Excess secretion of the counterregulatory hormones (acromegaly, Cushing syndrome, pheochromocytoma)
- Stress (via catecholamine release)

In addition, some patients have DM because of underlying disorders that should be considered at the time of the initial diagnosis:

- Hemochromatosis (iron overload)
- Pancreatic exocrine insufficiency (acute or chronic pancreatitis, pancreatectomy, cystic fibrosis)

DIAGNOSTIC EVALUATION

To make the diagnosis of DM, one of the following criteria must be present:

- Fasting glucose (FG) level >125 mg per dL (normal <100 mg per dL)
- Random glucose level >200 mg per dL with symptoms (polyuria, polydipsia, unexplained weight loss)
- 2-hour glucose level >200 mg per dL during a 75-g oral glucose tolerance test (OGTT)

To diagnose DM definitely, one of these criteria must be confirmed on a subsequent day. Impaired fasting glucose (defined by fasting glucose from 100 to 125 mg per dL) is a predictor of the progression to DM and should be formally diagnosed for patient education and intervention purposes. Impaired glucose tolerance is infrequently assessed in nonpregnant patients. Gestational DM has specific criteria based on a 100-g OGTT and is not discussed further in this chapter.

Once the diagnosis of DM is confirmed, glucose control may be assessed by self-monitoring of glucose and measuring the **glycosylated hemoglobin** (HbA1c). Normally, 3.8% to 6.3% of the total hemoglobin is glycosylated, and this proportion rises directly with the average blood glucose level. Given the average 120-day life span of a red blood cell (RBC), measurement of HbA1c gives an indication of the level of blood glucose over a 3-month period.

Initial laboratory evaluation of DM should include differential diagnostic assessments as indicated by the patient's history. Iron studies to assess hereditary hemochromatosis should be performed in whites and those with suggestive family histories. Cystic fibrosis is usually apparent by history. When chronic pancreatitis is suspected, abdominal computed tomography (CT) is often needed for confirmation.

Patients should be assessed for diabetic complications. Diabetic nephropathy is indicated by albuminuria. Because the urine dipstick test detects only marked albuminuria (>100 mg per day), a **urine microalbumin** and creatinine should be measured annually in all diabetic patients. Values over 30 mg of albumin per gram of creatinine are abnormal and require further treatment. Because diabetics should be offered aggressive medical control of cardiovascular risk factors, fasting lipids should be assessed.

TREATMENT

Diabetic management is twofold: **restore glycemic control** and **monitor for** and **treat complications** of long-term diabetes. An important development in the management of DM is the demonstration that achievement of normal glycemia (so-called tight control) lowers the rate of microvascular complications. This was first demonstrated in patients with type 1 DM in the Diabetic Control and Complications Trial (DCCT). The findings have been extended to type 2 DM in several follow-up studies. The effect of tight glucose control on macrovascular complications has been less impressive, and close attention to other vascular risk factors

(hyperlipidemia, BP, smoking) is advocated instead. Recent evidence suggests that very tight control (HbA1c 6%) in type 2 diabetic patients with established macrovascular disease may actually be harmful. Therefore, the risks of tight control, which include an increased risk of hypoglycemia (threefold in the DCCT), should be considered for each individual patient. The general goals for diabetic patients attempting tight control are a fasting glucose of 80 to 120 mg per dL and an HbA1c of <7%. In type 2 DM, these goals become increasingly more difficult to achieve over time; approximately 5% to 10% of type 2 DM patients fail to control their glucose on their oral agent each year. Patients who consistently have values greater than their goal should be offered additional treatment in the form of additional medication or education.

DIETARY THERAPY

In type 2 DM, dietary treatment combined with exercise and weight loss may be sufficient to achieve adequate glucose control. Close attention to dietary intake is also important in type 1 DM to avoid wide fluctuations in blood sugar and limit the total amount of insulin required. Previous dietary recommendations advocated restriction of carbohydrates, especially simple sugars such as sucrose. It is now recognized that complex carbohydrates and simple sugars have equal effects on postprandial blood glucose level and that excessive intake of fat and protein in a carbohydrate-restricted diet may lead to progression of atherosclerosis (from high fat intake) and nephropathy (from high protein intake). Therefore, a balanced diet of 55% carbohydrates, 15% protein, and 30% fat (saturated fats limited to 7%) is recommended. This is very similar to the standard recommendations for adults in the United States. For patients with type 2 DM, caloric restriction (1,500 to 2,000 kcal per day) is also important to achieve weight loss when appropriate. Consultation with a registered dietitian is highly recommended to enhance patient understanding and compliance.

ORAL HYPOGLYCEMICS

Patients with type 2 DM who are unable to regulate glucose by diet and exercise alone may be placed on an oral hypoglycemic after several months. Some experts recommend early initiation of medication even prior to a trial of diet and exercise.

The **biguanides** are "insulin-sensitizing" agents that are believed to lower blood glucose level by inhibiting hepatic gluconcogenesis and increasing peripheral uptake of glucose. Metformin is the most commonly prescribed biguanide in the United States. It has a very low incidence of lactic acidosis (3 per 100,000 patient-years) and is approved for initial monotherapy in the United States. Its efficacy is similar to that of the sulfonylureas (1.5% to 2% decrease in HbA1c), and metformin has the added benefit of decreasing circulating insulin levels and avoiding weight gain. There is no risk of hypoglycemia when metformin is used as monotherapy. For these reasons, metformin is generally preferred as first-line therapy in obese patients. Treatment should begin at the lowest dose of 500 mg once daily and be increased as needed over several weeks to a maximum of 850 mg three times daily. The most common side effects are gastrointestinal (GI) (abdominal discomfort and diarrhea), which often abate after 1 or 2 weeks. Metformin should not be used in patients with renal disease (estimated glomerular filtration rate [GFR] less than 50) or hepatic disease because of the increased risk of lactic acidosis in these patients. It should be discontinued temporarily in situations in which renal failure may occur (e.g., contrast dye studies, severe illness).

Sulfonylureas bind to specific sulfonylurea receptors on the pancreatic beta cells and stimulate insulin release. They are often chosen as first-line agents in nonobese patients, decreasing HbA1c by an average of 1.5% to 2%. However, approximately 15% of patients never respond to these agents and should be changed to another therapy. All sulfonylureas seem to have equal potency, although the second-generation agents (glyburide, glipizide, glimepiride) have become more popular in recent years. The lowest possible dose should be started and titrated upward on the basis of patient monitoring of glucose level over the next several weeks. Side effects include weight gain and hypoglycemia. Hypoglycemic reactions occur in approximately 4% of patients per year, but most are mild and do not require hospitalization. An initial concern that sulfonylureas increase mortality from coronary artery disease has not been confirmed in later studies.

The newer **meglitinides** repaglinide and nateglinide are nonsulfonylurea agents that also increase insulin secretion and appear to be equipotent to the sulfonylureas. Repaglinide is not renally secreted and is therefore preferred over sulfonylureas for diabetics with renal failure, but the meglitinides are more expensive than the older sulfonylureas.

The **thiazolidinediones** (pioglitazone, rosiglitazone) increase insulin sensitivity in the liver and muscle. They are slightly less potent (average reduction of 1% in HbA1c) and are more expensive than the older oral agents. More recently, the safety of thiazolidinediones (TZDs) has been questioned. These drugs increase the risk of heart failure and fluid retention, and a study of rosiglitazone increased the risk of myocardial infarction in high-risk patients. These agents are now reserved for patients who fail combination therapy with older agents and refuse insulin therapy. TZDs are associated with a low incidence of liver function abnormalities; liver tests should be monitored during the first year of therapy.

The **alpha-glucosidase inhibitors** (acarbose, miglitol) inhibit the absorption of carbohydrates by preventing the breakdown of oligosaccharides in the small intestine. The obvious side effects are bloating, diarrhea, and flatulence as these starches are delivered to the rest of the lower intestinal tract. They are not very effective as monotherapy but may be used in combination with other agents.

The **dipeptidyl peptidase-4 inhibitor**, sitagliptin, decreases the activity of dipeptidyl peptidase-4, which results in an increase in its substrate, glucagon-like peptide-1 (GLP-1). GLP-1 is produced by intestinal cells in response to glucose; it increases pancreatic beta cell production of insulin and decreases pancreatic alpha cell production of glucagon. Sitagliptin leads to small reductions in HbA1C (less than 1%), and therefore its use is limited to combination therapy. The long term benefits and safety of this drug have not been adequately studied.

INSULIN THERAPY

Subcutaneous insulin is required for all patients with type 1 DM and in many patients with type 2 DM. Insulin is classified by its pharmacokinetic properties, including rate of onset, peak effect, and length of duration (Table 49-1). Short-acting insulin (regular, lispro, aspart, and glulisine) is used for glycemic control around the time of meals (prandial insulin). Insulin lispro, aspart, and glulisine are very rapid acting, with an onset of action of 5 to 15 minutes. This insulin allows for matching of food intake with insulin administration. Intermediate insulin (NPH) and long-acting insulin (insulin glargine and detemir) are used to provide a basal insulin level throughout

■ TABLE 49-1 Pharmacokinetic Properties of Insulin Preparations

	Onset of Action	Peak of Action (hr)	Duration of Insulin Action (hr)
Lispro, aspart, glulisine	5 to 15 min	1 to 2	4 to 5
Regular	30 to 60 min	2 to 4	6 to 8
NPH	1 to 2 hr	5 to 7	12 to 18
Insulin glargine	2 to 4 hr	No peak	20 to 24
Insulin detemir	2 to 4 hr	No peak	6 to 24

the day and especially at night. Insulin glargine and detemir have no peak concentration and mimic continuous infusion of regular insulin.

Insulin may be delivered by multiple subcutaneous injections or continuous subcutaneous insulin infusion (CSII) through a pump. Any patient attempting intensive DM therapy for tight control requires multiple daily injections. Type 1 diabetics require short-acting insulin two or three times daily with meals and at least some basal insulin given before bedtime. An additional injection of basal insulin before breakfast is often desirable. Type 2 diabetics already have above-normal insulin levels, and therefore insulin therapy only provides a supplement. One strategy is to mimic type 1 diabetics with twice-daily intermediate-acting insulin and short-acting insulin before breakfast and dinner. Another strategy that controls glucose with less weight gain and lower insulin dose is a single injection of **bedtime NPH or insulin glargine**. This allows control of the increased nocturnal hepatic gluconeogenesis, which is responsible for the fasting hyperglycemia in most type 2 diabetics. The CSII pump is an option for motivated type 1 diabetics. These devices administer continuous low levels of regular or lispro insulin with boluses (either preprogrammed or manually entered) before meals.

OTHER INJECTABLE THERAPIES

Novel therapies for DM include mimetics of GLP-1 and amylin. Exenatide activates the GLP-1 receptor and is given as a subcutaneous injection (5 to 10 μg) twice daily. HbA1c reduction is modest (1%), but it has the added benefit of weight loss. Pramlintide, which is a synthetic amylin, is another injectable medication that is given prior to meals. Amylin is a

natural substance produced by pancreatic beta cells that reduces glucagon production. Pramlintide can be used in type 1 or type 2 DM, but the HbA1c reduction is small (less than 1%).

COMPLICATIONS

DIABETIC KETOACIDOSIS

DKA is generally seen in type 1 DM. It may be precipitated by infections, vascular events (stroke, myocardial infarction), cessation of insulin, or dehydration. The patient often presents with nausea and vomiting, perhaps in association with diffuse abdominal pain. Confusion or restlessness is seen in more severe cases. Examination may demonstrate Kussmaul respirations (deep respirations seen in acidosis) and signs of volume depletion. Laboratory studies show an anion gap acidosis (see Chapter 20), hyperglycemia, and positive ketone bodies in the urine and blood. Treatment consists of **volume repletion** and **insulin replacement** (Table 49-2). Volume replacement should be started urgently through IV infusion of normal saline. Insulin administration should be started with an IV bolus of approximately 7 to 10 U (in adults) followed by a continuous infusion of 0.1 U/kg/hour. Insulin therapy is adjusted based on the improvement in the anion gap. Glucose should be monitored every hour and often decreases below 250 mg per dL before the anion gap is normalized. In this instance, dextrose should be added to the IV solution while insulin is continued to treat the persistent ketosis. The insulin drip should be continued for several hours after the patient is given intermediate-acting subcutaneous insulin to allow for delay in onset of the intermediate

■ TABLE 49-2 Treatment of Diabetic Ketoacidosis

Therapeutics	Dosing Guidelines	Monitoring
Intravenous insulin	Start with 0.1 unit/kg bolus, then continue 0.1 unit/kg/hr	Adjust dose depending on anion gap
Subcutaneous insulin	Give NPH insulin once anion gap has normalized and patient eating	Must continue intravenous insulin for 4 hours after SC dose given (to allow onset of action)
Intravenous fluid	Normal saline 125 to 500 cc/hr; often need 1- to 2-liter bolus at presentation	Volume status, urine output
Intravenous dextrose	Add to IV fluid when glucose under 250 mg/dL and intravenous insulin still required	Also needed if patient not able to take po's
Potassium	Add to IV fluid when urine output established and potassium is less than 5.3 meq/L; 20 meq per hour often needed	Aggressively replete K+ less than 3.0 meq/L (may need central access).

insulin's action (see Table 49-1). Although serum potassium levels are often initially elevated (because of the acidosis and insulinopenia forcing potassium out of the intracellular space), patients with diabetic ketoacidosis (DKA) are always potassium depleted and should have potassium added to the replacement fluid as soon as urine output is established and serum potassium approaches normal levels. Intravenous sodium bicarbonate is controversial for DKA, and generally reserved for severe acidosis (pH less than 7.0).

HYPEROSMOLAR NONKETOTIC COMA

Hyperosmolar nonketotic coma is usually seen in patients with type 2 DM when progressive hyperglycemia leads to an osmotic diuresis and worsening dehydration. It usually is precipitated by a cardiovascular event (e.g., stroke) or infection that limits the patient's ability to maintain adequate hydration. Patients present with severe volume depletion and obtundation. Glucose is extremely high, in the 800 to 1,000 mg per dL range. Acidosis may be present as well but usually represents starvation ketosis and lactic acidosis rather than DKA. The mainstay of treatment is adequate hydration and aggressive treatment of the underlying precipitant. Hydration often decreases the glucose level significantly, but insulin can be used in addition. Because these individuals are often elderly patients with concomitant infections, mortality remains high (up to 50%).

HYPOGLYCEMIA

In general, the more intensive the chronic medical treatment, the greater the risk for induced hypoglycemia.

All diabetics who are on drug treatment, either insulin or oral hypoglycemics, should be instructed in self-monitoring of blood glucose level and be educated about the symptoms of hypoglycemia. Symptoms of hypoglycemia are divided into **adrenergic symptoms** from epinephrine release and **neuroglycopenic symptoms** from central nervous system (CNS) dysfunction. Adrenergic symptoms include tachycardia, diaphoresis, tremulousness, palpitations, and anxiety. Neuroglycopenic symptoms develop later and include headache, blurred vision, confusion, seizures, and loss of consciousness. Patients who have repeated episodes of hypoglycemia or autonomic neuropathy may experience **hypoglycemic unawareness**. In these instances, adrenergic symptoms are not seen, and only neuroglycopenic symptoms appear. Diabetics at risk for hypoglycemia should have sugar (in the form of candy or prepackaged high-glucose tablets) and glucagon (via injection pen) readily available.

MICROVASCULAR COMPLICATIONS

As mentioned previously, close glycemic control can limit the development of microvascular complications. However, even if these complications occur, additional treatment can slow progression or treat symptoms. **Retinopathy** occurs in the majority of patients having DM for >15 years. If retinopathy is detected early, laser photocoagulation can preserve vision. **Nephropathy** can be detected early by screening for microalbuminuria, as mentioned earlier. If microalbuminuria develops, treatment with an angiotensin-converting enzyme (ACE) inhibitor or angiotensin II receptor blocker decreases the rate of progression to overt nephropathy. There has been no convincing treatment other than glycemic control to delay the progression of **sensory neuropathy**. Amitriptyline and gabapentin are two agents used to treat painful neuropathy if it develops.

MACROVASCULAR COMPLICATIONS

Diabetics are at greatly increased risk for macrovascular disease (see Part I). Because of their risk for coronary heart disease, cerebrovascular disease, and peripheral vascular disease, all diabetics should be counseled on the benefits of smoking cessation, BP control, and lipid-lowering therapy (see Chapter 55). Prophylactic aspirin therapy (81 mg) and statin therapy should be given to diabetic patients over 40 years old, or to younger patients at above average risk for macrovascular disease. Metformin may reduce cardiovascular risk and should be considered early in oral hypoglycemic therapy.

KEY POINTS

- The diagnosis of DM is made when two separate blood tests confirm fasting glucose level >125 mg per dL or a random glucose level >200 mg per dL with symptoms. The 2-hour glucose tolerance test is now rarely used in the diagnosis of nonpregnant patients.

- Type 1 DM is a state of insulin deficiency, and patients are predisposed to DKA.

- Type 2 DM is a state of insulin resistance. Metformin and sulfonylureas are the mainstays to control blood glucose level, but many patients will require insulin.

- Microvascular complications of DM (nephropathy, retinopathy, and neuropathy) can be delayed by close control of blood glucose to near-normal levels.

- Glycosylated hemoglobin (HbA1c) and microalbumin are important monitoring tests for DM control and complications.

- DKA presents as nausea, vomiting, anion gap acidosis, and positive ketones in the blood and urine. Treatment is insulin, volume repletion, and potassium repletion.

Hypercalcemia

Under normal circumstances, serum calcium level is tightly regulated through a balance of parathyroid hormone (**PTH**), calcitonin, and vitamin D. PTH increases serum calcium by activating bone resorption and increasing renal tubular resorption of calcium. PTH also increases activation of **vitamin D**, which assists in increasing calcium reabsorption from the gut. In contrast, **calcitonin**, produced by thyroid parafollicular C cells, acts to reduce calcium levels through inhibition of bone resorption. Disorders involving increased bone destruction, decreased renal excretion, increased gastrointestinal (GI) absorption, unregulated secretion of PTH, and vitamin D abnormalities may manifest as hypercalcemia.

EPIDEMIOLOGY

Primary hyperparathyroidism is a disease of older adults, rarely occurring prior to 40 years and rising rapidly thereafter. It is more common in women than men. Prevalence is estimated at 0.1% to 0.5%. Hypercalcemia also occurs in up to 10% to 20% of cancer patients.

ETIOLOGY AND PATHOGENESIS

The two most common causes of hypercalcemia are **primary hyperparathyroidism** (HPTH) and **malignancy**, accounting for 90% of all cases.

Primary hyperparathyroidism occurs when increased PTH is secreted. Overfunction of the parathyroid gland with loss of normal calcium level feedback regulation leads to excessive calcium resorption from bone and distal renal tubules. Because PTH increases calcitriol [$1,25(OH)_2$ vitamin D] levels, calcium flux from the GI lumen to the blood is also increased. The etiologies of **primary HPTH** are:

- Solitary parathyroid adenoma (85% of cases of primary HPTH)
- Parathyroid hyperplasia (15% of cases; may be associated with hereditary causes, such as the multiple endocrine neoplasia [MEN] syndromes)
- Rare cases of multiple adenomas or parathyroid carcinoma

Malignancy may cause hypercalcemia by two mechanisms. In the first mechanism, malignancy leads to **direct bone destruction**, believed to be mediated by an osteoclast-activating factor. Cancers involved in bone destruction include breast cancer, nonsmall cell lung cancer, and multiple myeloma. In the second mechanism of malignant hypercalcemia, **humoral hypercalcemia of malignancy** (HHM), a PTH-related protein (PTHrP), is secreted by the tumor. Cancers most likely to cause HHM include:

- Lung cancer (especially squamous cell)
- Head and neck cancer
- Renal cancer
- T-cell leukemia (associated with the virus HTLV-1)

Less common causes of hypercalcemia include:

Vitamin D Mediated
- Increased vitamin D ingestion
- Granulomatous disease (e.g., sarcoid, tuberculosis)—granulomas activate vitamin D through production of α_1-hydroxylase
- Hodgkin disease and NHL

Increased Bone Turnover

- Hyperthyroidism
- Immobilization (usually in association with underlying high bone turnover, as seen in Paget disease)
- Vitamin A intoxication

Decreased Renal Excretion of Calcium

- Thiazide diuretics
- Milk-alkali syndrome

Milk-alkali syndrome may be caused by excessive ingestion of antacids or calcium supplements (mostly calcium carbonate). The resulting alkalosis leads to greater renal absorption of calcium, which in turn induces volume depletion and renal insufficiency. The cycle then continues, with more alkalosis and calcium reabsorption as long as ingestion persists, leading to increasing hypercalcemia.

Lithium intake and **familial hypocalciuric hypercalcemia** (FHH) are additional causes of mild to moderate hypercalcemia that involve increased PTH secretion (but are not primary hyperparathyroidism). FHH is an autosomal dominant disorder in which urine calcium excretion remains low (<100 mg per day) despite hypercalcemia. This is in contrast to primary hyperparathyroidism, where hypercalciuria occurs with the rising calcium levels. Both lithium and FHH involve a decreased activity in the calcium-sensing receptor, leading to elevated calcium levels in order to activate the receptor and decrease PTH secretion.

CLINICAL MANIFESTATIONS

HISTORY

Symptoms related to hypercalcemia are nonspecific and include **fatigue**, **anorexia**, and **drowsiness**; with higher elevations of calcium, confusion and stupor occur. GI complaints include nausea, vomiting, and constipation. Inhibition of renal-concentrating ability leads to polyuria. Patients with primary hyperparathyroidism and chronic hypercalcemia may give a history of recurrent nephrolithiasis or peptic ulcer disease (PUD). The simple hyperparathyroidism mnemonic "stones, bones, and groans" refers to nephrolithiasis, bone resorption, and constitutional/GI symptoms.

Diagnosis of the hypercalcemia etiology may be assisted by a history of weight loss and heavy tobacco use (malignancy), drug ingestion (lithium, thiazides, antacids), or excess vitamin ingestion (A or D). A positive family history may be discovered in MEN or FHH.

PHYSICAL EXAMINATION

Physical examination is usually unrevealing but should include a search for findings suggestive of malignancy, such as adenopathy or abnormal masses. Volume depletion may be present due to symptoms listed above.

DIAGNOSTIC EVALUATION

Calcium exists in three forms in the extracellular fluid: protein bound (40%), free ions (50%), and complexed with anions (10%). **Ionized calcium**, the free form, is the biologically active form and may be directly measured for an accurate assessment of calcium homeostasis. Acidemia decreases calcium binding to albumin, and therefore increases the ionized calcium. Hypophosphatemia is seen in hypercalcemia mediated through PTH or PTHrP.

The most helpful test in differentiating the cause of hypercalcemia is the **intact PTH assay**. If elevated, this points toward primary hyperparathyroidism. This is the cause in most (90%) asymptomatic patients, especially if the hypercalcemia is chronic. Other causes to consider with a normal to slightly high PTH include FHH and lithium ingestion (see earlier). If the PTH is low or undetectable, malignancy is most likely. PTHrP may be measured to confirm the diagnosis of HHM.

Malignancy is almost always apparent on initial selected testing for low PTH hypercalcemia, including:

- **Chest radiograph** (lung cancer)
- **Urine for red cells** (renal cancer)
- **Mammogram** (breast cancer)
- **Serum** and **urine immunoelectrophoresis** (multiple myeloma)

If these initial tests are unrevealing and cancer is still suspected, a CT of the chest or abdomen may be performed. Of note, primary hyperparathyroidism can coexist with malignancy, and therefore PTH levels should be investigated when hypercalcemia first presents in patients with known malignancies to determine if treatable benign hyperparathyroidism is present.

Radiographs in hypercalcemia may show either the consequence of the disease or the etiology. Metastatic cancer or myeloma may appear as lytic lesions on bone

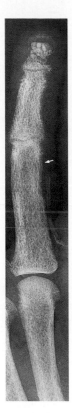

Figure 50-1 • Subperiosteal resorption in hyperparathyroidism (*arrow*).

films. Long-standing primary hyperparathyroidism may result in the following **bone manifestations**:

- Osteitis fibrosa cystica
- Subperiosteal resorption in phalanges (Fig. 50-1)
- Chondrocalcinosis with associated pseudogout (see Chapter 56)

Cardiac manifestations of hypercalcemia present as a **shortened QT interval** on electrocardiogram (ECG).

TREATMENT

The initial goal of treatment is to return the calcium level to normal range to prevent neurologic and cardiac dysfunction. The intensity of treatment depends on the level of calcium. After initially controlling calcium level, therapy is aimed at treating the underlying etiology.

The first treatment for moderate to severe hypercalcemia (>12 to 13 mg per dL) is **IV saline**, which restores the depleted intravascular volume and increases renal calcium excretion. Rates of infusion are often 200 to 400 mL per hour. Loop diuretics (e.g., furosemide) add little to further increase calcium excretion but are appropriate when volume overload is a concern.

After restoring volume and maximizing calcium excretion, sustained control of serum calcium via inhibition of bone resorption is the next priority. **Calcitonin** can be administered subcutaneously every 6 hours and reduces calcium levels within hours. However, continued use results in tachyphylaxis and limits the use of this drug. The **bisphosphonates** (alendronate, etidronate, pamidronate, and zoledronate) are synthetic analogues of pyrophosphate and inhibit osteoclast resorption of bone. They may be given IV and lower calcium over the following 2 to 3 days. Of the four agents, zoledronate (4 mg IV over 15 minutes) is preferred in patients with malignancy because of its rapid onset of action, its ease of infusion, and its prolonged induction of normocalcemia. The bisphosphonates maintain normocalcemia for several weeks after a single dose. Corticosteroids (e.g., dexamethasone) can treat hypercalcemia caused by hematologic malignancies or sarcoidosis.

Once calcium homeostasis is achieved, the focus turns to the underlying disease. In the case of drugs or vitamin D excess, the calcium level normalizes with removal of the offending agent. For malignancy-related hypercalcemia, cases of improvement have been reported after successful treatment of the cancer. Unfortunately, this is not usually possible because of the advanced nature of many of these cancers. Patients with malignancy-related hypercalcemia survive an average of 6 months after diagnosis of hypercalcemia. Because hypercalcemia causes sedation and pain relief and the prognosis for malignant hypercalcemia is poor, it is important to confer with cancer patients regarding their future wishes for or against hypercalcemia treatment once the diagnosis of malignant hypercalcemia is clarified.

For **symptomatic primary hyperparathyroidism** (HPTH), surgery should be performed. A single adenoma may be removed, or if hyperplasia is present, three and one-half glands are removed. In hereditary syndromes with parathyroid hyperplasia, remaining tissue is sometimes implanted in the forearm to ensure easy access in case of recurrent hypercalcemia.

For asymptomatic HPTH, surgery is recommended for patients younger than 50 years. For older patients, surgery should be recommended if there is:

- A calcium level >1.5 mg per dL above normal
- History of life-threatening hypercalcemia

- Nephrolithiasis or reduction in creatinine clearance
- Bone density two or more standard deviations below controls

If surgery is deferred, patients should be instructed to maintain adequate hydration. Calcium intake should be moderate. High intake could worsen hypercalcemia; a diet deficient in calcium could further stimulate PTH production and worsen bone loss.

A newer agent, cinacalcet, is a calcimimetic that stimulates the calcium-sensing receptor to decrease PTH production. It is approved for secondary hyperparathyroidism in renal failure, but may represent a nonsurgical approach to primary HPTH in the future.

If parathyroid surgery is performed, one must monitor for **postoperative hypocalcemia**. Signs of hypocalcemia include muscle twitching and spasm. Postoperative hypocalcemia may be secondary to:

- Hypoparathyroidism (too much gland removed or ischemic injury)

- "Hungry bone syndrome," rapid bone formation after gland removal that leads to excessive calcium loss from the bloodstream (usually seen only with severe osteitis fibrosa cystica)

KEY POINTS

- The two most common etiologies of hypercalcemia are primary hyperparathyroidism and malignancy.
- Measurement of parathyroid hormone can successfully discriminate these two etiologies.
- Immediate treatment consists of hydration with intravenous normal saline. Long-term control is achieved by treating the underlying disease or by using bisphosphonates.
- Primary hyperparathyroidism is treated surgically, most commonly with resection of a solitary parathyroid adenoma.

51 Adrenal Insufficiency

The **adrenal cortex** is responsible for the synthesis of three major steroid hormones:

- Glucocorticoids (e.g., cortisol): produced in the zona fasciculata
- Mineralocorticoids (e.g., aldosterone): produced in the zona glomerulosa
- Androgens (e.g., dehydroepiandrosterone [DHEA]): produced in the zona reticularis

The **adrenal medulla** produces catecholamines, primarily epinephrine and norepinephrine. The main stimulus for catecholamine secretion is the sympathetic nervous system.

Diseases of the adrenal gland consists of oversecretion of these substances, or deficiencies. Hyperaldosteronism and pheochromocytoma are discussed in Chapter 8, and Cushing syndrome is covered in Chapter 52. This chapter will focus on adrenal insufficiency (AI).

EPIDEMIOLOGY

Primary adrenal insufficiency (Addison disease) is rare, with a prevalence of 3 to 6 per 100,000 people. In contrast, secondary adrenal insufficiency related to therapeutic glucocorticoid use is relatively common. Patients with autoimmune etiologies of AI usually present between ages 20 and 50.

ETIOLOGY

Addison disease is usually related to an **autoimmune** etiology. It can be associated with other autoimmune diseases such as Hashimoto thyroiditis, type 1 diabetes mellitus, celiac sprue, and premature ovarian failure; this combination is known as the **polyglandular autoimmune syndrome type II**. Polyglandular autoimmune syndrome type I may also cause adrenal insufficiency, in association with hypoparathyroidism and mucocutaneous candidiasis. This disorder is inherited as an autosomal recessive trait and is caused by a mutation in the autoimmune regulator gene (AIRE) located on chromosome 21.

Other causes of Addison disease are **tuberculosis**, **human immunodeficiency virus (HIV) infection**, **metastatic carcinoma**, and **adrenal hemorrhage**. Adrenal hemorrhage may occur in the setting of anticoagulant therapy or sepsis. Adrenal vein thrombosis (seen in hypercoaguable states) may predispose to hemorrhage due to congestion of the adrenal glands. **X-linked adrenoleukodystrophy** is an inherited disorder of fatty acid metabolism, which leads to AI and demyelination in the central nervous system.

Secondary adrenal insufficiency (from pituitary suppression of adrenocorticotropin hormone [ACTH]) is commonly seen in patients on therapeutic doses of glucocorticoids. It can also occur as part of panhypopituitarism (see Chapter 53).

CLINICAL FINDINGS

HISTORY

The presentation of adrenal insufficiency is variable and often insidious; patients often have nonspecific symptoms such as fatigue, weight loss, nausea, anorexia, and abdominal pain.

Acute adrenal insufficiency (adrenal crisis) can occur in the patient with poor adrenal reserve who is exposed to surgery, infection, or injury. These patients may complain of nausea and abdominal pain, and appear ill.

PHYSICAL EXAMINATION

Orthostatic hypotension is associated with adrenal insufficiency, and overt shock occurs in adrenal crisis. **Hyperpigmentation**, due to excess production of proopiomelanocortin (the precursor to ACTH), is unique to the primary form of AI (usually autoimmune). Hyperpigmentation is often seen in skin folds and in scars. The patient should be examined for associated conditions such as thyroiditis (firm thyroid gland) and vitiligo.

DIFFERENTIAL DIAGNOSIS

Adrenal insufficiency can be difficult to differentiate from countless other conditions in the early stage because of the nonspecific constitutional symptoms, but the diagnosis should be suspected when constitutional symptoms are accompanied by **gastrointestinal (GI) distress**, **weight loss**, or a gradual increase of **skin pigmentation**.

DIAGNOSTIC EVALUATION

ELECTROLYTES

Primary adrenal insufficiency has the characteristic pattern of **hyperkalemia** and **hyponatremia**, due to the lack of mineralocorticoid production. In secondary AI, hyperkalemia is not present, but hyponatremia may occur as a manifestation of syndrome of inappropriate antidiuretic hormone (SIADH).

ADDITIONAL LABORATORY FINDINGS

The following abnormalities can be seen in adrenal insufficiency:

- Mild hypercalcemia
- Eosinophilia
- Normochromic, normocytic anemia
- Mild acidosis

COSYNTROPIN STIMULATION TEST

The cosyntropin (synthetic ACTH) stimulation test to diagnose glucocorticoid deficiency is described in Chapter 2. To confirm **primary** adrenal insufficiency (in addition to the submaximal ACTH stimulation), a high ACTH level (>52 pg/ml) or high plasma renin/low plasma aldosterone level (in the upright position) must be documented.

In patients with partial or recent ACTH deficiency, the cosyntropin test may be falsely normal. In these conditions, adrenal gland atrophy will not be present and the adrenal glands with respond to the supraphysiologic doses of ACTH used during testing. These patients can be detected by a suboptimal increase in ACTH after administration of corticotropin releasing hormone (CRH) or metyrapone (see Chapter 52).

TREATMENT

Maintenance therapy in patients with chronic adrenal insufficiency consists of **hydrocortisone** 15 to 25 mg daily in divided doses. Patients are monitored for improved appetite and general well-being to determine adequate dosing. ACTH or cortisol levels are not reliable to titrate dose. Excess replacement is avoided since side effects include osteoporosis, weight gain, and hyperglycemia. In patients with primary adrenal insufficiency, **fludrocortisone** is used for mineralocorticoid replacement. The average dose is 0.05 to 0.10 mg daily. Side effects include hypokalemia, hypertension, and fluid retention. Orthostatic vital signs and electrolytes are monitored to assess dosage.

CONTINUED CARE

Patients with adrenal insufficiency require stress-dose steroids at times of surgery or severe illness. The usual recommended dose is 50 to 100 mg of intravenous hydrocortisone three times daily. Hydrocortisone has mineralocorticoid activity at these high doses, so fludrocortisone is not routinely needed. High dose hydrocortisone should be maintained throughout the acute illness, and then tapered down as tolerated. For minor stressors (such as viral illness or minor surgery), the maintenance hydrocortisone dose can be doubled. All patients with AI should be provided with a medical alert bracelet indicating their condition.

KEY POINTS

- Primary adrenal insufficiency is usually autoimmune in etiology. It may be associated with other autoimmune disease (type 1 diabetes mellitus, hypothyroidism) as part of the type II polyglandular autoimmune syndrome.

- Secondary adrenal insufficiency is most often due to therapeutic glucocorticoid use.

- Adrenal insufficiency presents with weakness, weight loss, and abdominal pain. Hyponatremia and hyperkalemia are often present in primary adrenal insufficiency.

- The diagnosis of adrenal insufficiency is confirmed with a suboptimal one hour cortisol response to cosyntropin (cortisol less than 20 μg/dL).

- Treatment consists of hydrocortisone replacement (10 to 25 mg daily) with stress doses (100 to 300 mg) used for illness or surgery.

Chapter 52

Cushing Syndrome

Cushing syndrome is caused by excess levels of circulating cortisol. The normal regulation of cortisol is controlled by corticotropin-releasing hormone (CRH), which is produced by the hypothalamus. CRH stimulates adrenocorticotropic hormone (ACTH), which in turn stimulates cortisol secretion from the zona fasciculata of the adrenal cortex. Cortisol induces catabolism of fats and proteins and also has anti-inflammatory effects. Iatrogenic Cushing syndrome, seen with therapeutic use of glucocorticoids, is extremely common. Non-iatrogenic Cushing syndrome, may arise from the adrenal gland itself (15% of cases) or from stimulation by increased ACTH (85% of cases).

EPIDEMIOLOGY

In general, primary adrenal disorders are uncommon diseases. The annual incidence of endogenous Cushing syndrome is estimated at 2 to 5 per million individuals. In certain specialized populations (such as poorly controlled diabetics with hypertension), the prevalence may approach 2% to 5%. Cushing syndrome is more common in women.

ETIOLOGY AND PATHOPHYSIOLOGY

Overproduction of cortisol in Cushing syndrome can be either ACTH-dependent or ACTH-independent. Sources of ACTH production include:

- Pituitary adenomas (mostly from microadenomas), known as **Cushing disease**

- Ectopic ACTH production (usually from small cell lung cancer)

In the ACTH-independent Cushing syndrome, cortisol is autonomously produced by the adrenal glands. These diseases include:

- Adrenal tumor (adenoma or carcinoma)
- Micronodular adrenal disease

Cortisol's actions are seen throughout the body, due to the widespread distribution of the glucocorticoid receptor. After binding the receptor, cortisol enters the nucleus and regulates gene transcription. The effects are tissue dependent and include:

- Glucose metabolism—increased gluconeogenesis and decreased peripheral glucose uptake, leading to hyperglycemia
- Adipose tissue—increased lipolysis, although lipogenic effects of associated insulin release lead to central fat deposition
- Connective tissue—inhibition of fibroblasts, leading to skin atrophy and easy bruising, and increased breakdown of muscle protein
- Bone—Increased bone resorption, inhibition of intestinal calcium absorption, and increased urinary calcium excretion
- Immunologic function—decreased prostaglandin synthesis and neutrophil migration
- Kidney—Increased sodium retention through the mineralocorticoid activity of cortisol (cortisol is usually metabolized to inactive cortisone by 11 β-hydroxysteroid dehydrogenase type 2, but this enzyme is overwhelmed in Cushing syndrome)

CLINICAL FINDINGS

HISTORY

The patient with Cushing syndrome can present with the following complaints:

- Weight gain, especially central obesity
- Muscle weakness
- Easy bruising
- Depression or mood changes
- Irregular menses, impotence or decreased libido

Since many of these symptoms are common in the population, further suspicion is raised if metabolic abnormalities are seen or specific physical findings are detected.

PHYSICAL EXAMINATION

Central (or truncal) obesity is nearly universal in Cushing syndrome, occurring in 90% to 100% of patients. Rounded (or moon) facies and facial plethora are also seen. Excess fat deposition can occur on the cervical spine (buffalo hump) and supraclavicular fossae.

Other skin findings include **purple striae**, which are usually wide (>1 cm) and located on lateral abdomen, axillae, or internal thighs.

Muscle atrophy results in proximal limb weakness, and **hypertension** is seen in most patients.

DIFFERENTIAL DIAGNOSIS

Excess cortisol production is also seen in alcoholism and obesity, which can mimic some of the physical findings of Cushing syndrome.

DIAGNOSTIC EVALUATION

Cushing syndrome is characterized by excess cortisol production, lack of response to usual feedback mechanisms, and lack of normal circadian rhythm of cortisol (see Fig. 52-1). Initial diagnostic testing focuses on these features. **Urine free cortisol** (in a 24-hour urine collection) is usually 3 to 4 times higher than the upper limit of normal (normal limit is about 100 µg/day). The **overnight dexamethasone suppression test** is easier to perform. In healthy individuals, administration of 1 mg of dexamethasone at midnight suppresses the next morning's (8 AM) cortisol to less than 5 µg per dL. To avoid missing Cushing syndrome, the cut-off is further reduced to 1.8 µg per dL. Failure to suppress cortisol occurs in Cushing syndrome, but false-positive tests also occur in obesity, depression, and alcoholism. A newer test is the **late-night salivary cortisol**. The patient may sample saliva at home around 11 PM, when cortisol production is usually at a nadir.

After initial testing, equivocal cases can be confirmed with a low-dose dexamethasone suppression test (0.5 mg dexamethasone every 6 hours for 48 hours) combined with CRH stimulation. Failure to suppress plasma cortisol indicates Cushing syndrome.

Once hypercortisolism is confirmed, a **serum ACTH level** distinguishes between primary (i.e., adrenal) and secondary (i.e., pituitary or ectopic) causes of hypercortisolism. ACTH is suppressed (less than 5 pg/ml) in adrenal causes and high (more than 20 pg/ml) in pituitary (Cushing disease) and ectopic etiologies. Intermediate values may require CRH stimulation to assess the ACTH response.

When ACTH is not suppressed, a **high-dose dexamethasone suppression test** (2 mg every 6 hours) can differentiate between a pituitary adenoma (which suppresses cortisol in response to dexamethasone) and an ectopic source of ACTH production (which does not suppress cortisol). However, high-dose dexamethasone testing will not suppress cortisol in about 20% of pituitary tumors, and some ectopic ACTH secreting tumors express glucocorticoid receptors and will suppress cortisol production to dexamethasone. Therefore, in ACTH-dependent Cushing syndrome, definitive localization may require **inferior petrosal sinus sampling**. In this interventional procedure, catheters are placed in the inferior petrosal sinuses (which contain the venous drainage of the pituitary) and simultaneous sampling of the petrosal sinus and peripheral blood are obtained for ACTH levels. A ratio of 2 or more (3 or more after CRH administration) is diagnostic for a pituitary source of ACTH.

IMAGING STUDIES

Computed tomography (CT) of the abdomen usually locates the adrenal masses in adrenal adenomas and adrenal carcinomas. Because asymptomatic adrenal masses ("incidentalomas") are quite common (2% to 4% of normal individuals), an abdominal CT should

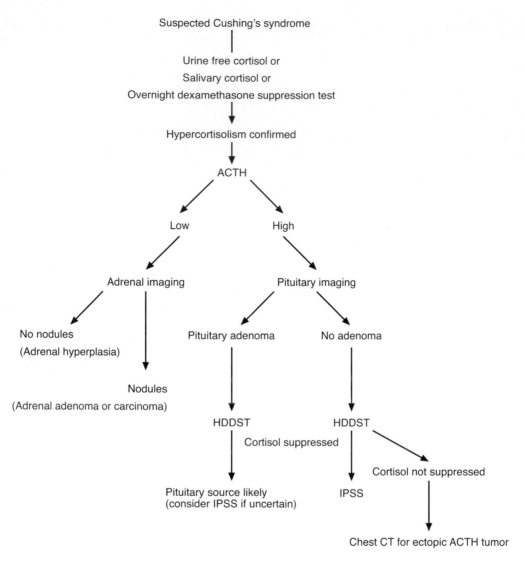

HDDST - High-dose dexamethasone suppression test, IPSS = inferior petrosal sinus sampling

Figure 52-1 • Diagnostic evaluation of Cushing syndrome.

not be ordered routinely unless ACTH-independent Cushing syndrome is confirmed biochemically. **Magnetic resonance imaging** (MRI) of the brain is the test of choice for detecting pituitary adenomas in Cushing disease, and a chest radiograph or CT may be needed in ectopic ACTH production to look for a small cell carcinoma or bronchial carcinoid tumor.

TREATMENT

SURGICAL RESECTION

Surgical resection is the treatment of choice for most causes of Cushing syndrome. Transsphenoidal sur-

gery for Cushing disease results in remission in 60% to 80% of patients. In long-term follow-up, about 20% of these patients will relapse. Patients with adrenal nodules should have a unilateral adrenalectomy. Patients with ectopic Cushing syndrome often have unresectable tumors (e.g., small cell lung carcinoma), but if resection of the tumor is possible, it should be attempted.

ADRENALECTOMY

In patients who fail initial surgery, bilateral adrenalectomy will eliminate Cushing syndrome. However, the patient then requires lifelong glucocorticoid and mineralocorticoid replacement (see Chapter 51). In addition, a patient with a pituitary adenoma may have continued enlargement of the adenoma due to lack of feedback (Nelson syndrome).

MEDICAL THERAPY

Adrenal blocking drugs are used as temporary treatments while awaiting surgery. These drugs include the adrenal enzyme inhibitors (ketoconazole, metyrapone, and aminoglutethimide) and mitotane (which is toxic to the adrenal gland). Side effects, especially to mitotane, limit the usefulness of these drugs. In addition, cortisol secretion can usually escape from enzyme inhibition, so the effect is limited. The dopamine agonist, cabergoline, has shown some benefit in pituitary Cushing disease.

CONTINUED CARE

After treatment for Cushing syndrome, adrenal insufficiency may persist for months. Patients should be given glucocorticoid and mineralocorticoid replacement, and tested for adrenal insufficiency every 3 months.

KEY POINTS

- Excess cortisol production in Cushing syndrome can be ACTH-dependent (pituitary and ectopic ACTH) or ACTH independent (adrenal).
- Physical examination findings suggestive of Cushing syndrome include moon facies, truncal obesity, "buffalo hump," proximal muscle weakness, and wide purple striae.
- Initial diagnostic work-up includes measurement of urine free cortisol or late-night salivary cortisol. Overnight dexamethasone suppression (1 mg) of cortisol can also be used.
- ACTH levels determine the source of cortisol production and guide the diagnostic imaging that follows.
- Transsphenoidal surgery is effective in achieving remission in 60% to 80% of the cases of Cushing disease.

53 Pituitary Disease

The anterior pituitary gland produces six hormones; the posterior pituitary gland stores and releases two hormones. Table 53-1 lists these hormones and their major functions. The anterior pituitary hormones are stimulated by hormones produced in the hypothalamus. The one exception is prolactin, which is chronically inhibited by **dopamine**. Drugs that block dopamine elevate prolactin levels.

Diseases of the pituitary may be classified as disorders of oversecretion or undersecretion of these hormones. Oversecretion of pituitary hormones occurs in **pituitary adenomas**. Undersecretion of all anterior hormones occurs in **panhypopituitarism**, and undersecretion of vasopressin produces **diabetes insipidus** (DI).

EPIDEMIOLOGY

Pituitary adenomas are uncommon diseases, with an annual incidence of 1 in 100,000 individuals. A pituitary adenoma is classified by the predominant hormone secreted. Most pituitary adenomas are nonfunctioning (although they produce the alpha subunit common to luteinizing hormone [LH], follicle-stimulating hormone [FSH], and thyroid-stimulating hormone [TSH]). The most common functioning adenomas are **prolactinomas**, followed by adenomas that produce growth hormone (leading to **acromegaly**) and those that produce adrenocorticotropin hormone (ACTH; causing **Cushing disease**).

RISK FACTORS

Pituitary adenomas may occur in association with **multiple endocrine neoplasia (MEN) syndrome** type I. Associated diseases in MEN type I include parathyroid hyperplasia and pancreatic islet cell tumors. Radiation treatment of CNS tumors may lead to panhypopituitarism.

CLINICAL FINDINGS

HISTORY

Hypogonadism (amenorrhea in women; impotence in men) along with **galactorrhea** may be seen in prolactin-secreting adenomas. Galactorrhea is defined as milk production outside of the postpartum period; it is not usually seen in men. Amenorrhea may also be seen in other hormone excesses (such as ACTH and growth hormone) and in hypopituitarism.

The physical changes related to excess growth hormone are slow to develop and often go unnoticed by the patient. Instead, complaints in acromegaly are nonspecific, such as fatigue, arthralgias (especially large joints), or headaches. Hypersomnolence (related to sleep apnea) and increased sweating can also be seen.

Symptoms of Cushing disease are discussed in Chapter 52. Nonfunctioning adenomas and gonadotropin-producing adenomas usually produce local, not systemic, symptoms such as **visual defects** and **headaches**. Thyroid-stimulating hormone (TSH)-producing adenomas are very rare and mimic symptoms of hyperthyroidism (see Chapter 47).

Symptoms of **hypopituitarism** are related to the lack of pituitary hormones. Loss of axillary and pubic hair, impotence, fatigue, and weight loss or gain are all seen. Polyuria and polydipsia suggest DI. Lack of lactation following pregnancy may be the

■ **TABLE 53-1** Hormones and Their Major Functions

Hormone	Function
GH	Regulation of growth and metabolism
ACTH	Controls secretion of glucocorticoids
Luteinizing hormone (LH)	Controls gonadal function
Follicle-stimulating hormone (FSH)	Controls gonadal function
Prolactin	Necessary for lactation
TSH	Regulates thyroid function
Oxytocin	Necessary for milk secretion in lactation
Vasopressin	Regulates water secretion

first suspicion of **Sheehan syndrome** (postpartum infarction of the pituitary, often caused by hypotension during delivery).

PHYSICAL EXAMINATION

Hypertension is often seen in acromegaly and Cushing disease. Orthostatic hypotension may be seen in panhypopituitarism.

Skin examination is notable for:

- Hirsutism (Cushing disease, acromegaly)
- Skin tags and moist, doughy skin (acromegaly)
- Wide purple striae (Cushing disease)

Widening of the spaces between teeth, macroglossia, and coarse facial features are seen in acromegaly.

The proximity of the pituitary to the optic chiasm may result in visual field deficits because of compression from a large adenoma. By compressing the chiasm itself, the adenoma primarily affects the optic fibers that cross over the midline (temporal visual fields), resulting in the classic **bitemporal hemianopia**.

DIFFERENTIAL DIAGNOSIS

Causes of **hypopituitarism** include:

- Large (nonfunctioning) pituitary adenomas (by mass effect on normal pituitary)
- Pituitary apoplexy (usually hemorrhagic infarction of pituitary adenoma)

- Sellar tumors (e.g., craniopharyngioma)
- Granulomatous disease (sarcoidosis, tuberculosis)
- Postpartum necrosis (Sheehan syndrome)
- Radiation
- Infiltrative diseases (hemochromatosis, amyloidosis)

Always remember to rule out pregnancy in women with amenorrhea. In the patient with **amenorrhea** and **hirsutism**, consider:

- Pituitary disorders (Cushing disease, acromegaly)
- Polycystic ovary syndrome
- Congenital adrenal hyperplasia

Galactorrhea is a common symptom of prolactinoma but should be differentiated from the unilateral and sometimes bloody discharge caused by breast cancer.

DIAGNOSTIC EVALUATION

PITUITARY ADENOMAS

Prolactin levels are elevated in patients with prolactinomas, usually levels above 150 µg per L. Mild elevations in prolactin may be seen with nonfunctioning pituitary adenomas (because of stalk compression), dopamine antagonists (such as phenothiazines), other medications (tricyclic antidepressants, opiates), pregnancy, and hypothyroidism. GH is difficult to measure because of its pulsatile secretion, and therefore **insulin-like growth factor 1** (IGF-1), produced by the liver in response to GH, is measured instead. Elevated levels of IGF-1 (also known as somatomedin C) are found in acromegaly. Cushing disease may be screened for by an **overnight dexamethasone suppression test** and confirmed by elevated levels of free cortisol in the urine (see Chapter 52).

Magnetic resonance imaging (MRI) with gadolinium enhancement is the radiologic test of choice for pituitary abnormalities (see Fig. 53-1). The pituitary and the optic chiasm are well visualized. Pituitary tumors are classified as microadenomas (<10 mm) and macroadenomas (>10 mm). Some functioning adenomas may not be seen on MRI. Sampling of the inferior petrosal venous sinus, which drains the pituitary, has been used in Cushing disease to confirm the diagnosis.

PANHYPOPITUITARISM

Laboratory studies reveal deficiencies in multiple peripheral hormones (thyroxine, testosterone or

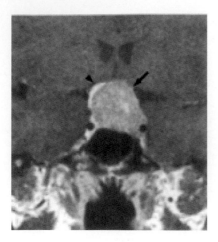

Figure 53-1 • A pituitary macroadenoma (*arrow*) with displacement of the optic chiasm (*arrowhead*).

estrogen, cortisol) without an increase in the respective pituitary hormones. These patterns include:

- Low free T_4 (thyroxine) and T_3 (triiodothyronine) in the setting of low or low-normal TSH
- Low testosterone or estrogen with low FSH and LH
- Suboptimal ACTH stimulation test (may still be normal in hypopituitarism of recent onset, such as Sheehan syndrome or pituitary apoplexy; however, an unstimulated morning serum cortisol of less than 5 μg per dL is highly suggestive of adrenal insufficiency)

Note that because prolactin secretion is under chronic inhibition, prolactin level may be normal or slightly elevated in hypopituitarism.

DIABETES INSIPIDUS

DI is suggested by **low urine osmolality** in the setting of **high serum osmolality**. Under direct supervision, the patient is restricted from fluid intake until serum osmolality is >295 mOsm per kg. The urine osmolality fails to increase; improvement with administration of vasopressin confirms a central etiology (pituitary or hypothalamic) of the disorder.

TREATMENT

PITUITARY ADENOMAS

Management of adenomas is directed at correcting the oversecretion of hormone and mass effects.

Nonfunctioning microadenomas or asymptomatic prolactin microadenomas do not need immediate treatment and may be closely followed.

Symptomatic prolactin adenomas should be medically treated. Both microadenomas and macroadenomas respond dramatically to **dopamine agonists**. Bromocriptine (2.5 mg orally two or three times a day) is the oldest dopamine agonist and considered a standard agent, but it requires multiple daily doses and causes side effects of orthostasis, nausea, and vomiting. **Cabergoline** (0.5 mg once or twice weekly) has a longer half-life and fewer side effects so is now a preferred dopamine agonist. Side effects can be limited by starting at a very low dose of medication. With medical treatment, gonadal function (and fertility) returns in most patients. Surgery is required in patients with refractory disease.

For pituitary adenomas secreting hormones other than prolactin, surgery is indicated. **Transsphenoidal surgery** is the standard of care and, if performed well, can lead to remission in 70% to 80% of patients. Surgery is less successful for larger tumors. Medical treatment is required for GH-secreting tumors that recur after surgery. Somatostatin analogues (octreotide and lanreotide) inhibit GH and can be used for patients who are not cured surgically. They can be given by injection once monthly. A GH receptor antagonist (pegvisomant) has recently been used as adjunct therapy. Dopamine agonists also have some effect in GH-secreting adenomas.

Conventional **radiation therapy** has been used in the past, but the side effect of hypopituitarism and the overall lack of efficacy have relegated this technique to an adjunctive role in refractory patients. Newer techniques, such as gamma knife and heavy particle therapy, show higher success rates.

PANHYPOPITUITARISM

Most patients have irreversible causes for panhypopituitarism, and treatment consists of hormone replacement therapy. Daily medications include hydrocortiosone (15 to 25 mg in divided doses) and levothyroxine (0.05 to 0.15 mg). Replacement of estrogen in women and testosterone in men relieves symptoms of hypogonadism. Cortisol should be the first hormone replaced, and stress doses (up to three times maintenance dose) are indicated during illness or surgery. Adrenal crisis should be treated with an initial dose of 100 mg hydrocortisone intravenously.

Replacement of growth hormone in adults is of uncertain benefit.

DIABETES INSIPIDUS

Patients with DI and hypernatremia need replacement of free water, either orally or with a hypotonic IV solution such as D5W. **Desmopressin acetate (DDAVP)**, a synthetic vasopressin, is used to control polyuria in central DI. It is given intranasally, subcutaneously, or orally twice daily.

CONTINUED CARE

Patients with pituitary macroadenomas need a formal examination of visual fields, and those with deficits are followed closely for worsening. Blood levels of hormones are followed during treatment or after surgery to assess response. Patients undergoing pituitary surgery or radiation should be monitored for the development of hypopituitarism or DI. Patients with resected Cushing disease are typically adrenally insufficient for several months and need cortisol replacement until normal adrenal function returns. Patients with acromegaly have an increased rate of colonic polyps and should be screened with colonoscopy every 3 to 5 years.

KEY POINTS

- Most pituitary adenomas are nonfunctioning; the most common functioning adenomas are prolactinomas.

- Prolactinomas often present as amenorrhea and galactorrhea in women. Diagnosis is confirmed by the combination of an elevated prolactin level (>150 μg per L) and pituitary mass. Treatment in most cases is a dopamine agonist.

- Acromegaly (excess GH) often presents as fatigue and arthralgias, sometimes in association with common disorders such as diabetes mellitus (DM), hypertension, or carpal tunnel syndrome. IGF-1 levels are elevated.

- Hypopituitarism is suspected in patients with hypogonadism who have low levels of FSH and LH. TSH is also low or normal. Causes include large (nonfunctioning) pituitary adenomas, radiation exposure, and granulomatous disease.

Nutritional Disorders

Vitamins and minerals compose the micronutrients needed for normal functions of metabolism. **Vitamins** are organic compounds that serve as cofactors for enzymes or (in the case of vitamin A) prosthetic groups needed for a functional molecule. They are often classified as the fat-soluble vitamins (A, D, E, and K) and the water-soluble vitamins (B and C). **Minerals** are inorganic compounds that are important components of enzymes and proteins. Minerals present in body fluids at concentrations of less than 1 μg per g wet weight are known as **trace elements** and are discussed in this chapter. These include cobalt, copper, iron, manganese, selenium, and zinc.

In general, humans are unable to synthesize vitamins and minerals independently and rely on dietary intake to provide adequate amounts of these compounds. Some exceptions that can be synthesized in low levels are vitamin D, which is synthesized from cholesterol; niacin, which is synthesized from tryptophan; and vitamin K, which is synthesized from intestinal microorganisms. The **recommended daily allowance** (RDA) is defined as the minimum amount of a vitamin or mineral needed to prevent a gross deficiency syndrome in most individuals. However, recent research has started to explore the benefit of vitamin supplementation above the RDA for prevention and treatment of disease. Table 54-1 lists disorders associated with vitamin deficiency and excess.

EPIDEMIOLOGY AND RISK FACTORS

Vitamin D deficiency is common, affecting as many as half of older adults or hospitalized patients who have low sun exposure, and even younger people can be mildly vitamin D deficient at the end of the winter months. Vitamin B_{12} deficiency is also more common in elderly patients. Other vitamin deficiencies are only rarely seen in clinical practice, even in developing countries, because of supplementation of processed foods. Still, malnourished patients and food faddists are at risk for developing deficiencies. Alcoholics are susceptible to deficiencies of thiamine, folic acid, and vitamin B_{12}. Also, patients dependent on total parenteral nutrition (TPN) may develop deficiencies if not carefully monitored. Patients with disorders of fat absorption, such as cystic fibrosis and cholestatic liver disease, may preferentially develop deficiencies of the fat-soluble vitamins.

FAT-SOLUBLE VITAMINS

Vitamin A

Vitamin A forms the prosthetic group of carotenoid proteins in the retina necessary for retinal excitation. It may be obtained directly through ingestion (liver, dairy products, eggs) or synthesized from beta-carotene (found in green leafy vegetables and carrots). Vitamin A deficiency is manifested as night blindness, followed by corneal ulceration and permanent damage. Xerosis (dry skin) and scaling of skin are also seen. Acute vitamin A toxicity (usually as a result of excess vitamin supplement intake) causes increased nausea and vomiting, malaise, and headache. Chronic excessive intake results in hepatosplenomegaly, ataxia, joint pain, and alopecia. Excessive intake of carotene does not cause hypervitaminosis A (because of regulation), but carotene can cause yellowing of the skin.

■ TABLE 54-1 Classic Syndromes of Vitamin Deficiency or Excess

Vitamin	Deficiency	Excess/Toxicity	Therapeutic Use
B_1 (thiamine)	Beriberi (high-output heart failure); Wernicke-Korsakoff syndrome	None	None
B_6 (pyridoxine)	Dermatitis, stomatitis, glossitis, peripheral neuropathy; may be precipitated by INH	Sensory neuropathy reported with very high doses	Supplementation lowers homocysteine levels (benefit unknown)
B_{12} (cobalamin)	Megaloblastic anemia, posterior column neuropathy	None known	None
Folate	Megaloblastic anemia	None known	Supplementation reduces neural tube defects (proven benefit) and lowers homocysteine levels (benefit unknown)
Niacin	Pellagra (diarrhea, dementia, dermatitis)	Flushing, pruritus, GI disturbances, hyperuricemia	Large (gram) doses useful to treat hyperlipidemia
C (ascorbic acid)	Scurvy (easy bruising, purpura, bleeding gums, poor wound healing)	GI discomfort, predisposition to form oxalate stones	
A (retinoic acid)	Night blindness, corneal ulceration	Central nervous system (CNS) effects (headaches, increased intracerebral pressure, papilledema) acutely; chronic excess can cause alopecia, hepatosplenomegaly, joint pain	None
E (tocopherol)	Ataxia, ophthalmoplegia, and loss of proprioception	Predisposition to bleeding in patients on warfarin	Antioxidant benefit in coronary artery disease and cancer prevention unproven
D (cholecalciferol)	Osteomalacia, hypocalcemia	Hypercalcemia	Supplementation in high-risk individuals prevents fractures
K	Bleeding disorder	None known	None

Vitamin D

Vitamin D is important in calcium absorption and bone formation. It may be synthesized in the skin from its precursor when exposed to ultraviolet light. Vitamin D is then hydroxylated in the liver to 25 (OH) vitamin D. Conversion to the active form (1,25 [OH]$_2$ vitamin D) occurs in the kidney and is tightly regulated by parathyroid hormone. Dietary sources include all dairy products and fortified cereals.

Vitamin D deficiency is the most common of all the deficiencies, and it is especially prevalent in the elderly and the chronically ill. It is manifested as hypocalcemia and osteomalacia, which leads to fractures. Vitamin D supplementation (800 U daily) along with calcium prevents fractures in high-risk groups. Because the formation of 1,25 (OH)$_2$ vitamin D is tightly regulated, vitamin D toxicity occurs only in the setting of massive ingestion or iatrogenic toxicity through use of calcitriol (synthetic 1,25 [OH]$_2$

vitamin D). This can lead to hypercalcemia (see Chapter 50).

Vitamin E

Vitamin E consists of a group of compounds known as tocopherols; the most common form is α-tocopherol. Vitamin E serves as an antioxidant and is widely distributed in foods, including grains and green leafy vegetables. Deficiency of this vitamin is rare, but hemolytic anemia in children has been reported. Also, an autosomal recessive mutation leading to vitamin E deficiency is associated with ataxia, posterior column neuropathy, and ophthalmoplegia. Vitamin E toxicity is not seen, although patients may have easy bruisability, and a patient on an oral anticoagulant may have an increased prothrombin time from the antagonism of vitamin K by excess vitamin E.

Vitamin K

Vitamin K consists of a quinone ring and is an important cofactor in the γ-carboxylation of clotting factors II, VII, IX, and X (see Chapter 66). It is found in green vegetables and is also produced by intestinal bacteria. Deficiency manifests as a bleeding disorder and is most commonly iatrogenic through the use of warfarin. Broad-spectrum antibiotics may destroy normal intestinal flora and lead to deficient vitamin K production if dietary intake is poor. Newborn infants are also vitamin K deficient at birth and are commonly given supplementation. There does not seem to be a clear syndrome of toxicity.

WATER-SOLUBLE VITAMINS

Thiamine (B$_1$)

Thiamine pyrophosphate is the active form of thiamine and serves as a cofactor in several enzymes in carbohydrate and protein catabolism. It is found in grains and legumes. Thiamine deficiency is seen most often in alcoholics, a result of overall malnutrition and alcohol's direct effects on thiamine. Deficiency syndromes are classified into cardiovascular (wet beriberi) and nervous system (Wernicke-Korsakoff syndrome) dysfunction. **Wet beriberi** presents with high-output cardiac failure, peripheral vasodilation, and edema. **Wernicke encephalopathy** is the acute neurologic presentation of thiamine deficiency, with delirium, ataxia, nystagmus, and ophthalmoplegia. This may be reversed with thiamine, but the chronic

deficiency often results in **Korsakoff syndrome**, which is notable for anterograde amnesia (inability to form new memory) and confabulation. In susceptible patients, a glucose load (such as IV dextrose) may precipitate Wernicke encephalopathy by using the little remaining thiamine with glucose catabolism. Alcoholics and malnourished patients should always receive thiamine first to avoid this complication. Toxicity with thiamine is not seen.

Pyridoxine (B$_6$)

Pyridoxine is an important cofactor in numerous enzyme reactions, including amino acid catabolism, heme synthesis, and glycogen breakdown. It is found in white meats (chicken, pork, fish), bananas, and grains. Severe deficiency results in angular stomatitis, glossitis, and dermatitis. Subclinical deficiency results in increases in homocysteine, a potential risk factor for coronary artery disease (see later). In addition, there are genetic disorders that require increased amounts of pyridoxine to avoid complications. These include pyridoxine-dependent seizures and some sideroblastic anemias. INH inhibits the function of pyridoxine and may cause deficiency symptoms in susceptible patients. Ingestion of several grams daily (a thousand times the RDA) has resulted in neuropathy.

Niacin

Niacin is an essential component of the coenzymes nicotinamide adenine dinucleotide (NAD) and nicotinamide adenine dinucleotide phosphate (NADPH) that are important in the body's reduction-oxidation reactions. It is widely distributed in foods and may also be synthesized from tryptophan. **Pellagra**, the classic niacin deficiency syndrome, was previously common in areas with a high intake of maize (American corn) or millet (sorghum). Although present in these foods, niacin is apparently biologically unavailable. Symptoms of deficiency include diarrhea, dermatitis, and dementia. Large doses (grams) of niacin, such as those given to lower cholesterol, cause flushing, hyperuricemia, and liver dysfunction.

Folate

Folate serves an important role in the transfer of one-carbon fragments between organic compounds. These reactions are important in purine and pyrimidine synthesis as well as in methionine production from homocysteine. Folate is found in high amounts in fortified cereals, citrus fruits, and legumes. Folate deficiency results in megaloblastic anemia (see Chapter 63) but also has been implicated in neural tube birth defects. Supplementation with 400 µg of folate is recommended for all women of childbearing years, and supplementation should increase to 1,000 µg daily during active attempts at conception and during pregnancy. Like pyridoxine, subclinical deficiency also leads to elevated homocysteine levels. Toxicity has not been reported, but there are concerns that excessive supplementation may mask the hematologic effects of B_{12} deficiency (leading to irreversible neurologic damage).

Vitamin C

Vitamin C, or ascorbic acid, is important for the synthesis of collagen and acts as an antioxidant. It is found in citrus fruits, tomatoes, and green leafy vegetables. **Scurvy**, the classic vitamin C deficiency seen in sailors with poor diets, is characterized by bleeding gums, loosening of the teeth, easy bruisability, poor wound healing, and hyperkeratotic perifollicular papules. It is still seen in impoverished areas of the United States. Large doses of vitamin C, often used to prevent colds and probably ineffective, do not seem to cause adverse effects. Vitamin C improves the absorption of iron and can be used to assist in iron repletion.

Other Water-Soluble Vitamins

Deficiency of riboflavin, a component of coenzyme flavin adenine dinucleotide (FAD), results in angular cheilitis and glossitis. Deficiency of biotin, an important cofactor in carboxylases, presents as a perioral rash and alopecia. Raw egg whites bind biotin and can result in a deficiency in individuals who consume large amounts of this food. Vitamin B_{12} (cobalamin) is found only in animal products; its deficiency causes megaloblastic anemia (see Chapter 63).

TRACE ELEMENTS

Deficiency of the trace elements is related either to inadequate dietary intake or to an increased loss in body fluids (e.g., gastrointestinal [GI] bleeding, pancreatic fistula). The use of TPN has helped elucidate the role and the importance of some of these trace minerals.

Iron

Iron is a key component of the oxygen-carrying proteins in the body, hemoglobin and myoglobin. Iron

sources include enriched grains, meats, poultry, and legumes. Iron deficiency is usually secondary to blood loss, although poor dietary intake or malabsorption can also lead to deficiency (see Chapter 63 for further details). Excessive iron ingestion remains an important cause of pediatric poisonings and can cause diarrhea and vomiting. In severe poisoning, cardiovascular collapse and seizures can occur. Treatment is gastric lavage because activated charcoal is ineffective at binding the cationic iron. Chronic iron toxicity is seen in hemochromatosis (see Chapter 42).

Zinc

Zinc is integral to the function of numerous proteins and enzymes (including RNA polymerase) throughout the reproductive, neurologic, GI, and immune systems. It is abundant in meats and shellfish. Zinc deficiency can result from chronic malabsorption and manifests as diarrhea, dermatitis, and growth retardation.

Copper

Copper is important to the function of numerous enzymes involved in connective tissue synthesis, iron transport, and energy production. It is available in organ meats, shellfish, and nuts. Copper deficiency is rare but can be caused by excessive zinc supplementation, which decreases copper absorption. Symptoms are similar to iron deficiency. Copper excess is seen in the autosomal recessive Wilson disease (see Chapter 42).

Therapeutic Use

There has been a recent interest in using vitamin supplementation at or above the RDA levels to prevent disease. As stated previously, vitamin D (800 U) in postmenopausal women and patients older than 65 years appears effective in slowing osteoporosis. Folate supplementation (800 to 1,000 µg) decreases neural tube defects if taken in the first trimester of pregnancy. Although observational studies showing that diets high in antioxidants decrease coronary artery disease (CAD) and cancer, trials using vitamin supplements have been unable to confirm a benefit, and the increased risk of bleeding related to high doses of vitamin E have led to a decline in its use. Homocysteine, a suggested risk factor for CAD, can be lowered by supplementation with folate, B_{12}, and B_6, but studies have not demonstrated a decrease in cardiovascular events.

KEY POINTS

- Vitamins are organic compounds that serve as cofactors and are obtained primarily through diet. Deficiency syndromes can be seen in alcoholics, malnourished individuals, and patients with malabsorption.

- Vitamin D deficiency is common and should be considered in elderly, hospitalized, or disabled patients.

- Minerals are inorganic compounds that are common components of enzymes and proteins. Iron deficiency is commonly seen with malabsorption or blood loss.

- Therapeutic uses of vitamins include vitamin D supplementation to prevent osteoporosis, folate supplementation to prevent neural tube defects, and niacin treatment to lower cholesterol. The role of antioxidants (vitamins A, C, and E) in decreasing coronary disease or cancer remains unproved.

Dyslipidemia

The following serum lipids are measured in the blood:

- Low-density lipoproteins (LDLs): "L for Lousy" cholesterol, most closely associated with cardiac disease
- High-density lipoproteins (HDLs): "H for Healthy" cholesterol, involved in removing cholesterol from tissues and protecting against coronary heart disease (CHD)
- Triglycerides: Used as a proxy measure for very low-density lipoproteins (VLDLs) in the fasting state

Dyslipidemia consists primarily of elevated LDL cholesterol, elevated triglyceride levels, or low HDL. Other forms of dyslipidemia, for example, apoB or Lp(a), are not addressed in this chapter. Hypercholesterolemia has been unequivocally associated with premature coronary artery disease (CAD). Hypertriglyceridemia has a weaker association with heart disease but at high levels leads to pancreatitis. Recommendations on screening and treatment in this chapter are based primarily on the National Cholesterol Education Program (NCEP) Adult Treatment Panel III (ATP III) expert panel consensus statement.

EPIDEMIOLOGY

Cholesterol levels rise with age by approximately 2 mg per dL each year. Women have lower cholesterol levels than men until menopause, when values become more equivalent. Hypercholesterolemia is extremely common, with more than 20% of adults having cholesterol levels greater than 240 mg per dL.

ETIOLOGY

Genetic factors play a role in the development of dyslipidemia, mostly through polygenic mechanisms. A few autosomal disorders account for a small number of individuals with extreme elevations in lipids. **Familial hypercholesterolemia** is characterized by a defective hepatic LDL receptor, resulting in LDL elevations. **Familial combined hyperlipidemia** is a more common disorder that may present with elevation in cholesterol, triglycerides, or both.

Dietary factors that may increase cholesterol include a high intake of saturated fats and exogenous cholesterol. Alcohol increases triglycerides by inhibiting their metabolism.

RISK FACTORS

Evaluation of dyslipidemia involves assessing for additional **risk factors for CHD**:

- Men older than 45 years or women older than 55 years
- Family history of premature CAD (men younger than 55 or women younger than 65)
- Current smoking
- Hypertension (blood pressure [BP] >140/90 or on medication)
- Diabetes mellitus (DM)
- Low HDL cholesterol (<40 mg per dL)

High HDL cholesterol (>60 mg per dL) is considered a protective factor; patients with high HDL are considered to have one less risk factor.

CLINICAL MANIFESTATIONS

HISTORY

The history should concentrate on obtaining additional risk factors for CHD (see earlier) and co-morbid factors that may influence treatment decisions, such as a history of DM, peptic ulcer, or gout. A dietary history should be obtained.

PHYSICAL EXAMINATION

Physical examination is almost always normal in dyslipidemia, except in cases of extreme elevation of cholesterol, as seen in hereditary disorders. Physical findings include:

- **Tendinous xanthomas** (subcutaneous painless nodules located on extensor tendons or Achilles tendon)
- **Eruptive xanthomas** (smaller yellowish papules occurring on buttocks and pressure-sensitive surfaces)
- **Xanthelasmas** (yellowish plaques located on eyelids)

DIFFERENTIAL DIAGNOSIS

Once the diagnosis of dyslipidemia is made, always consider other disorders that may **increase lipid levels**, such as:

- Hypothyroidism
- Nephrotic syndrome or chronic renal failure
- DM
- Cholestatic liver disease
- Drugs (thiazides, oral contraceptives)

DIAGNOSTIC EVALUATION

The initial screening test in healthy patients is a **fasting lipid profile** (total, HDL, LDL, and triglycerides). In a fasting analysis, LDL is calculated by the following equation:

$$LDL = \text{Total Cholesterol} - \text{HDL} - (\text{Triglycerides} \div 5)$$

This calculation is accurate only in the fasting state and if the triglyceride level is <400 mg per dL. A total cholesterol of <200 mg per dL and an HDL >40 mg per dL are desirable values. All other patients should be managed according to the LDL

■ TABLE 55-1 Levels of LDL at Which to Begin Treatment

Risk Factors	LDL Goal	Dietary Rx	Drug Rx
0 to 1	<160	>160	>190
2 or more RF CHD risk[a] <10%	<130	>130	>160
2 or more RF CHD risk 10–20%	<130	>130	>130
Known CHD[b] or CHD risk >20%	<100	>100	>130

[a]CHD risk is the 10-year risk as calculated by the Framingham risk score.
[b]Patients with DM and peripheral vascular disease are also in this group. Statins are strongly recommended regardless of LDL level.

level and the associated risk factors. In addition, the latest recommendations of the NCEP call for a risk assessment (via the Framingham risk score*) in patients with two or more of the risk factors just listed. Patients with a Framingham risk score suggesting their 10-year coronary event risk is >20% are considered to be "CHD equivalent." Such high-risk patients should be aggressively treated as though they have presumed cardiovascular disease.

Laboratory tests to rule out secondary causes include thyroid-stimulating hormone (TSH; hypothyroidism), fasting glucose (DM), creatinine (chronic renal failure), liver function tests (LFTs; cholestasis), and UA for protein (nephrotic syndrome).

TREATMENT

Treatment for dyslipidemia is directed at lowering the risk of CHD. Intensity of treatment depends on the patient's individual risk for CHD (as determined by the Framingham risk score) and the level of LDL (Table 55-1). Treatment may be divided into non-pharmacologic measures (diet, exercise, smoking cessation) and pharmacologic measures. Weight loss, smoking cessation, and aerobic exercise are a few of the techniques to raise HDL.

Overall, treatment is most aggressive in patients with known CHD. The NCEP ATP III goal for LDL in these patients is <100 mg per dL, and further evidence supports lowering LDL down to 70 for

*The Framingham risk calculator is available at http://hp2010 .nhlbihin.net/atpiii/calculator.asp?usertype%20=%20prof.

patients with recent cardiac events. Treatment goals are similar in patients with DM or peripheral vascular disease (PVD), who are also at high risk for cardiovascular events. Statin treatment decreases cardiovascular risk in these groups regardless of baseline LDL; therefore, medication should be initiated and increased to meet the LDL goal. Conversely, drug therapy should be delayed in men younger than 35 years and in premenopausal women because of the low incidence of CHD in these populations. However, patients with a strong family history and high cholesterol level may have a hereditary disorder requiring more intense treatment.

Dietary therapy limits the intake of cholesterol and saturated fats. Current dietary recommendations include reduced cholesterol intake (<200 mg daily), reduced saturated fat (<7% of calories), and limited intake of *trans*-fatty acids. Patients have varied responses to dietary intake. Those who already have well-balanced diets may show no change in their cholesterol values. On average, cholesterol decreases by 5% to 10% of total value with dietary measures. The largest decrease in total cholesterol through diet is probably approximately 20% to 25%; therefore, if a greater decrease is desired, drug therapy may be considered early. Referral to a dietitian is recommended.

Drug therapy in dyslipidemia consists of five main classes of drugs. The drugs differ in their side effects, potency, and lipid-lowering properties (Table 55-2).

The **HMG-CoA reductase inhibitors** (statins) have the most convincing effect on reducing cardiovascular events both in patients without known CHD (primary prevention) and in established disease (secondary prevention). These agents inhibit the rate-limiting step in cholesterol synthesis and reduce LDL levels by an average of 35%. The amount of LDL reduction depends on the specific drug and the dose. Lovastatin, pravastatin, fluvastatin, and simvastatin achieve approximately 25% reduction in LDL,

with a maximum of 40% at the highest dosages. Atorvastatin and rosuvastatin are more potent drugs, with 50% to 60% reductions in LDL at the maximal dosages. Important side effects include myopathy (especially when taken with niacin or fibric acid derivatives) and elevated LFTs (in 1% to 2% of patients). With rosuvastatin, serious myopathy and rhabdomyolysis has been reported at high doses; people of Asian descent are increased risk. Patients who complain of muscle pain or cramping on these medications should be examined and have creatine kinase levels checked.

Niacin was previously considered a first-line therapy to lower LDL and raise HDL (through an unknown mechanism). However, this drug is limited by its side effects, most notably flushing. To avoid these side effects, begin with low-dose niacin (100 mg thrice daily), use prophylactic aspirin (325 mg daily) to counteract flushing for the first few weeks, and advance the niacin dose slowly, doubling every 2 weeks until reaching 500 to 1,000 mg thrice daily. Even with these efforts, up to 50% of patients discontinue the medication. Time-release preparations may be better tolerated but some have an increased risk of hepatotoxicity. Other side effects include aggravating peptic ulcer disease, gout, and hyperglycemia (in diabetics).

Bile acid sequestrants (cholestyramine, colestipol, colesevelam) are nonabsorbable drugs that bind bile acids and prevent enterohepatic circulation of cholesterol. Side effects include bloating and constipation, binding of certain drugs (e.g., digoxin, thyroxine, warfarin), and aggravation of preexisting hypertriglyceridemia. Colesevelam may have fewer side effects.

Fibric acid derivatives (gemfibrozil, fenofibrate) are reserved for lowering triglycerides by increasing VLDL metabolism. HDL cholesterol usually increases (10%) when triglycerides are lowered. Gemfibrozil (300 to 600 mg twice daily) is limited by GI side effects and may increase the risk of gallstones. Fenofibrate (145 mg every day) offers easier dosing, and fewer side effects. Plasma creatinine may increase when taking fenofibrate.

Ezetimibe (10 mg per day) is a newer agent that reduces cholesterol dietary absorption. Although it is effective in lowering LDL when used alone, it is most commonly used with a statin to provide additional LDL lowering benefit to achieve stricter LDL goals. However, controlled trials have not proven this strategy to be more effective in lowering cardiovascular events. Ezetimibe can cause myalgias as well, but can still be used in patients intolerant of statins.

■ **TABLE 55-2** Drug Effects on Lipid Profiles			
	LDL	**HDL**	**Triglycerides**
HMG-CoA reductase inhibitors	↓	↑	—
Niacin	↓	↑↑	↓
Bile acid resins	↓	—	↑
Fibric acid derivatives	↓↑	↑	↓↓
Ezetimibe	↓	—	—

Patients should have a fasting lipid analysis and LFTs 1 to 3 months after a change of therapy. Failure to achieve LDL goal leads to increasing dietary restrictions and adding or increasing medication. Given the risk of myopathy when niacin or fibric acid derivatives are added to statin therapy, the statins are best combined with ezetimibe or bile acid resins when combination therapy is required.

TREATMENT OF ISOLATED HYPERTRIGLYCERIDEMIA

Triglycerides may be markedly elevated in the presence of reasonable LDL values. Although there is less direct evidence that triglyceride lowering improves cardiovascular outcomes, triglyceride levels over 500 mg/dL should be lowered to prevent pancreatitis. NCEP ATPIII guidelines recommend a target triglyceride level of less than 200 mg/dL.

In addition to the fibrates mentioned above, weight reduction, glucose control, and limiting excess alcohol can help to lower triglycerides. Fish oil (omega-3 fatty acids) in doses of 1,000 to 2,000 mg daily have lowered triglycerides in controlled trials, but the effect on cardiovascular events is less certain.

 KEY POINTS

- Screening for dyslipidemia consists of a fasting total cholesterol, HDL, and calculated LDL; desirable values are based on the total CHD risk factor profile.
- Secondary causes of dyslipidemia include DM, liver disease, chronic renal failure, nephrotic syndrome, and hypothyroidism.
- Treatment is initially dietary restriction when <25% LDL reduction is needed.
- Drug treatment includes the statin drugs, ezetimibe, niacin, bile acid sequestrants, and fibric acid derivatives. Statin drugs have the most evidence for prevention of cardiovascular events and are the first-line agents.
- Patients with known CHD have a goal of LDL below 100 mg per dL or lower (as low as 70 mg per dL).

Part 7

Rheumatology

Acute Monoarticular Arthritis

Acute monoarticular arthritis is an inflammatory process that develops in a single joint, usually over several days. Rapid assessment is required to rule out bacterial infection, which quickly leads to irreversible joint damage if not treated. Accurate diagnosis requires joint aspiration and examination of synovial fluid.

DIFFERENTIAL DIAGNOSIS

The differential diagnosis can be divided into several categories:

Infection
- Gonococcal (GC)
- Non-GC bacterial (most commonly *Staphylococcus aureus*)
- Lyme disease

Crystalline disease
- Gout
- Pseudogout

Trauma
- Cruciate ligament or meniscal tear (knee)
- Osteoarthritis
- Hemarthrosis

Rheumatologic disease
- Rheumatoid arthritis
- Seronegative spondyloarthropathy
- Systemic lupus erythematosus (SLE)

Rheumatologic disease is often polyarticular but may present with solitary joint involvement in atypical cases. These diseases are discussed in detail in Chapters 58, 59, and 60.

CLINICAL MANIFESTATIONS

HISTORY

Duration of symptoms assists in differentiating the cause of joint inflammation. Extremely rapid onset, especially when associated with a "pop" or "snap," implies torn menisci or ligaments. Gout and bacterial infection usually develop over hours to days, whereas pseudogout may take several days to develop. Rheumatologic causes are often more subacute, occurring over weeks. Disseminated gonorrhea often has an initial syndrome of fever and **migratory polyarthralgia** before a predominant joint becomes affected.

A past history of monoarticular arthritis may suggest a crystalline or rheumatologic disease. **Risk factors for gout** include diabetes mellitus, hypertension, obesity, hyperlipidemia, alcohol intake, and thiazide use. A history of a tick bite strongly raises the suspicion of Lyme disease. Unlike the acute presentation of the typical rash (erythema migrans), Lyme arthritis occurs weeks to months after the tick bite. Bacterial infection is more common in diabetics and IV drug users. Swelling of a prosthetic joint is of great concern for infection. Patients on anticoagulation drugs (heparin, warfarin) or with an inherited defect in coagulation (hemophilia) are at increased risk for hemarthrosis with minor trauma.

PHYSICAL EXAMINATION

The presence of **fever** is an important sign because most patients with bacterial infection are febrile.

However, gout and rheumatologic disease may also cause an increase in temperature.

Skin examination should concentrate on searching for the typical rashes of GC infection or Lyme disease. **Skin lesions in GC** are found on the extremities. They begin as small papules and then quickly become pustular with a necrotic center. **Erythema migrans** (Lyme disease) is a round or oval lesion that is well demarcated and usually has a central clearing. The diameter of the lesion is >5 cm and median size is 15 cm. The rash of Lyme disease has often resolved before the presentation of monoarthritis. Other findings to look for on skin examination include gouty tophi (subcutaneous nodules found on extensor surfaces), needle track marks (as seen in IV drug users), and psoriatic plaques (suggesting spondyloarthropathy).

Joint examination reveals a warm and tender joint. Painful limitation of motion is almost always present with articular involvement but may sometimes be present in non-articular causes of joint pain (e.g., cellulitis, tendinitis). The **knee joint** is the most common joint affected in bacterial infection, Lyme disease, pseudogout, and traumatic causes. Gout primarily affects the **first metatarsal joint** or **ankle joint** but may involve the knee as well. **Tenosynovitis**, usually in the tendons of the hands and fingers, is present in the majority of patients with disseminated GC infection.

DIAGNOSTIC EVALUATION

Arthrocentesis is the definitive diagnostic procedure. Septic arthritis has a predilection for damaged joints; therefore, joint aspiration still needs to be performed in patients with a past history of osteoarthritis or crystalline-induced arthritis. Aspiration of some joints (e.g., hip) requires fluoroscopic or ultrasonographic guidance and should be performed by a specialist. Fluid appearance is sometimes helpful in determining etiology. The presence of frank blood on aspiration confirms hemarthrosis; cloudy or turbulent fluid is likely to be secondary to infection or crystalline disease.

Leukocyte count should be performed to determine the inflammatory nature of the effusion. Table 56-1 shows general guidelines in interpreting the leukocyte count. **Fluid culture** and **Gram stain** are mandatory when infection is a possibility. Gram-positive cocci are seen on Gram stain in 80% of *S. aureus* infected joints. *Neisseria gonorrhea* is rarely seen on Gram stain.

Crystal examination should be performed on synovial fluid to rule out gout (needle-shaped, negatively

TABLE 56-1 General Guidelines for Interpreting Leukocyte Count	
WBC Count (cells/mm³)	**Interpretation**
<200	Normal fluid
<2000	Noninflammatory (e.g., osteoarthritis)
2000 to 50,000	Mild to moderate inflammation (rheumatologic, crystalline)
50,000 to 100,000	Severe inflammation (sepsis or gout)
>100,000	Sepsis until proven otherwise

birefringent crystals) or pseudogout (rhomboid, weakly positive birefringence) (see Color Plates 16 and 17). The presence of crystals does not exclude infection because damaged joints are more susceptible to infection.

Urethral, pharyngeal, cervical (in women), and rectal specimens should be sent to the laboratory for culture on all patients with suspected GC infection. Blood cultures may be positive for GC early in the course of the disease. Activated partial thromboplastin time (aPTT) is elevated in patients with hemophilia. Radiographs of the affected joint may show chondrocalcinosis in pseudogout or an associated fracture in traumatic causes. The presence of osteoarthritis may be noted, but this does not rule out other causes, such as crystalline disease or infection.

Uric acid level is **not** useful in acute gouty arthritis because it is normal in 30% to 40% of patients. Lyme antibody cannot distinguish between active and inactive infection, but a negative result argues against Lyme arthritis.

TREATMENT

INFECTION

Patients with suspected or confirmed bacterial infection should receive parenteral antibiotic therapy as soon as cultures are sent. **Vancomycin** (1 g every 12 hours) is the drug of choice for most patients to cover *S. aureus*. IV drug users or diabetic patients should be covered for gram-negative organisms as well. Repeated drainage is needed in all patients with confirmed non-GC septic arthritis to avoid joint damage. In the patient with suspected GC infection (especially a young patient with rash or tenosynovitis), **ceftriaxone** is the drug of choice, although most disseminated GC infections are sensitive to penicillin. Lyme arthritis is treated with doxycycline, 100 mg twice daily for 1 to 2 months. Lyme disease with meningitis or severe carditis should be treated with IV ceftriaxone.

CRYSTALLINE DISEASE

Gout and pseudogout should be treated with a **non-steroidal anti-inflammatory drug** (NSAID) such as indomethacin, 50 mg three times daily. **Colchicine** (0.6 mg twice daily) may also be used but is limited by its side effects (diarrhea and myelosuppression). It may be used in patients unable to take NSAIDs (e.g., peptic ulcer disease [PUD]) but should be avoided in patients with hepatic or renal disease. Intra-articular steroid injection is an alternative if oral therapy is contraindicated and infection has been excluded. In recurrent gout, **allopurinol** (a xanthine oxidase inhibitor) may be given to decrease uric acid levels. It should not be started during an acute flare, and NSAIDs or colchicine should be given as prophylaxis when starting allopurinol. **Probeniecid** increases uric acid excretion, and is an alternative to allopurinol in patients with normal renal function who are not taking high-dose aspirin (which blocks probeniecid's effect).

TRAUMATIC CAUSES

General principles include rest, ice, elevation, and anti-inflammatory agents. Osteoarthritis may be treated with acetaminophen or NSAIDs. Active patients with possible ligament or meniscal tears should be referred to an orthopedic surgeon to consider arthroscopic repair.

KEY POINTS

- Acute monoarticular arthritis should be promptly evaluated because history and physical are unable to definitively rule out bacterial infection, which will lead to irreversible damage if untreated.

- Gout often occurs in the first metatarsal or ankle joint. Diabetes, hypertension, obesity, and alcohol intake increase risk for gout. Treatment consists of NSAIDs or colchicine.

- GC infection is a common cause of monoarticular arthritis in young individuals. Associated findings include pustular rash and tenosynovitis. Fluid Gram stain and synovial cultures are often negative. Treatment is with ceftriaxone.

- Bacterial infection should be ruled out by Gram stain and culture. Suspicion is high when the fluid leukocyte count is >100,000 cells per mm^3.

Low Back Pain

Low back pain affects approximately 70% of people at some time in their lives. Evaluation may not result in a specific diagnosis, but because most patients have resolution of the symptoms in 2 to 6 weeks, diagnostic testing can be limited to those patients with worrisome historical or physical findings.

DIFFERENTIAL DIAGNOSIS

Differential diagnosis can be divided into several categories:

Musculoskeletal causes
- Musculoligamentous injury
- Herniated intervertebral disk
- Spinal stenosis
- Vertebral compression fracture
- Spondylolysis or spondylolisthesis

Systemic causes
- Malignancy (most commonly metastasis from breast, lung, prostate, kidney carcinoma, or multiple myeloma)
- Vertebral osteomyelitis
- Epidural abscess
- Spondyloarthropathy

Referred pain
- Aortic dissection or aneurysm
- Pyelonephritis or nephrolithiasis
- Prostatitis
- Pancreatic carcinoma or pancreatitis

CLINICAL MANIFESTATIONS

The evaluation of low back pain is focused on two key aspects: evidence of systemic disease and evidence of nerve compression.

HISTORY

Although many patients with musculoskeletal injury have pain radiating to the buttocks or thighs, only true **sciatica** from nerve root compression radiates below the knee to the foot. Back pain without sciatica is rarely caused by disk herniation. A history of low back pain with morning stiffness in a younger person raises the question of **ankylosing spondylitis**. The patient with **spinal stenosis** often presents with back or leg pain that worsens with walking (pseudo-claudication) and with prolonged standing.

Important "**red flags**" to obtain from the history are past history of malignancy, fever, weight loss, bladder or bowel dysfunction, and "saddle anesthesia." Patients with a previous diagnosis of cancer should be presumed to have back pain secondary to malignancy until proved otherwise. Patients with back pain due to malignancy often do not experience relief of pain with supine position (in contrast to musculoskeletal causes). **Fever** associated with back pain raises the suspicion of osteomyelitis or epidural abscess.

Age is an important risk factor for worrisome etiologies of back pain. Compression fractures, malignancy, and spinal stenosis increase in incidence with age. Additional information to obtain includes relation of the back pain to litigation or workers' compensation. These nonmedical factors may influence the patient's desire for testing and recovery.

PHYSICAL EXAMINATION

Physical examination focuses on elucidating signs of **nerve root compression**. Disk herniation occurs at the L4 to L5 level or L5 to S1 level in 95% of all disk herniations. Weakness of dorsiflexion occurs in L5 root compression, and weakness of plantar flexion occurs in S1 root compression. **Cauda equina syndrome** is an extremely uncommon occurrence in disk herniation but is a "must-not-miss" diagnosis. Sensory examination in these patients may reveal saddle anesthesia (decreased sensation over buttocks, perineum, and posterior thighs) due to compression of sacral nerves. Table 57-1 lists these syndromes associated with disk herniation.

Straight leg raising should also be performed in patients with suspected disk herniation. With the patient supine, the extended leg is raised off the table. A positive sign reproduces sciatica at 30 to 60 degrees of elevation. A more specific (but less sensitive) sign is pain that is reproduced when the contralateral leg is raised.

Paraspinal tenderness is often seen in musculoskeletal strain but is difficult to reproduce. Focal vertebral tenderness is often seen in osteomyelitis or epidural abscess, but it is not specific. Although pain may limit range of motion in many cases of back pain, limited flexion is also seen in ankylosing spondylitis.

Overreaction during the examination, superficial tenderness, and back pain with "axial loading" (pressing on patient's head) all suggest a psychological component to the back pain.

DIAGNOSTIC EVALUATION

Most patients with low back pain and no worrisome clinical features need no further evaluation beyond history and physical examination, and most patients improve in <4 weeks. Unnecessary testing may demonstrate radiologic findings such as spondylolisthesis or disk protrusion that are common in asymptomatic individuals and may mislead the physician.

Patients older than 50 years or those with a history of weight loss, significant trauma, malignancy, or chronic steroid use should have a **lumbar spine film** to look for compression fractures or malignant lesions. An erythrocyte sedimentation rate (ESR), although not specific or sensitive, may be elevated in infections or malignancies that cause back pain.

Further testing depends on the response to treatment. **Treatment strategy for nonworrisome low back pain** consists of the following:

- Nonsteroidal anti-inflammatory drugs (NSAIDs,) such as ibuprofen or naproxen
- Continuation of usual activity with avoidance of bending or twisting. Bed rest should be limited for periods of severe pain because prolonged bed rest may lead to deconditioning and a worse outcome
- Ice to affected area for first 24 hours, followed by warm compresses
- Back exercises that extend and flex back muscles after the acute pain subsides

Magnetic resonance imaging (MRI) and/or **surgical referral** should be obtained for sciatica that fails to improve after 4 to 6 weeks, progressive neurologic deficit, findings suspicious for epidural abscess, and bilateral neurologic deficits or urinary retention (suggesting cauda equina syndrome). The cauda equina syndrome requires urgent evaluation.

Spinal cord compression may initially present with back pain alone. Therefore, early MRI is necessary for

■ **TABLE 57-1** Findings of Herniated Disks				
Disk Location	**Nerve Root Involved**	**Pain Radiation**	**Neurologic Deficits**	**Additional Features**
L4 to L5	L5	Anterolateral leg and great toe	Dorsiflexion (ankle and great toe)	
L5 to S1	S1	Posterior leg and lateral toes	Plantar flexion (ankle)	Decreased ankle reflex
Midline disk herniation	Cauda equina	Bilateral leg numbness	Saddle anesthesia	Urinary retention

any patient with a known malignancy who develops new-onset back pain. If not treated early in its course, cord compression may progress to irreversible neurologic injury.

Patients with a history or physical findings worrisome for malignancy should have testing performed for common malignancies that metastasize to the vertebrae (lung, prostate, breast). A new compression fracture without risk factors (e.g., steroid use) should raise the suspicion of multiple myeloma; **serum and urine immunoelectrophoresis** may be performed to rule out this diagnosis.

 KEY POINTS

- Most patients with back pain do not receive a definitive diagnosis and are labeled with musculoskeletal strain; 80% of these patients improve with conservative treatment in <6 weeks.

- Patients at risk for compression fractures or malignancy should receive an initial lumbar spine film; MRI should be reserved for selected patients.

- Treatment consists of short-term rest, ice, NSAIDs, and back exercises. Psychological factors may impede the patient's recovery.

- Cauda equina syndrome presents with back pain, leg weakness, saddle anesthesia, and urinary retention. Urgent MRI is required for evaluation.

58 Rheumatoid Arthritis

Rheumatoid arthritis (RA) is a symmetric inflammatory peripheral polyarthritis characterized by lymphocytic infiltration of the synovial joints and granulomatous extra-articular nodules. The inflammatory process is generally progressive and despite intermittent remissions, ongoing joint destruction can be debilitating.

EPIDEMIOLOGY AND RISK FACTORS

RA affects 1% of the adult population, with a peak onset most often between 40 and 50 years of age. Women are more affected than men (3:1). The prevalence of RA in women older than 65 years is as much as 5%, making RA a significant cause of morbidity.

There appears to be a genetic predisposition to RA, with a strong linkage to certain HLA-DR alleles. First-degree relatives of RA patients have a fourfold higher risk of developing the disease. The increased prevalence in women compared to men has led to theories of predisposing hormonal states, but as yet a direct hormonal stimulus is not apparent. Theories about infectious agents precipitating RA have not been proved. Of note, smoking has been associated with increased RA risk, but data remain controversial.

PATHOGENESIS

It is not yet clear how the pathologic inflammatory process is initiated in RA. However, it is clear that synovial T cells become activated, leading to a cascade of inflammation that causes the synovial lining to become invasive, causing erosion and destruction of the joint cartilage. Inflammation is accompanied by angiogenesis, with new blood vessel formation in the inflamed synovium. Analysis of synovial tissue in RA reveals high levels of tumor necrosis factor alpha (TNF-α) and interleukin-1 (IL-1). These factors upregulate the production of metalloproteinases, which are believed to be responsible for joint destruction. Blockade of the effects of TNF-α and IL-1 has an important role in RA treatment.

CLINICAL MANIFESTATIONS

HISTORY

Patients often present with gradual onset of **pain** and **swelling** in peripheral joints, usually polyarticular and symmetric. **Morning stiffness** (>1 hour) is a key feature. Constitutional symptoms such as weight loss, fatigue, and anorexia may also occur and even precede the onset of joint symptoms.

PHYSICAL EXAMINATION

Most often involved are the proximal interphalangeal, metacarpophalangeal, and wrist joints. Knee joints may be affected, with inflammatory knee joint synovium resulting in a Baker cyst. Examination of the joints reveals an inflammatory synovitis (warmth, tenderness, and swelling). Late presentations include joint deformities such as ulnar deviation of the phalanges, swan neck, or boutonnière deformities (Fig. 58-1). Axial joints are less often involved than peripheral joints, with the cervical spine the most likely axial joints involved. Cervical spine synovial and bursa inflammation can cause atlantoaxial subluxation, a

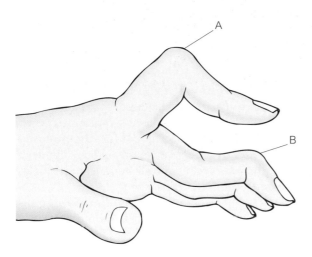

Figure 58-1 • (A) Boutonnière deformity. **(B)** Swan neck deformity.

potentially serious complication that can cause spinal cord compression with associated findings.

Subcutaneous nontender **rheumatoid nodules** may be found on the extensor surfaces of the forearm and elbow or Achilles tendon. Splenomegaly may be found in RA, and, when associated with leukopenia, the triad is known as **Felty syndrome**.

RA may also be associated with a severe **vasculitis**, presenting with digital infarcts, palpable purpura, and mononeuritis multiplex.

DIFFERENTIAL DIAGNOSIS

The differential diagnosis involves other etiologies of arthritis or joint pain, including:

- Osteoarthritis (more distal interphalangeal joint involvement, non-inflammatory examination)
- Psoriatic arthritis (look for psoriasis of the skin and nail changes)
- Gout or pseudogout (best diagnosed with synovial fluid analysis)
- Connective tissue diseases such as systemic lupus erythematosus (SLE; less deforming and lacks subcutaneous nodules)
- Septic arthritis (more likely monoarticular, with erythema and likely fever)
- Reactive arthritis (recent history of gastrointestinal [GI] or GU disease, asymmetric lower extremity arthritis)
- Lyme disease (usually monoarticular knee arthritis with preceding rash and fever)

DIAGNOSTIC EVALUATION

Table 58-1 shows an abbreviated version of the American Rheumatism Association's diagnostic criterion for RA. Most criteria are achieved through clinical examination and history. Two additional criteria are **rheumatoid factor** (RF) and **plain films**. RF is an autoimmune antibody to IgG and is positive in 70% to 80% of patients with RA. However, it is not specific for RA and by itself does not confirm the diagnosis. The following conditions may have a positive **RF** in the absence of **RA**:

- Older age
- Other autoimmune diseases (SLE, sarcoid, etc.)
- Infective endocarditis
- Liver disease (especially hepatitis C)
- Chronic infections (syphilis, leprosy, parasites)
- Hyperglobulinemic states

Because of the lack of specificity, other antibody testing may be used in combination with RF. Antibodies to citrulline-containing proteins (anti-CCP) are seen in RF patients, with sensitivity for RA approximating that of RF. However, anti-CCP has much greater specificity (90% to 96%). Although anti-CCP is not yet included in the American Rheumatism Association's diagnostic criterion for RA, initial anti-CCP testing (as well as antinuclear antibody and hepatitis testing) is frequently performed for initial diagnosis. Plain films of the hands may demonstrate periarticular osteopenia or erosions, usually in more advanced disease.

■ **TABLE 58-1** Criteria for Diagnosis of Rheumatoid Arthritis*a*
Morning stiffness of joints >1 hr for at least 6 wk
Arthritis (soft tissue swelling) of three or more joints for at least 6 wk
Arthritis includes wrist, metacarpophalangeal, or proximal intraphalangeal joints
Arthritis is symmetric
Rheumatoid nodules
Elevated serum rheumatoid factor
Hand or wrist films showing erosions or periarticular osteopenia

aFour or more criteria are necessary for definite diagnosis.

Other laboratory findings measure the inflammatory nature of the disease, such as an increased erythrocyte sedimentation rate (ESR) or C-reactive protein (**CRP**). Joint aspiration is usually performed to rule out other causes, such as infection or gout. See Chapter 56 for a discussion of the joint fluid examination.

Chest radiograph may reveal extra-articular disease such as rheumatoid nodules, interstitial lung disease, or pleural effusions. Pulmonary nodules should be tested in the usual manner (see Chapter 19). Effusions that are tapped show an exudative pattern, usually with a low fluid glucose level.

Patients with RA may also have atlantoaxial subluxation discovered on cervical spine films. This must be ruled out before manipulation of the patient's neck, as in endotracheal intubation.

TREATMENT

The primary goal of treatment in RA is to achieve a complete remission, defined as absence of symptoms or objective synovitis, no radiographic progression, and a normal erythrocyte sedimentation rate (ESR)/CRP. Early administration of **disease-modifying antirheumatic drugs** (DMARDs) is advocated to accomplish this goal. When remission is unable to be achieved, management focuses on pain control, maintenance of function, and slowing irreversible joint destruction. Patients with positive RF, erosions on hand films, or extra-articular manifestations tend to have a more severe disease course; however, there is no reliable way to predict a poor prognosis.

Symptom relief in RA may initially rely on analgesics including **NSAIDs**. Examples include ibuprofen, ketoprofen, and naproxen. NSAIDs do not significantly influence synovial inflammation or joint destruction. **Side effects of NSAIDs** are numerous and include:

- Peptic ulcers/gastritis
- Renal dysfunction
- Increased liver enzymes
- Rash

COX-2 inhibitors such as celecoxib are NSAIDs that selectively inhibit the cyclooxygenase-2 enzyme (involved in inflammation) and not the cyclooxygenase-1 enzyme (involved in gastric mucosa protection). These are reserved for use in selected patients at high risk for GI because they are expensive, and COX-2 inhibitor use is associated with an increased risk of cardiovascular disease. Celecoxib is a sulfonamide derivative and is avoided in patients with a history of severe sulfa allergy. As an alternative to COX-2 inhibitors, use of traditional NSAIDs with a proton pump inhibitor or the prostaglandin analogue misoprostol offers GI bleeding protection.

Corticosteroids should be used sparingly in RA. Prednisone is effective to relieve symptoms, but the numerous side effects (osteoporosis, immunosuppression, hyperglycemia) make this choice less desirable over the long term. Corticosteroids may be used as a bridge to the DMARDs.

DMARDs have the added benefit of slowing disease progression in RA. DMARDs should be started early (within 3 months) in almost all patients with RA to prevent further joint destruction. Typical DMARDs and their common side effects are:

- Methotrexate (bone marrow toxicity, hepatic fibrosis, pneumonitis, stomatitis)
- Sulfasalazine (rash)
- Antimalarials, such as hydroxychloroquine (retinopathy)
- Leflunomide (diarrhea, rash)
- Minocycline (hyperpigmentation)
- Azathioprine (immunosuppression)

With a multitude of choices, older agents such as gold and penicillamine have been abandoned due to serious side effects (bone marrow toxicity, proteinuria).

Methotrexate is used as a first-line DMARD in many patients with RA. Methotrexate has a high clinical response rate and an acceptable treatment adherence rate. It is given in low doses (7.5 to 15 mg) in weekly intervals. The dose should be increased up to 25 mg weekly when patients fail to respond. A unique feature of methotrexate is that rheumatoid nodules may increase with initiation of treatment. Liver biopsy for cirrhosis was once recommended for all patients on treatment but now is reserved for persistent liver function abnormalities. Alcohol should certainly be avoided to minimize the risk of liver damage. GI symptoms may be decreased with oral folate supplements. An alternative to methotrexate therapy is leflunomide, a pyrimidine synthesis inhibitor. The dosage is 10 to 20 mg daily, and its efficacy is similar to methotrexate. DMARDs can be used in combination, but an optimal combination therapy is not yet clear.

In patients with uncontrolled disease on the agents just described, **biologic anticytokine agents** are promising newer DMARDs. Monoclonal antibodies against TNF-α (infliximab and adalimumab) and soluble TNF receptors (etanercept) have been effective in decreasing disease activity for up to 12 months in trials. An IL-1 receptor antagonist (anakinra) can be used for patients who fail therapy with anti-TNF-α agents. It requires daily subcutaneous injection and can lead to injection site irritant reactions.

Two additional biologic agents given by intravenous infusion are rituximab and abatacept. **Rituximab** is a chimeric human/mouse monoclonal antibody against CD20 (found on mature B cells). **Abatacept** is a recombinant fusion protein of cytotoxic T-lymphocyte antigen 4 (CTLA-4) and immunoglobulin. Abatacept mimics the action of CTLA-4, which is released by T-cells and leads to downregulation of T cell activation. Both agents have demonstrated decreased disease activity in patients who have failed standard DMARDs.

All biologic agents can increase the risk of reactivation of tuberculosis or lead to serious bacterial infections. Purified protein derivative (PPD) testing should be performed prior to initiating treatment, and any fever or acute illness should be carefully evaluated.

Monitoring in RA consists of following the patient's symptoms and examining joints for improvement. Other monitoring includes hand and/or foot films for disease progression, CRP for inflammation, liver and renal function tests (especially for patients on NSAIDs or methotrexate) and regular retinal evaluation (if on hydroxychloroquine). All patients should be maintained on calcium (1,000 to 1,500 mg daily) and vitamin D (400 to 800 units daily), and the bone density should be routinely monitored for osteoporosis.

KEY POINTS

- RA is an inflammatory disease characterized by symmetric peripheral polyarthritis, most commonly affecting the wrist and the metacarpophalangeal and proximal interphalangeal joints. Morning stiffness is a key feature.

- RF is positive in 70% to 80% of patients with RA. RF is not a specific test, and false positives occur in the elderly and in patients with other autoimmune diseases, liver diseases, and chronic infections. Antibodies to citrulline-containing proteins (anti-CCP) are more specific.

- Extra-articular manifestations of RA include rheumatoid nodules, pleural effusions, vasculitis, and Felty syndrome (associated splenomegaly and leukopenia). Associated conditions include atlantoaxial subluxation and Baker cysts.

- Treatment consists of analgesia and early institution of DMARDS such as methotrexate, leflunomide, sulfasalazine, or hydroxychloroquine. Biologic agents against TNF-α or IL-1 are useful adjuncts for refractory cases but increase risk for infection.

Seronegative Spondylo-arthropathies

The seronegative spondyloarthropathies are an inter-related group of inflammatory disorders affecting the spine, joints, and periarticular structures. The **spondyloarthropathies** include:

- Ankylosing spondylitis (AS)
- Psoriatic arthritis
- Enteropathic arthritis (associated with inflammatory bowel disease [IBD])
- Reactive arthritis

See Table 59-1 for a comparison of the spondyloarthropathies.

EPIDEMIOLOGY

Reactive arthritis and AS are **more common in men** than in women (two of the few rheumatologic diseases that show a male predominance). The other disorders (enteropathic arthritis and psoriatic arthritis) are equally prevalent in men and women. Spondyloarthropathies usually occur in patients younger than 40 years, and their combined prevalence is around 1% (approximately equal to rheumatoid arthritis).

ETIOLOGY

The spondyloarthropathies have varying degrees of association with **human leukocyte antigen (HLA) B-27**. The strongest is AS; 90% of patients are HLA B-27 positive. Family members positive for B-27 who have a first-degree relative with AS have a 10% to 20% chance of developing the disease.

Reactive arthritis appears to be precipitated by **enteric infection** (caused by *Salmonella*, *Shigella*, *Campylobacter*, or *Yersinia*) or **genitourinary infection** (*Chlamydia*). Arthritis usually occurs 1 to 3 weeks after infection.

CLINICAL MANIFESTATIONS

HISTORY

Chronic **low back pain** with morning stiffness in a young adult is the typical presenting symptom for AS. The subacute nature (worsening over several months) of the pain and its improvement with exercise distinguish AS from the more common mechanical etiologies of back pain. Alternating buttock pain is another presenting feature.

Enthesopathy (inflammation of ligaments and tendons) is a key feature of all spondyloarthropathies, often affecting the Achilles tendon or plantar fascia. Heel pain may be the presenting symptom in reactive arthritis.

Eye involvement occurs in approximately 20% of spondyloarthropathy cases. Conjunctivitis can be seen in reactive arthritis, but also occurs in the other diseases. Uveitis (inflammation of pigmented structures: iris, ciliary body) can present as pain, photophobia, or decreased vision.

PHYSICAL EXAMINATION

Sacroiliac involvement in AS may show pain on compression of the pelvis, limitation of lumbar spine forward flexion, extension and lateral flexion, loss of normal lumbar lordosis, and tenderness to palpation around spinous processes and iliac crests.

■ TABLE 59-1 Comparison of the Spondyloarthropathies

	Ankylosing Spondylitis	Reactive Arthritis	Psoriatic Arthritis	Enteropathic Arthritis
Sex distribution	Male > female	Male > female	Female = male	Female = male
Spinal involvement	Always	Occasional	Occasional	Infrequent (10%) and does not correlate with bowel disease
Frequency of HLA-B27 positivity	90%	70%	20%	10% (mostly patients with sacroiliac disease)
Skin involvement	None	Circinate balanitis, keratoderma	Psoriatic plaques, nail pitting	Erythema nodosum, pyoderma gangrenosum
Eye involvement	Uveitis (25%)	Uveitis (20%), conjunctivitis	Uveitis (10%): often insidious onset and bilateral	Uveitis (10%): often insidious onset and bilateral
Natural history	Chronic	Self-limiting (75%)	Chronic	Peripheral arthritis flares with bowel disease, spinal disease chronic

Inflammation of tendons in reactive and psoriatic arthritis causes diffuse swelling of fingers or toes, leading to the typical "**sausage digit**" appearance. Peripheral arthritis is often asymmetric and localized to lower extremities (knees, ankles, metatarsophalangeal joints). Peripheral arthritis in IBD flares around the same time as the bowel symptoms and often improves with resection of diseased bowel. Spinal disease in IBD does not show this correlation.

In addition, certain **skin lesions** are helpful (although not always present) in differentiating the spondyloarthropathies. Psoriasis is characterized by erythematous scaly lesions, usually seen on extensor surfaces of the extremities, and nails may show pitting or onycholysis. The classic skin lesion in reactive arthritis is **keratoderma blennorrhagica**. This is a hyperkeratotic papular rash on the soles of the feet that mimics pustular psoriasis (Color Plate 22). Reactive arthritis also is associated with **balanitis circinata**, which appears as shallow painless ulcers on the penis.

DIFFERENTIAL DIAGNOSIS

In the patient who presents with **low back pain**, the differential diagnosis includes:

- Lumbar strain
- Herniated vertebral disk

- Spinal stenosis
- Malignancy

In the patient with **inflammatory peripheral arthritis**, consider:

- Septic arthritis (including gonococcal arthritis)
- Gout
- Lyme disease
- Rheumatoid arthritis
- Connective tissue disease (e.g., systemic lupus erythematosus [SLE])
- Sarcoidosis

DIAGNOSTIC EVALUATION

Blood tests show signs typical of an inflammatory process, including an **elevated erythrocyte sedimentation rate** (ESR) and **C reactive protein** in about half the patients. In addition, these diseases are seronegative for rheumatoid factor and antinuclear antibody, hence the name **seronegative** spondyloarthropathies.

HLA typing for B-27 may be useful in cases that are atypical and in which the diagnosis is uncertain. Because 5% of whites are positive for B-27, this is not specific for spondyloarthropathies and not recommended as a screening test.

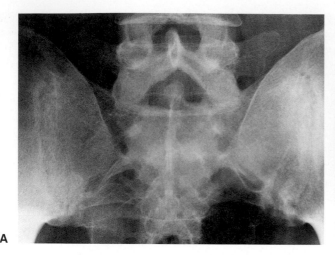

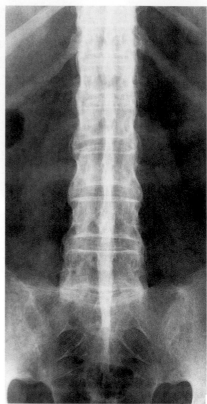

Figure 59-1 • (A) Sacroiliitis. The joints have an irregular fuzzy outline. **(B)** Bamboo spine in ankylosing spondylitis. The vertebrae have become fused, and there is ossification of the longitudinal ligament.

Spinal and pelvic films may be normal in early disease but are often helpful. **Radiograph features of ankylosing spondylitis** include:

- Sacroiliitis (erosions of iliac bone lead to "pseudowidening" of the joint, followed by sclerosis and obliteration) (see Fig. 59-1A)
- Squaring of vertebrae on lateral view of the spine
- Ossification of ligaments between vertebral bodies ("bamboo spine") (see Fig. 59-1B)

Hand films in advanced psoriatic arthritis may reveal erosion of the distal interphalangeal joint, giving the "pencil in cup" appearance on radiograph.

In cases of suspected reactive arthritis, **stool cultures** for pathogens should be sent, but often are negative by the time the patient presents with arthritis. A **urethral chlamydial (and gonococcal) DNA probe** should be performed to rule out infection in cases of suspected urethritis. Urinalysis may show a sterile pyuria.

TREATMENT

The **natural history** of the spondyloarthropathies varies for each specific disease. AS is a lifelong disease and may remain localized or may ascend to the thoracic and cervical spine. The life span of patients with AS is usually normal.

Reactive arthritis is often self-limited but may become chronic or relapsing in 20% to 30% of patients; in severe cases it resembles AS. Active chlamydial infection associated with reactive arthritis should be treated with azithromycin or doxycycline. Long-term antibiotics do not appear to have additional benefit. Antibiotics do not have a role in enteric reactive arthritis.

Psoriatic arthritis and enteropathic arthritis may regress with treatment of the underlying disease. Enteropathic arthritis has improved with sulfasalazine or bowel resection. Psoriatic arthritis has been reported to respond when skin disease is treated with methotrexate, psoralen ultraviolet therapy, or tumor necrosis factor (TNF) inhibitors. Otherwise, treatment is directed at symptoms. Anti-inflammatory medications are effective in most patients. Back extension exercises and hydrotherapy appear useful in maintaining mobility with sacroiliitis.

First-line therapy in the spondyloarthropathies remains **NSAIDs**, usually indomethacin 50 mg thrice daily (see Chapter 58 for side effects). In refractory cases, **sulfasalazine**, 1 g thrice daily, even in the absence of known IBD, has been tried with some success. Sulfasalazine is preferred in enteropathic arthritis since NSAIDs have been associated with flares in inflammatory bowel disease. Anti-TNF-α therapies (see Chapter 58) have also improved symptoms in severe AS and psoriatic arthritis. Glucocorticoids have not been effective and are generally not recommended. However, topical steroids may be used to treat associated uveitis.

Patients with chronic disease (such as AS) are at risk for complications many years after diagnosis.

Spinal fractures may occur with minor trauma and should be suspected in the previously stable patient with an increase in back pain. Atlantoaxial subluxation may also occur, presenting as occipital pain with or without signs of cord compression.

Approximately 10% of patients with AS may have **cardiac complications**, such as aortic insufficiency or conduction disease.

In patients with reactive arthritis related to chlamydial infection, prevention of recurrence by education and use of condoms is important. Recurrent attacks may be more severe than the primary occurrence.

KEY POINTS

- Spondyloarthropathy should be suspected in younger individuals complaining of back pain with stiffness or asymmetric lower extremity arthritis. Peripheral arthritis often appears as "sausage digits." Eye involvement (conjunctivitis or uveitis) is also a key feature.

- Reactive arthritis can occur after infectious diarrhea or urethritis.

- Patients with spondyloarthropathies have an increased incidence of HLA B-27 and are negative for rheumatoid factor and antinuclear antibodies.

- Complications in ankylosing spondylitis include spinal fractures, atlantoaxial subluxation, aortic insufficiency, and cardiac conduction disease.

Connective Tissue Diseases

The term *connective tissue disease* (CTD) refers to one of a heterogeneous group of diseases that target the connective tissues of the body. Some are inherited (e.g., Marfan syndrome, Ehlers-Danlos syndrome), and some are acquired. The acquired CTDs used to be described as **collagen vascular diseases**. These diseases are characterized by **alterations in immune function**, often leading to the production of **autoantibodies**. Autoantibodies are immunoglobulins that are specific for self-antigens, often components of the cell nucleus.

The connective tissue diseases discussed in this chapter include:

- Systemic lupus erythematosus (SLE)
- Systemic sclerosis (SSc), also known as scleroderma
- Polymyositis/dermatomyositis (PM/DM)
- Sjögren syndrome
- Mixed connective-tissue disorder (MCTD)

Rheumatoid arthritis (Chapter 58) is also classi-fied as a CTD. Patients who have features of two or more CTDs are often diagnosed with MCTD or an "overlap syndrome."

EPIDEMIOLOGY

CTDs occur predominantly (>75%) in **women** with a peak incidence in the fourth and fifth decades of life. African Americans have a fourfold risk of SLE compared to whites. In addition, there are **genetic predispositions** to the development of a CTD. Many of these predispositions are related to inheritance of particular alleles of the major histocompatibility complex (MHC) genes, often MHC class II alleles. Deficiencies of complements C1, C2, or C4 increase the risk of SLE.

ETIOLOGY AND PATHOGENESIS

The etiology and pathogenesis of the CTDs are poorly understood. As already mentioned, many CTDs are associated with inheritance of particular MHC class II alleles. Because the MHC class II gene products are important in the **presentation of anti-gens** to the immune system, abnormalities in this function may result in the production of autoanti-bodies. The autoantibodies produced may be the cause of the disease manifestations or simply an epiphenomenon of altered immune function. These autoantibodies are not required for the development of disease.

The **pathology** encountered in CTD is diverse:

- Immune complex deposition: Most often seen in SLE. Circulating immune complexes may deposit in the kidney, resulting in glomerulonephritis, or in the skin.
- Vascular damage: CTDs may have vascular inflam-mation that resembles the pathology seen in the primary vasculitides (see Chapter 61). Abnormal immune responses (ranging from unregulated cyto-toxic T-cell responses to antibody-mediated inflam-mation) are believed to be responsible.
- Overproduction and accumulation of extracellular matrix (ECM) components: Following vascular damage, deposition of collagen and other compo-nents of the ECM can occur. This is a key patho-logic feature of SSc and results in fibrosis of the skin and other organs.
- Altered immune responses: The widespread dis-turbances in immune function can lead to an im-munosuppressed state, predisposing patients to

viruses and encapsulated bacteria. Immuno-suppressive agents used to treat CTDs may exacerbate this problem.

CLINICAL MANIFESTATIONS

HISTORY

Patients often present with diffuse complaints consistent with the systemic nature of these diseases. Myalgias, arthralgias, fever, and rash are common presenting symptoms in SLE. Dry mouth and dry eyes are seen in Sjögren syndrome. Patients with polymyositis complain of muscle weakness, usually involving proximal muscles. Although Raynaud phenomenon can be seen in all CTDs, it is often the earliest symptom of SSc. **Raynaud phenomenon**, a disorder of vasospasm in small blood vessels, is characterized by changes in hand/foot color with cold

exposure or stress. The classic "tricolor" pattern consists of pallor (white), followed by cyanosis (blue), and resolving with hyperemia (red). However, Raynaud phenomenon can also be seen in up to 10% of healthy young women who do not have an underlying CTD ("primary" Raynaud). Patients with Ssc often have esophageal hypomotility, which leads to symptoms of acid reflux or dysphagia. Additional symptoms in CTDs depend on organ involvement (see later).

PHYSICAL EXAMINATION

Table 60-1 summarizes physical examination findings. The **malar ("butterfly") rash** of SLE is an erythematous rash over the cheeks and nose, which is present in approximately half of patients (Color Plate 21). The **heliotrope rash** of dermatomyosis (DM) is a purple-colored rash in a similar

■ **TABLE 60-1** Features of the Connective Tissue Diseases			
Disease	**Musculoskeletal Findings**	**Dermatologic Findings**	**Other Organ System Involvement**
SLE	Arthritis of predominantly small joints, usually symmetric, may be deforming; myopathy (40%)	Malar rash, photosensitivity (70%), discoid rash (erythematous plaques with scale), alopecia	Oral ulcers, pericarditis/pleuritis, Liebman-Sacks endocarditis, glomerulonephritis, interstitial lung disease, seizures, cognitive dysfunction
Scleroderma	Arthralgias of small and large joints, flexion contractures; swelling of hands/fingers and Raynaud phenomenon (early findings)	Skin thickening/induration, telangiectasias, calcinosis	Esophageal hypomotility, pulmonary fibrosis or hypertension, scleroderma renal crisis
Polymyositis/dermatomyositis	Proximal limb muscle weakness, myalgias	Heliotrope rash, Gottron papules, telangiectasias (skin findings occur in dermatomyositis only)	Congestive heart failure, arrhythmias, interstitial lung disease, dysphagia
Sjögren syndrome	Polyarthralgias, Raynaud phenomenon	None specific	Xerostomia (dry mouth) and dry eyes, corneal ulcerations, salivary or lacrimal gland enlargement, autoimmune thyroiditis, interstitial nephritis, interstitial lung disease

distribution but may also involve eyelids and chest (in a V-neck distribution). **Gottron papules** are papular lesions on the dorsal interphalangeal joints that are seen in approximately a third of patients with DM. The characteristic skin finding in SSc is thickened, indurated skin with loss of folds. This may be limited to the distal extremities and face, or it may spread to involve arms and trunk. The limited scleroderma patients are more likely to develop pulmonary hypertension, but the diffuse scleroderma patients are at higher risk for visceral organ involvement. Patients with limited scleroderma are also more likely to have calcinosis (subcutaneous calcium deposits) and telangiectasias, lending itself to the acronym **CREST syndrome** (calcinosis, Raynaud, esophageal dysmotility, sclerodactyly, and telangiectasia).

DIFFERENTIAL DIAGNOSIS

Because of the extensive overlap of the diseases, the main differential diagnosis consists of other CTDs, including rheumatoid arthritis as well as the spondyloarthropathies. The vasculitides may share some of the systemic manifestations as well. Viral illnesses (such as Epstein-Barr virus [EBV] and acute HIV infection) can mimic CTDs with arthritis, pericarditis, fever, and myalgias. The parotid and lacrimal involvement of sarcoidosis may sometimes be confused with Sjögren syndrome. Polymyositis must be distinguished from metabolic myopathies (e.g., glycogen storage diseases) and neuromuscular diseases (e.g., myasthenia gravis).

DIAGNOSTIC EVALUATION

The diagnosis of CTDs relies predominantly on clinical examination and a constellation of features indicating systemic disease. Routine laboratory studies tend to show nonspecific markers of inflammation: elevated erythrocyte sedimentation rate (ESR), normocytic anemia, decreased albumin, and elevated globulin. However, certain **autoantibodies** may assist in confirming the diagnosis (see Table 60-2). The most common autoantibody in CTD is the **antinuclear antibody** (ANA). The test involves incubating the patient's serum with a human tumor cell line (HEp-2) and then adding fluorescent anti-immunoglobulin. The fluorescent pattern on the nucleus is then described (homogeneous, speckled, rim, nucleolar) and quantified (by dilution). None of the autoantibodies is 100% specific, so indiscriminate testing of patients with a low likelihood of CTD generate false-positive results. In general, the lower titers (1:40) are less specific. Further testing for specific nuclear antibodies may assist in diagnosis. However, these antibodies are less sensitive for the CTDs. For example, although anti-topoisomerase I (anti-Scl-70) and anticentromere antibodies are specific for scleroderma, both antibodies are negative in approximately 40% of patients with scleroderma. The presence of antibodies to the U1-ribonucleoprotein (anti-RNP) is a criterion for the diagnosis of mixed connective-tissue disorder (MCTD), although these antibodies are also found in other CTDs. Antihistone antibodies are seen in drug-induced SLE (as seen with the antiarrhythmic drug, procainamide).

■ TABLE 60-2 Autoantibodies in Connective Tissue Diseases

Disease	ANA-Positive Cases (%)	Typical ANA Pattern	Specific Autoantibodies (% of Cases Positive)
SLE	98	Homogeneous > speckled	Anti-Sm (15%), anti-dsDNA (60%)
Diffuse scleroderma	90	Speckled	Anti-Sci-70 (40%)
Limited scleroderma (CREST variant)	90	Speckled > nucleolar	Anticentromere (60%)
Polymyositis/dermatomyositis	90	Speckled > nucleolar	Anti-Jo-1 (25%)
Sjögren syndrome	95	Speckled > homogeneous[a]	

[a]There are no specific autoantibodies in Sjögren syndrome; however, anti-Ro and anti-La antibodies, which are also seen in SLE, are present in approximately 70% of patients.
ANA, antinuclear antibody; CREST, calcinosis, Raynaud, esophageal dysmotility, sclerodactyly, and telangiectasia.

Finally, patients with SLE may have several other laboratory abnormalities when the disease is active. **Immune complex glomerulonephritis** (see Chapter 24) may be present, with red cell casts and dysmorphic red cells in the urine. Complement (C3 and C4) is decreased in this setting. **Leukopenia** is an expected finding in SLE, and **autoimmune hemolytic anemia** (see Chapter 64) is also possible.

The **antiphospholipid antibody syndrome** (APS) occasionally seen in SLE may present with thrombocytopenia and an elevated PTT. However, this is a hypercoagulable state, not a bleeding disorder. Patients may have thromboembolic events (arterial or venous) and recurrent pregnancy loss. The antiphospholipid antibody in APS is often directed at the antiphospholipid binding protein, beta-2 glycoprotein I. APS and SLE are known to cause false positive tests (rapid plasma reagin [RPR]) for syphilis.

TREATMENT

SYSTEMIC LUPUS ERYTHEMATOSUS

Because SLE is a chronic rheumatic disease, treatment is aimed at inducing and then maintaining remissions. The clinical course is extremely variable; patients with nephritis tend to have a worse overall prognosis. Milder disease (arthritis and serositis) may be controlled with **NSAIDs**. Involvement of visceral organs (lungs, heart, kidneys) requires increased immunosuppression, starting with **prednisone**. Treatment for lupus nephritis is more complicated but generally involves the addition of immunosuppressants such as cyclophosphamide, mycophenolate, or azathioprine. Antimalarials, such as hydroxychloroquine (200 mg twice daily), are effective drugs for the skin manifestations of SLE. Arterial or venous thrombosis from APS requires lifelong anticoagulation with warfarin.

SYSTEMIC SCLEROSIS

No single agent has demonstrated a clear benefit in treating the underlying disease in SSc. Treatments aimed at preventing endothelial damage, platelet activation, or fibroblast proliferation have yielded disappointing results. **Methotrexate** may have some benefit in the treatment of early diffuse scleroderma, but **d-penicillamine** is no longer recommended because of its toxicity. Most treatment is directed toward ameliorating organ damage. **IV epoprostanol**, a vasodilator, is used in pulmonary hypertension as well as in cases of severe Raynaud phenomenon. **Bosentan** (125 mg twice daily), an oral endothelin receptor antagonist, can also improve hemodynamics and symptoms in pulmonary hypertension. Antireflux agents and prokinetic agents may be helpful in esophageal dysmotility. The use of **angiotensin-converting enzyme (ACE) inhibitors** in scleroderma renal crisis has dramatically improved survival in this disorder. Scleroderma renal crisis is characterized by oliguric renal failure and malignant hypertension.

POLYMYOSITIS/DERMATOMYOSITIS

The primary treatment of PM/DM is **high-dose prednisone** (1 to 2 mg/kg/day). Response is monitored by following muscle strength and muscle enzymes (creatine phosphokinase [CPK]). Prednisone can be gradually weaned, although many patients require maintenance therapy. In patients who are refractory to corticosteroids, azathioprine and methotrexate have been used.

SJÖGREN SYNDROME

No treatment has been able to reverse the underlying disease in Sjögren syndrome. Artificial tears and saliva are used to relieve mucosal dryness. Thyroid disease should be treated as appropriate, and corticosteroids may benefit patients who develop interstitial lung disease or interstitial nephritis.

CONTINUED CARE

The **risk of malignancy** is increased in PM/DM and Sjögren syndrome. Patients with PM/DM are at a twofold risk of malignancy, and evaluation should focus on careful history and physical examination in addition to standard cancer screening (mammography, colonoscopy, etc.). Sjögren syndrome is associated with a higher incidence of B-cell neoplasms, including lymphomas and Waldenström macroglobulinemia. Rapid enlargement of salivary glands may be the first manifestation of an underlying lymphoma.

Patients with SLE are at increased risk of atherosclerosis, which may be related to the underlying disease or the treatment prescribed. Therefore, patients with SLE presenting with symptoms of vascular insufficiency may have atherosclerosis, vasculitis, or APS. Aggressive preventative therapy (including statin treatment) should be considered in patients with SLE.

Patients maintained on prednisone for long periods of time should be evaluated for osteoporosis and placed on trimethoprim/sulfamethoxazole prophylaxis for *Pneumocystis* pneumonia.

 KEY POINTS

- SLE is characterized by small joint arthritis, rashes, and leukopenia. Serositis and glomerulonephritis can also be present.

- ANAs are present (usually in titers >1:80) in almost all (98%) of patients with SLE. Anti-Sm and anti-dsDNA antibodies are specific for SLE. Low complement levels can indicate active disease.

- Limited scleroderma, with skin thickening of hands and face, is associated with anticentromere antibody (present in 60% of patients) and the CREST syndrome.

- Scleroderma renal crisis, presenting as oliguric renal failure and hypertension, is seen in patients with diffuse scleroderma, and it should be treated quickly with ACE inhibitors.

- The mainstay of treatment for CTDs is glucocorticoids in SLE and PM/DM, with less effective treatment options for SSc and Sjögren syndrome. Severe nephritis requires cyclophosphamide or mycophenolate.

Vasculitis

The vasculitides, diseases involving inflammation of blood vessels, are syndromes characterized by the size of the blood vessel involved and the predominant organs affected. These **vasculitides** include:

- Polyarteritis nodosa (PAN)
- Churg-Strauss disease (allergic angiitis and granulomatosis)
- Wegener granulomatosis (WG)
- Takayasu arteritis
- Temporal arteritis
- Hypersensitivity vasculitis (including Henoch-Schönlein purpura)
- Microscopic polyangiitis (MPA)

Kawasaki disease is a vasculitis with a predilection for coronary arteries. It is predominantly a disease of young children and not discussed further here.

EPIDEMIOLOGY

Most vasculitides occur in middle-age individuals (mean, 40 to 45 years of age), with men affected slightly more often (ratio 1.3:1). Exceptions include temporal arteritis (elderly), Henoch-Schönlein purpura (mostly children and adolescents), and Takayasu arteritis (adolescents and young women). As a group, however, the vasculitides are rare.

ETIOLOGY

Many cases of vasculitis, such as hypersensitivity vasculitis, may be associated with immune complex deposition. Other diseases (WG, Churg-Strauss) have a more prominent granulomatous involvement, suggesting cell-mediated pathology.

Hypersensitivity vasculitis may involve an offending drug or associated disease. Certain drugs may cause "serum sickness," occurring 7 to 10 days after primary exposure. Diseases associated with hypersensitivity vasculitis include **systemic lupus erythematosus (SLE), rheumatoid arthritis, and bacterial endocarditis. Chronic hepatitis B and C** are associated with MPA and PAN. In addition, chronic hepatitis C may lead to essential mixed cryoglobulinemia, which can cause a hypersensitivity vasculitis.

CLINICAL MANIFESTATIONS

HISTORY

Many patients with vasculitis present with nonspecific findings such as **fever, weight loss, malaise,** and **arthralgias.** Organ-specific manifestations are more common in certain diseases. PAN affects the visceral arteries and may present with **abdominal pain.** The GI symptoms of Henoch-Schönlein purpura (abdominal pain and bleeding) may precede the typical rash. Churg-Strauss disease presents as **recurrent asthma** attacks. WG often involves the lungs and upper airways, presenting as **recurrent sinusitis, dyspnea, cough,** and/or **hemoptysis. New-onset headache, scalp tenderness,** and **jaw claudication** in the elderly are seen in temporal arteritis. Takayasu arteritis, which affects large vessels such as the carotid arteries, may cause **syncope** and **stroke.**

PHYSICAL EXAMINATION

Physical examination may often reveal skin changes, most notably **palpable purpura**. These raised lesions are red to purple, do not blanch, and usually appear on the lower extremities. Skin involvement is predominant in hypersensitivity vasculitis (and often the skin is the only organ affected). Purpura can be seen in the other vasculitides as well, although it is most common in Churg-Strauss disease.

Hypertension is seen in those diseases involving the renal vasculature: PAN, MPA, WG, Takayasu arteritis, and Henoch-Schönlein purpura. Involvement of the subclavian arteries in Takayasu arteritis (also known as "pulseless disease") leads to diminished peripheral pulses. Temporal arteries may be tender to palpation and thickened in temporal arteritis.

Eye examination may reveal episcleritis or uveitis. Examination of the nose in WG may reveal septal ulceration and "saddle-nose" deformity. Signs of congestive heart failure are seen if there is cardiac involvement in Churg-Strauss disease. Neurologic manifestations include **mononeuritis multiplex** and **cranial nerve palsies.**

DIFFERENTIAL DIAGNOSIS

Vasculitis presenting with fever, skin lesions, and weight loss must be differentiated from **subacute bacterial endocarditis.** Other causes of palpable purpura include **disseminated meningococcal** or **gonococcal infection** and **Rocky Mountain spotted fever.**

Eosinophilia with pulmonary infiltrates (as in Churg-Strauss disease) is also seen in **allergic bronchopulmonary aspergillosis, Loeffler syndrome** (often parasitic), and **chronic eosinophilic pneumonia.**

In the patient with WG presenting with pulmonary and renal disease, one must consider **Goodpasture syndrome** (antiglomerular basement membrane [GBM] disease).

DIAGNOSTIC EVALUATION

Elevated erythrocyte sedimentation rate (ESR) is almost always seen with active vasculitis, often >100 mm per hour. Other signs of inflammation include a normochromic, normocytic anemia and thrombocytosis. Leukocytosis can also be seen, leading to a search for an infectious etiology. **Eosinophilia** is the hallmark of Churg-Strauss disease. Although hypersensitivity vasculitis may also have increased eosinophils in the blood, the history of recurrent asthma is not present. Thrombocytopenia is unusual in the vasculitides and suggests an alternative diagnosis.

Chest radiograph may reveal pulmonary infiltrates in both WG and Churg-Strauss disease; the former may also show cavitary lesions or nodules. A widened aorta may be seen in Takayasu arteritis or temporal arteritis. Because bacterial infections can mimic vasculitis, blood cultures should be obtained on initial evaluation.

Antineutrophil cytoplasmic antibody, specifically the cytoplasmic type (C-ANCA), is diagnostic for WG in the setting of a compatible clinical picture. The antigen responsible for C-ANCA is proteinase-3 (PR3). A perinuclear staining pattern (perinuclear antineutrophil cytoplasmic antibody [P-ANCA]), produced by antibodies to myeloperoxidase (MPO), is seen in microscopic polyangiitis, Churg-Strauss disease, and in 10% of WG. High titers of **rheumatoid factor** (RF) may be seen in rheumatoid vasculitis, although RF is also positive in mixed cryoglobulinemia. **Hepatitis C antibody** is found in most patients with mixed cryoglobulinemia, and **hepatitis B surface antigen** is seen in 30% of patients with PAN.

Renal disease may occur with all vasculitides but is most notable in WG, MPA, and Henoch-Schönlein purpura. Glomerulonephritis and its manifestations are discussed in Chapter 24.

Biopsy remains the definitive test to document inflammation and destruction of the vessels. Table 61-1 shows the sizes and types of blood vessels affected and the predominant microscopic appearance. However, because vasculitis tends to be segmental and focal, biopsy may miss an affected area.

In cases where biopsy may be difficult to perform, **angiography** is used to confirm the diagnosis. Angiography of the mesenteric arteries in PAN shows a "beaded" appearance of aneurysms and segmental stenosis. In Takayasu arteritis, the aorta and subclavian arteries can show irregular vessel walls, stenosis, and poststenotic dilation. Magnetic resonance angiography has been used to diagnose and follow progression of Takayasu arteritis.

TREATMENT

Treatment is directed at the underlying disease for those vasculitides with known causes. Withdrawal of the offending drug in serum sickness and treatment of hepatitis C with interferon and ribavirin in mixed cryoglobulinemia are two such strategies. Henoch-Schönlein purpura often remits on its own. In the other diseases, immunosuppression is the mainstay of treatment. These treatments have led to

▪ TABLE 61-1 Biopsy Results in the Vasculitides

Vasculitis	Vessels Involved	Appearance
Hypersensitivity vasculitis	Arterioles and venules	Leukocytoclastic vasculitis, IgA present in Henoch-Schönlein purpura
Churg-Strauss disease	Various sizes, including venules	Granulomas with eosinophils
Microscopic polyangiitis	Small arteries and veins	Mononuclear or polymorphonuclear lymphocytes, necrotizing
Wegener granulomatosis	Small arteries and veins	Granulomas
Polyarteritis nodosa	Small to medium arteries	Mononuclear or polymorphonuclear lymphocytes, necrotizing
Temporal arteritis	Medium arteries (temporal)	Granulomas
Takayasu arteritis	Large arteries (aorta, subclavian)	Usually not biopsied

major improvements in survival for PAN and WG, which previously had 5-year mortality rates of 85% to 100%.

Prednisone (1 mg/kg/day) and cyclophosphamide (2 mg/kg/day) are the first-line therapy for WG, MPA, and PAN. Prednisone is usually continued for approximately 6 months and then tapered off to avoid long-term side effects such as cataracts and osteoporosis. Cyclophosphamide is continued for approximately 1 year. Complications of cyclophosphamide include hemorrhagic cystitis, bladder cancer, myelodysplasia, and infertility. To avoid cyclophosphamide-related complications, methotrexate or azathioprine can be substituted after 3 to 6 months. Plasma exchange has been used for life-threatening WG.

Prednisone (1 mg per kg) is required for temporal arteritis and Churg-Strauss disease. After improvement, a steroid taper may be attempted. Prednisone is also used for severe cases of Henoch-Schönlein purpura.

Takayasu arteritis is treated with steroids and, in more severe cases, methotrexate. Aggressive surgical repair with grafting of affected arteries has markedly improved survival.

KEY POINTS

- Palpable purpura is a common finding in the vasculitides, especially hypersensitivity vasculitis (including Henoch-Schönlein purpura) and Churg-Strauss disease. Purpura is also seen in life-threatening infections (gonococcemia, meningococcemia, and Rocky Mountain spotted fever).

- Pulmonary involvement occurs in both Wegener granulomatosis and Churg-Strauss disease. The latter is also characterized by eosinophilia and asthma.

- Antibody to proteinase 3 (which produces a C-ANCA pattern) is highly specific for WG, although it may be absent when disease is limited to the lungs.

- New-onset headache with an elevated ESR in an elderly patient is highly suggestive of temporal arteritis. Scalp tenderness and jaw claudication may be present. With a high suspicion, prednisone can be instituted and a prompt temporal artery biopsy obtained.

62 Amyloidosis

Amyloidosis is a systemic disorder characterized by extracellular deposition of amyloid, a fibrous protein, in one or more sites of the body. Although amyloid fibrils can be made from many different proteins, all types of amyloid share the following common characteristics on **pathologic examination**:

- Amorphous, eosinophilic, extracellular deposition
- Green birefringence under polarized light after staining with Congo red dye
- Protein structure is a beta-pleated sheet

EPIDEMIOLOGY

Amyloidosis tends to be a disease of older individuals; less than 1% of patients are younger than 40 years. It occurs in equal frequency in men and women.

ETIOLOGY

Amyloidosis may be either primary (i.e., no apparent cause) or secondary to an ongoing disease. The most common forms of amyloidosis are **AL amyloidosis** caused by immunoglobulin light chain deposition and **AA amyloidosis** caused by deposition of the serum amyloid-A protein. In the United States, AL is the most common cause. Causes of AL and AA amyloidosis include:

AL Amyloidosis: Immunoglobulin Light Chain Deposition
- Primary amyloidosis
- Multiple myeloma

AA Amyloidosis: Serum Amyloid-A Deposition
- Rheumatoid arthritis
- Chronic infection or inflammation
- Familial Mediterranean fever

There are numerous other, less common forms of amyloidosis. Of the more than 20 other amyloidosis syndromes, the following amyloid proteins deserve note:

- β_2-Microglobulin (hemodialysis)
- Transthyretin (familial amyloid polyneuropathy)

PATHOGENESIS

Precursor proteins undergo conformational changes, causing the soluble precursor to form insoluble amyloid subunits that then polymerize into amyloid fibrils. The amyloid fibril depositions themselves may contribute to clinical pathology, but the soluble oligomer intermediates of fibril formation may also be pathogenic.

CLINICAL MANIFESTATIONS

Clinical findings in amyloidosis depend on the numerous organs the disease affects. Table 62-1 lists the major syndromes seen in amyloidosis by organ system. Because AL and AA amyloid are the most common forms, patients generally present with impairment of the organs affected by AL or AA amyloid: kidney, heart, and liver.

■ **TABLE 62-1** Organ Involvement in Amyloidosis	
Organ Systems	**Syndromes**
Neurologic	Autonomic dysfunction Carpal tunnel syndrome Distal polyneuropathy
Cardiac	Restrictive cardiomyopathy Conduction disturbance
Renal	Nephrotic syndrome Renal tubular acidosis
GI	Malabsorption Motility disorders Macroglossia
Hepatic	Intrahepatic cholestasis
Rheumatologic	Symmetric arthritis
Hematologic	Acquired factor X deficiency

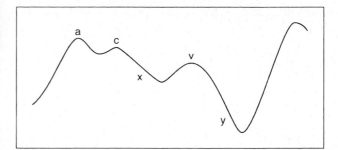

Figure 62-1 • Rapid y descent in the JVP seen in restrictive cardiomyopathy.

HISTORY

Amyloidosis often presents with generalized non-specific symptoms, such as **fatigue** and **weight loss**. The weight loss is often marked and averages approximately 15 to 20 pounds. Other symptoms may signify specific organ damage from amyloid. These include the edema and dyspnea of heart involvement or the paresthesias and light-headedness of neurologic involvement.

PHYSICAL EXAMINATION

Vital signs may reveal bradycardia from cardiac conduction disturbances, or orthostatic hypotension from autonomic failure. Fever suggests an infectious etiology, such as osteomyelitis, leading to secondary amyloidosis.

Neurologic involvement may be manifested by carpal tunnel syndrome or distal polyneuropathy.

Cardiac amyloidosis appears as a **restrictive cardiomyopathy** on physical examination. Increased jugular venous pressure (JVP) is present along with Kussmaul sign (JVP increases instead of decreases with inspiration) or rapid y descent of the JVP (Fig. 62-1).

Skin examination may show signs of easy bruising, including periorbital ecchymoses. Amyloid deposition in the skin appears as **raised waxy papules**.

Gastrointestinal (GI) involvement may be indicated by **macroglossia** or **hepatomegaly**.

DIFFERENTIAL DIAGNOSIS

Amyloidosis is often considered when the patient presents with fatigue and weight loss, suggesting a chronic wasting illness. Other etiologies, such as malignancy or chronic infections, may resemble amyloidosis or may cause amyloidosis. Amyloidosis should be suspected when additional systemic features (nephrotic syndrome, orthostatic hypotension, or restrictive cardiomyopathy) are present.

Amyloidosis is distinguished from light chain deposition disease, which is caused by tissue deposition of immunoglobulin light chains but without associated fibril formation. With light chain deposition disease, renal failure with nephritic syndrome is prominent, whereas cardiac or liver involvement is less common.

DIAGNOSTIC EVALUATION

Infiltration of the heart can be noted on the electrocardiogram (ECG) as **conduction disturbances** (atrioventricular block) and **low-voltage QRS**. On echocardiogram, there is a characteristic "sparkling" of the myocardium, and the ventricular wall is often thickened (especially compared with the low voltage on the ECG). Elevated cardiac troponin or B-natriuretic peptide is correlated with a poor prognosis.

Urinalysis often shows proteinuria from nephrotic syndrome. Of note, light chain excretion is not detected by a dipstick, which only detects albuminuria. Immunoelectrophoresis of the urine or serum often reveals a monoclonal spike in primary amyloidosis or multiple myeloma. Serum free light chains may also be elevated in AL amyloidosis.

Other nonspecific laboratory findings may include increased alkaline phosphatase (cholestasis from liver infiltration), decreased albumin (malabsorption and nephrotic syndrome), and increased prothrombin time (acquired factor X deficiency).

Diagnosis of amyloidosis requires a biopsy that shows the characteristic **Congo red staining**. Although affected organs, such as liver or kidney, often show amyloid on pathology, biopsy may be dangerous because of the high rate of bleeding. Therefore, diagnosis is preferentially made by **abdominal fat pad aspirate** or **rectal biopsy**. The abdominal fat pad aspirate is easy to perform and reported to be 70% to 80% sensitive. Amyloidosis is also detected in bone marrow biopsies, which are often performed to rule out multiple myeloma.

TREATMENT

Once the diagnosis of amyloidosis is made, treatment focuses on supportive care. There is no effective treatment for amyloidosis itself, although treatment aimed at the underlying etiology may be effective (see later). Diuretics may be used for symptomatic relief of heart failure and edema, but digoxin is often avoided because of increased cardiotoxicity in these patients. Dialysis has been used in certain patients who have progressed to end-stage renal disease.

The prognosis in amyloidosis remains poor (average, 1 year) and depends on the extent of organ involvement. Patients presenting with congestive heart failure (CHF) survive a median of 6 months, whereas patients presenting with peripheral neuropathy alone have median survivals of approximately 56 months.

Treatment directed at the underlying etiology may improve survival in amyloidosis. The most dramatic example is AA amyloidosis caused by familial Mediterranean fever, which is successfully treated with colchicine. Prophylactic colchicine not only reduces symptomatic episodes in familial Mediterranean fever, but also appears to prevent the development of amyloidosis. In AL amyloidosis, either of primary origin or related to multiple myeloma, melphalan and prednisone (or dexamethasone) may be used to prolong survival. Use of autologous stem cell transplantation for amyloidosis is limited by a high rate of therapy-related death and did not show a survival benefit in a recent randomized trial.

KEY POINTS

- Amyloidosis is a systemic disorder characterized by extracellular deposition of an amorphous eosinophilic protein that stains positive with Congo red stain.

- Diagnosis may be made by biopsy of any affected organ but is easiest and safest with an abdominal fat pad aspirate.

- Cardiac involvement appears as a conduction disturbance and/or restrictive cardiomyopathy. Echocardiogram reveals a classic "sparkling" pattern. Patients may be extremely sensitive to digoxin toxicity.

- Development of signs of amyloidosis (such as carpal tunnel syndrome or polyneuropathy) in a patient on long-term hemodialysis should raise the suspicion of β_2-microglobulin-mediated amyloidosis.

- Amyloidosis should be included in the differential diagnosis of elderly patients with fatigue and weight loss.

- Treatment is supportive, with the exception of colchicine for amyloidosis secondary to familial Mediterranean fever and chemotherapy for multiple myeloma or for selected patients with primary amyloidosis.

Part 8

Hematology/
Oncology

Anemia is a reduction in the total red blood cell (RBC) mass, as defined by the number of RBCs, hemoglobin level in the blood, or percentage of red cell volume (hematocrit). Lower limits of normal hemoglobin vary among laboratories, but the general criteria for anemia are a hemoglobin level <13 g per dL in men and <12 g per dL in women.

Anemia itself is not considered a disease but rather is a sign of an underlying disease. Anemia is the result of one of the following mechanisms:

- Decreased RBC production
- Increased red cell destruction (hemolysis)
- Blood loss

Red cell destruction and blood loss result in an increased production of immature red cells, known as **reticulocytes**. Thus, these two causes of anemia, which have a high reticulocyte count (RC), are differentiated from decreased production, which has a low RC (see "Diagnostic Evaluation"). Hemolytic anemias are discussed in Chapter 64.

DIFFERENTIAL DIAGNOSIS

The differential diagnosis of anemia is classified by its mechanism as well as the size of the RBCs. **Microcytosis** is defined by a mean corpuscular volume (MCV) <80 μm^3, and **macrocytosis** is an MCV >100 μm^3. An approach to the evaluation is diagrammed in Figure 63-1.

High Reticulocyte Count
- Acute blood loss (trauma, gastrointestinal [GI] bleeding)
- Hemolysis

Low Reticulocyte Count (Decreased Production)
Microcytic
- Iron deficiency
- Thalassemia
- Anemia of chronic disease
- Sideroblastic anemia (usually hereditary)

Macrocytic
- B_{12} (cobalamin) deficiency
- Folate deficiency
- Alcohol abuse
- Liver disease
- Myelodysplastic syndrome
- Hypothyroidism, severe
- Sideroblastic anemia (acquired)
- Drug effects

Normocytic
- Anemia of chronic disease
- Anemia of renal failure
- Aplastic anemia
- Multiple myeloma
- Myelophthisis
- Hypothyroidism

Anemia of chronic disease (ACD) is caused by iron trapping in the reticuloendothelial system and suppression of erythropoiesis, perhaps mediated by cytokines such as interleukin-1. The three major categories of disease associated with ACD are **infection**, **malignancy**, and **inflammatory disease** (e.g., rheumatoid arthritis).

Sideroblastic anemia has multiple etiologies, including alcohol abuse, lead poisoning, isoniazid use, and pyridoxine deficiency. The characteristic feature is the presence of ringed sideroblasts in the bone marrow, which represents abnormal iron

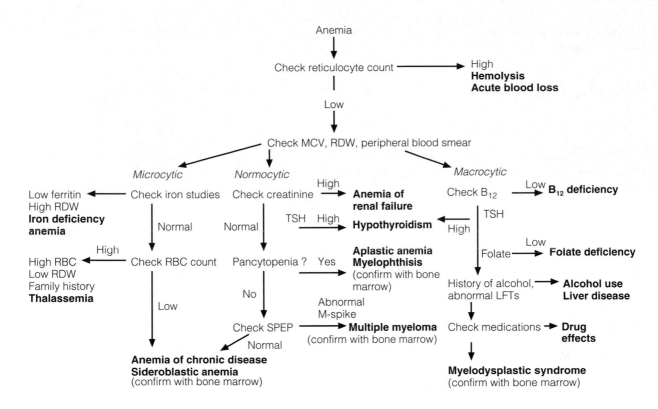

Figure 63-1 • An approach to the evaluation of anemia.

accumulation in the mitochondria. Hereditary sideroblastic anemia may respond to pyridoxine supplementation.

Myelodysplastic syndrome (MDS) is a stem cell disorder characterized by an arrest in maturation of all blood cells, usually presenting as a pancytopenia. It occurs most often in the elderly.

Myelophthisis refers to extensive marrow infiltration that inhibits bone marrow function, usually leading to a pancytopenia. It may be secondary to metastatic carcinoma, leukemia, or chronic infection (e.g., tuberculosis). Idiopathic myelofibrosis may also present in this manner. (See Color Plate 18.)

Thalassemia is an inherited defect in either the α- or the β-globin gene. Mutations result in lack of, or decreased production of, a globin chain. Lack of one of the two β genes or two of the four α genes leads to the **thalassemia trait**, usually an asymptomatic microcytic anemia. More severe defects present in childhood. Patients of Mediterranean, Middle Eastern, or Southeast Asian descent are at increased risk for β-thalassemia; α-thalassemia is seen in these groups as well as in African Americans.

Drug effects that cause anemia include chemotherapy of any type (through myelosuppression) and folate antagonists, such as methotrexate and trimethoprim.

CLINICAL FINDINGS

HISTORY

Patients with anemia are usually asymptomatic, unless the decrease in hematocrit is sudden or severe. General symptoms include:

- Fatigue
- Dyspnea
- Dizziness

Alcohol consumption should be determined in all patients. There are multiple causes of anemia in alcoholic patients. Folate deficiency, liver disease, sideroblastic anemia, and alcohol itself cause macrocytic anemias.

Patients should be assessed for potential sites of blood loss. In premenopausal women, menstrual bleeding is the most common cause of anemia. GI bleeding may present with a history of dark, tarry stools or bright red blood from the rectum.

PHYSICAL EXAMINATION

Most patients with mild anemia have a normal physical examination. However, when hemoglobin is <11 g per dL, patients may have pallor of the nail beds, palmar creases, and conjunctivae. Fever raises the suspicion of a hemolytic anemia.

Findings seen in marked **iron deficiency anemia** include:

- Atrophic glossitis
- Angular cheilitis (scaling at corners of mouth)
- Koilonychia (spoon nails)

Glossitis and **peripheral neuropathy** may be seen in vitamin B_{12} deficiency. The posterior columns of the spinal cord are involved, affecting position and vibratory sense. Almost all patients should be evaluated for occult blood loss from the GI tract with stool guaiac testing. Signs of liver disease are detailed in Chapter 42.

DIAGNOSTIC EVALUATION

The key to the diagnostic workup is to classify the anemia by the red cell indexes (micro-, macro-, or normocytic) and RC. The RC must be corrected for the level of anemia:

$$\text{Corrected RC} = \text{RC} \times (\text{Patient's Hematocrit} \div \text{Expected Hematocrit})$$

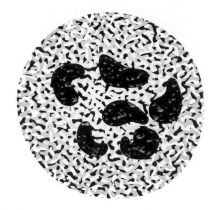

Figure 63-2 • Hypersegmented neutrophil.

A corrected RC of ≤2% or less suggests the diagnosis of decreased RBC production, whereas a value >3% indicates hemolysis or blood loss.

The next important step is to examine the **peripheral smear**. The blood smear is used to decide if there is a single morphology of cells or two different populations (dimorphic). An anemia that has a dimorphic population also has a high **red (blood cell) distribution width** (RDW). This automated measure of red cell variation may assist in distinguishing two common types of microcytic anemia: iron deficiency anemia (high RDW) and thalassemia (low RDW).

Table 63-1 lists classic findings on peripheral smear (see also Figs. 63-2 to 63-6).

MICROCYTIC ANEMIA

All pure microcytic anemias are associated with a low RC. The most useful initial tests are **iron studies**.

■ TABLE 63-1 Peripheral Smear Findings

Finding on Smear	Likely Etiologies
Hypersegmented PMNs	Megaloblastic anemia
Ovalocytes	Megaloblastic anemia
Target cells	Liver disease, thalassemia, hemolysis
Bilobed PMNs	Myelodysplastic syndrome
Teardrop cells	Myelophthisis
Schistocytes	Microangiopathic hemolytic anemia

PMN, polymorphonuclear lymphocyte.

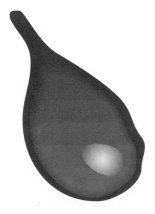

Figure 63-3 • Teardrop cell.

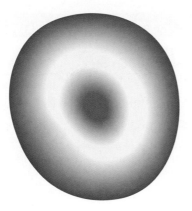

Figure 63-4 • Target cell.

Figure 63-6 • Sickle cell.

Ferritin is the storage form of iron; transferrin is the transport protein and the main determinant of the total iron-binding capacity. Table 63-2 lists the common patterns of iron studies in microcytic anemia.

It is often difficult to distinguish between anemia of chronic disease and iron deficiency anemia because both can lower iron levels. Because ferritin (an acute-phase reactant) may be elevated with inflammation, some state that a normal ferritin level does not rule out iron deficiency in the presence of chronic disease. However, iron deficiency is extremely uncommon when the ferritin level is >150 µg per L. An elevated RBC count in the presence of a microcytic anemia is suggestive of thalassemia. β-Thalassemia is confirmed by an elevated level of hemoglobin A_2 (an alternative form of hemoglobin, $\alpha_2\delta_2$).

MACROCYTIC ANEMIA

A high RC should be ruled out in these patients. Macrocytic anemias are then subclassified into those

with impaired deoxyribonucleic acid (DNA) synthesis (megaloblastic anemias) and those without impairment. Megaloblastic anemias include B_{12} deficiency, folate deficiency, and drug effects. Table 63-1 lists the characteristics of megaloblastosis.

Folate and **B_{12}** levels should be checked in all patients with a megaloblastic picture. Low levels confirm deficiency. Drug effects from chemotherapy and folate antagonists should be excluded as well. Patients with myelodysplasia often have extremely high B_{12} levels. **Lactate dehydrogenase** (LDH) may be elevated in all megaloblastic anemias because of ineffective erythropoiesis. LFTs and TFTs should be sent as well. The MCV is rarely >110 in patients with hypothyroidism or liver disease.

NORMOCYTIC ANEMIA

A high RC should be ruled out in these patients. Anemia of chronic disease is the most common cause of normocytic anemia. Aplastic anemia is characterized by pancytopenia and a zero RC. The anemia of renal failure may be present in a patient with an estimated glomerular filtration rate (GFR) less than 50.

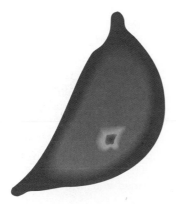

Figure 63-5 • Schistocyte.

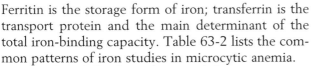

■ **TABLE 63-2** Common Patterns in Microcytic Anemias			
	Iron	**TIBC**	**Ferritin**
Iron deficiency	↓	↑	↓
Thalassemia	N	N	N
Anemia of chronic disease	↓	↓	↑
Sideroblastic anemia	↑	N	N/↑
N, normal; TIBC, total iron binding capacity; ↑, increased; ↓, decreased.			

Erythropoietin in these patients is inappropriately low or normal. A serum protein electrophoresis and free light chains should be sent to look for a monoclonal gammopathy consistent with multiple myeloma. Patients with no known chronic disease and no apparent cause of the anemia are candidates for **bone marrow biopsy** to rule out myelophthisis or another bone marrow process.

IRON DEFICIENCY ANEMIA

Menstruating or pregnant women have known losses of iron, and therapy is empirically begun in these patients. However, in postmenopausal women and in men, iron deficiency should be further investigated. The most worrisome cause of iron deficiency in the elderly is due to gastrointestinal blood loss, particularly colon cancer. These patients should be evaluated for an etiology of bleeding, preferably by endoscopy. Symptoms, such as constipation or heartburn, may direct the initial endoscopic evaluation. Patients with iron deficiency and no apparent source of blood loss may have intestinal malabsorption, such as is seen in celiac sprue.

B$_{12}$ DEFICIENCY

The body stores enough B$_{12}$ to last for years, so most causes of B$_{12}$ deficiency are not from poor diet. Elderly patients with atrophic gastritis may not be able to liberate B$_{12}$ from food, resulting in the so-called food-cobalamin malabsorption. **Pernicious anemia** is related to the lack of intrinsic factor (IF), produced by the stomach and necessary for B$_{12}$ absorption. Anti-IF antibody is found in approximately 60% of patients with pernicious anemia and is highly specific. The B$_{12}$-IF complex is absorbed by the terminal ileum, so patients with ileal disease (e.g., Crohn disease) are also at risk for B$_{12}$ deficiency. Bacterial overgrowth, as seen in the **blind intestinal loop syndrome**, reduces the B$_{12}$ available for absorption.

A **Schilling's test** is the classic approach to determine the etiology of B$_{12}$ deficiency. After loading the body with IM B$_{12}$, a radioactive dose of B$_{12}$ is ingested and excretion through the kidney is measured. Failure to excrete the radioactive B$_{12}$ indicates lack of absorption. The next part of the test involves administering B$_{12}$ and IF together; excretion of B$_{12}$ during this part confirms that the deficiency is caused by a lack of IF (pernicious anemia). Failure to absorb and then excrete B$_{12}$-IF complex suggests malabsorption as a

cause. Correction of this malabsorption after antibiotics suggests blind loop syndrome. Table 63-3 summarizes these results.

■ TABLE 63-3 Schilling's Test Results	
Able to Absorb B$_{12}$ After Oral Administration of:	**Likely Etiology**
B$_{12}$ only	Inadequate diet
B$_{12}$ and intrinsic factor	Pernicious anemia
B$_{12}$ after administration of antibiotics	Blind loop syndrome
Failure to absorb B$_{12}$ in all of above tests	Ileal disease

BONE MARROW BIOPSY

A bone marrow biopsy is an invasive procedure, but it is occasionally necessary to determine the etiology of the anemia. Some indications for bone marrow biopsy are:

- Pancytopenia (suggesting aplastic anemia or marrow infiltration)
- Macrocytic anemia of unknown etiology (to rule out myelodysplasia)
- Findings suggestive of sideroblastic anemia or myelophthisis

 KEY POINTS

- Anemia is caused by increased RBC destruction, blood loss, or decreased production. An RC is a useful initial test to determine the underlying mechanism.

- Iron deficiency is a common cause of microcytic anemia. Although usually a benign condition in premenopausal women, it may be related to occult GI malignancy in men and postmenopausal women.

- In healthy patients, a normal ferritin level almost always excludes iron deficiency. Although ferritin may be elevated in inflammatory conditions, it rarely rises higher than 150 μg per L with associated iron deficiency.

- B$_{12}$ deficiency may present with a macrocytic anemia and peripheral neuropathy. The most common cause of B$_{12}$ deficiency is pernicious anemia, which may be confirmed with a positive intrinsic factor antibody.

Hemolytic Anemia

Hemolysis is the premature destruction of red blood cells (RBCs). The decreased survival of the RBCs results in an increase in the production of immature RBCs (reticulocytes). Thus, hemolytic anemia is characterized by a decreased hemoglobin level and an increase in reticulocyte count. Acute blood loss may mimic this pattern, but an obvious site of bleeding is usually identified. Hemolysis may be caused by **extraerythrocytic factors** (usually acquired) or **intrinsic defects** in the RBC (often inherited). In addition, hemolysis can occur in the intravascular space or in the extravascular space (mainly the spleen and liver).

Intravascular hemolysis results in release of hemoglobin, which is quickly bound to the serum protein **haptoglobin**. Next, the hemoglobin–haptoglobin complex is cleared by the reticuloendothelial (RE) system, and the haptoglobin level rapidly falls to low or undetectable levels. Once intravascular hemoglobin overloads the haptoglobin capacity, it is filtered by the kidney and reabsorbed in the proximal tubule. These tubular cells are sloughed off into the urine and are detected as **urine hemosiderin**. Finally, when proximal tubular reabsorption is overwhelmed (only in severe hemolysis), **hemoglobinuria** can be detected. This is suggested by a positive occult blood reading on urine dipstick, but no RBCs are seen on urinalysis. In **extravascular hemolysis**, RBCs are removed by the spleen and RE system; therefore, little hemoglobin is released into the bloodstream. Haptoglobin may be low, but urine hemosiderin and hemoglobinuria are usually not present.

DIFFERENTIAL DIAGNOSIS

Extraerythrocytic Factors
Microangiopathic hemolytic anemia (MAHA) (Intravascular)
- Disseminated intravascular coagulation (DIC)
- Hemolytic uremic syndrome (HUS)
- Thrombotic thrombocytopenic purpura (TTP)
- Cardiac valve hemolysis

Immune-Mediated Hemolytic Anemia
- Warm antibody (hematologic malignancy, connective tissue disorders, drugs) (extravascular)
- Cold antibody (lymphoma, mycoplasma, mononucleosis) (intravascular)

Infections (Intravascular/Extravascular)
- Malaria (see Color Plate 19)
- Babesiosis
- Clostridial toxin

Splenomegaly (Extravascular)
- Infiltrative diseases
- Portal hypertension

Red Blood Cell Defects
Hemoglobinopathies (Extravascular)
- Sickle cell disease

Enzyme Defects (Intravascular)
- Pyruvate kinase deficiency
- Glucose-6-phosphate dehydrogenase (G6PD) deficiency

Membrane Defects
- Hereditary spherocytosis and elliptocytosis (extravascular)
- Paroxysmal nocturnal hemoglobinuria (intravascular)

Sickle cell disease is an autosomal recessive disease that occurs in people of African descent (prevalence is about 0.2% in African Americans). A mutation in the beta hemoglobin chain results in production of hemoglobin S, which polymerizes in the deoxygenated state and causes red cells to form sickle-shaped cells. This leads to vaso-occlusion in the microvasculature, which causes pain and organ dysfunction.

G6PD deficiency is an X-linked trait (and therefore affects predominantly men) that occurs in people of Mediterranean and African descent. G6PD is the enzyme responsible for generation of NADPH in the red blood cell, which protects against oxidative stress. Loss of this enzyme leads to oxidation of hemoglobin and hemolysis.

Paroxysmal nocturnal hemoglobinuria (PNH) is a unique RBC defect because it is acquired. It is a stem cell disorder that involves a mutation in the PIG-A gene, which results in lack of a glycosylphosphatidylinositol (GPI) anchor in RBCs. Lack of certain GPI dependent receptors leads to an increased sensitivity to complement-mediated hemolysis.

CLINICAL FINDINGS

HISTORY

No specific symptoms are associated with hemolytic anemia. However, the history may lead to a suspected etiology of the hemolysis. A **history of travel** to Africa, Asia, or Central America may suggest malaria. A **family history** of hemolytic anemia may be found in any patient with an RBC defect (see earlier).

Certain **drugs** are associated with warm-antibody hemolytic anemia:

- Methyldopa
- Quinine
- Sulfonamides
- Penicillin

An oxidative stress often precedes the hemolysis in G6PD deficiency. This stress can be an infection, in-

gestion of fava beans, or certain drugs. Drugs that can induce hemolysis in persons with **G6PD deficiency** include:

- Sulfonamides
- Nitrofurantoin
- Methylene blue
- Dapsone
- Primaquine

PHYSICAL EXAMINATION

Fever suggests the presence of an infectious or microangiopathic etiology. Scleral icterus (from hyperbilirubinemia) may be seen in severe cases. Splenomegaly may be the cause of the hemolysis or a result of the hemolysis (in extravascular cases). It is not helpful in distinguishing etiologies.

DIAGNOSTIC EVALUATION

Figure 64-1 provides an algorithm for the evaluation of hemolytic anemia. The key **laboratory features of hemolysis** include:

- Elevated indirect bilirubin
- Elevated lactate dehydrogenase (LDH)
- Increased reticulocyte count
- Decreased haptoglobin

Note that elevated LDH and indirect bilirubin may also be seen in patients with ineffective hematopoiesis (e.g., B_{12} deficiency). However, the reticulocyte count is low in these patients. **Thrombocytopenia** may be seen in many causes but is most prominent in the microangiopathic etiologies (TTP, HUS, and DIC). **PT** is elevated in DIC but is normal in TTP and HUS. Renal failure is an important feature of HUS but is also seen in other microangiopathic etiologies.

The next important step is examination of the **peripheral smear**. Figures 63-4, 63-5, and 63-6 (see preceding chapter) demonstrate examples of abnormal red cells in hemolysis. The hemolysis itself commonly results in target cells and spherocytes. However, large numbers of spherocytes are limited to hereditary spherocytosis and warm-antibody hemolysis. Elliptocytes are seen in hereditary elliptocytosis and severe iron deficiency. The presence of schistocytes (more than five per high-power field) confirms the diagnosis of MAHA.

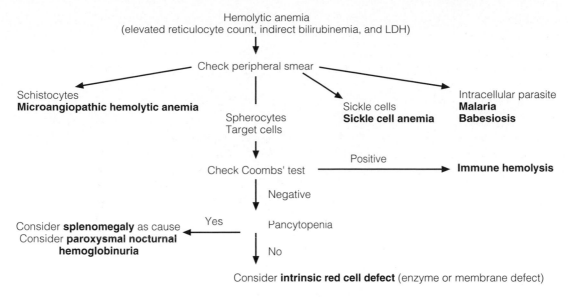

Figure 64-1 • An approach to the evaluation of hemolytic anemia.

Once examination of the smear eliminates MAHA or intraerythrocytic infections, a **Coombs' test** should be performed to evaluate for immune-mediated hemolysis. An **indirect** Coombs' test looks for an antibody in the patient's serum that can agglutinate normal RBCs. However, a **direct Coombs' test** is the definitive test for immune-mediated hemolysis, searching for the presence of the antibody directly on the patient's own RBCs.

A direct Coombs' test may be further classified by the type of antibody associated with the hemolysis. Most warm-antibody hemolysis is mediated by immunoglobulin (Ig)G, and therefore IgG and C3 will be detected on the RBC surface. Cold-antibody hemolysis is mostly IgM mediated. IgM binds to the RBC and fixes complement at lower temperatures but then dissociates from the RBC. Therefore, only C3 will be detected on the cell surface.

FURTHER DIAGNOSTIC TESTS

The **osmotic fragility test** is used to look for membrane defects, such as a hereditary spherocytosis. The abnormal cells lyse more easily than normal RBCs. Paroxysmal nocturnal hemoglobinuria (PNH) is diagnosed by **flow cytometry** to detect cells deficient in the GPI anchor protein. The sucrose lysis test and the acidified serum lysis (Ham) test to activate the complement pathway have been largely abandoned for the diagnosis of PNH.

Enzyme deficiencies may be diagnosed by testing for the specific enzyme in the patient's RBCs. The **fluorescent spot test**, which measures generation of the reduced form of nicotinamide adenine dinucleotide phosphate (NADPH), is a reliable measure for G6PD deficiency. In cases of severe hemolysis, the most deficient cells will already have been destroyed, resulting in a falsely normal test. The assay should be repeated at a later time. Sickle cell disease may be confirmed by a **hemoglobin electrophoresis**, which demonstrates hemoglobin S.

KEY POINTS

- Hemolytic anemia is characterized by an indirect hyperbilirubinemia, an elevated LDH, and decreased haptoglobin. Urine hemosiderin may be present (especially with intravascular hemolysis).

- Schistocytes and thrombocytopenia indicate microangiopathic hemolytic anemia. Causes include DIC, HUS, and TTP.

- A direct Coombs' test is positive in immune-mediated hemolysis. Hemolysis related to warm antibodies (IgG) demonstrates both IgG and complement (C3) on the red cell surface, whereas hemolysis related to cold antibodies (IgM) only detects C3.

Adenopathy often represents a benign self-limited process. However, more serious diseases such as lymphoma or HIV infection may also present with enlarged lymph nodes. In normal individuals, lymph nodes range from 0.5 to 2 cm. Lymph nodes >1 cm are often evaluated further; the age of the patient and the characteristics of the node should be considered in this decision.

CLINICAL MANIFESTATIONS

HISTORY

Adenopathy that persists after a few weeks is less likely to be infectious in origin. **Associated symptoms** may suggest certain etiologies:

- Weight loss, night sweats (lymphoma, metastatic cancer, tuberculosis)
- Sore throat (mononucleosis, pharyngitis)
- Genital lesion (syphilis, chancroid)
- Pets, especially cats (cat-scratch disease, toxoplasmosis)
- History of travel to the southwestern United States (coccidioidomycosis) or the midwestern United States (histoplasmosis)
- History of IV drug use or high-risk sexual behavior (HIV)

Age is also an important consideration. Individuals older than 50 years have a malignant etiology 50% of the time; those younger than 30 years have a benign etiology 80% of the time. When considering lymphoma as a cause of adenopathy, inquire about

phenytoin (Dilantin) use, which may cause a pseudolymphoma syndrome.

PHYSICAL EXAMINATION

The **location** of the adenopathy often leads to the diagnosis (see Differential Diagnosis). Tender erythematous nodes are consistent with lymphadenitis, whereas firm rubbery adenopathy may be found in lymphoma. Metastatic disease tends to present with hard fixed nodes. Erythema nodosum (tender, red subcutaneous nodules) with hilar adenopathy is highly suggestive of sarcoidosis; a maculopapular rash involving palms and soles is seen in syphilis.

DIFFERENTIAL DIAGNOSIS

The evaluation of adenopathy is best categorized by the **location of the adenopathy**.

Generalized
- HIV infection
- Lymphoma
- Hypersensitivity reaction (including phenytoin)
- Systemic lupus erythematosus (SLE)
- Toxoplasmosis
- Secondary syphilis

Cervical
- Mononucleosis
- Lymphoma
- Pharyngitis
- Toxoplasmosis
- Sarcoidosis

Inguinal
- Syphilis
- Herpes simplex
- Lymphogranuloma venereum
- Chancroid

Supraclavicular
- Mediastinal or pulmonary malignancy (right)
- Abdominal malignancy (left)

Hilar adenopathy
- Sarcoidosis (bilateral)
- Lymphoma
- Tuberculosis
- Bronchogenic carcinoma (unilateral)
- Fungal infection (bilateral)

Two additional clinical scenarios deserve mention. **Secondary syphilis** may present with bilateral epitrochlear adenopathy; **cat-scratch disease** presents with unilateral adenopathy proximal to the cat bite or scratch (usually epitrochlear or axillary).

DIAGNOSTIC EVALUATION

In the young patient with cervical adenopathy, infectious mononucleosis is the primary consideration. A **complete blood count (CBC) with differential** should be sent. Lymphocytosis, with atypical lymphocytes, is almost always seen. A **heterophile antibody** confirms the diagnosis of mononucleosis, although it may be negative early in the disease.

If inguinal adenopathy is present, urethral or cervical cultures should be obtained to rule out a sexually transmitted disease (STD; see Chapter 28).

In the older patient with supraclavicular adenopathy, a **chest radiograph** should be obtained to rule out bronchogenic carcinoma or lymphoma. However, these patients are likely to proceed to biopsy given the concern for malignancy. A **mammogram** should be obtained in all women with axillary adenopathy (if not infectious in origin).

Asymptomatic hilar adenopathy with symptoms consistent with sarcoidosis may be observed if tuberculosis and fungal disease are not considerations. Patients with hilar adenopathy related to lymphoma or bronchogenic cancer usually have associated symptoms. If the adenopathy is associated with a mass or effusion, it must be investigated further.

Lymph node biopsy remains the definitive diagnostic test. Often the adenopathy resolves after a **period of observation**, making biopsy unnecessary. **Early biopsy** should be considered when the following features are present:

- Lymph node >2 to 3 cm in diameter without findings suggestive of mononucleosis
- Adenopathy in association with an abnormal chest radiograph (hilar adenopathy, pulmonary mass or cavity)
- Supraclavicular adenopathy (especially in the older patient)
- Axillary adenopathy without signs of upper extremity infection (consider breast malignancy in women and lymphoma in both sexes)

Additional tests that may be performed to assist in diagnosis if indicated include:

- Purified protein derivative (PPD) skin test for tuberculosis
- Toxoplasma titers
- HIV antibody testing
- Rapid plasma reagin (RPR) to rule out syphilis

Biopsy is diagnostic for malignancy and will show noncaseating granulomas in sarcoidosis. Special stains can reveal certain organisms: Warthin-Starry stain for the small bacilli of *Bartonella henselae* (cat-scratch disease) and the acid fast stain for *Mycobacterium tuberculosis*. Biopsy may be nondiagnostic in approximately 30% of patients who eventually undergo biopsy. These patients should be carefully followed because some will eventually prove to have lymphoma.

KEY POINTS

- Location of the adenopathy is a key feature in determining etiology. Cervical adenopathy in a young patient is often mononucleosis; asymptomatic hilar adenopathy is often related to sarcoidosis.

- A period of observation is often indicated in the young patient with adenopathy; many of these patients have a reactive adenopathy that will resolve.

- Supraclavicular adenopathy may represent malignancy. The left supraclavicular node (Virchow's node) drains the abdominal cavity and therefore may be enlarged in gastric, colon, or ovarian cancer.

Hemostasis is accomplished after vascular injury via the interplay of the proteins composing the clotting cascades and a variety of cells, including platelets, leukocytes, and endothelial cells. Normal function of these elements after vascular injury leads to the **formation of a clot**, composed of **fibrin** and **platelets**. Fibrin is produced by the cleavage of **fibrinogen** by the protease **thrombin** (Fig. 66-1). The **thrombolytic system**, in which the fibrin-cleaving protein **plasmin** is a central component, is responsible for remodeling and removing existing fibrin clots. The thrombolytic system is activated from the time the coagulation system begins clot formation, providing close regulation of hemostasis.

Defects in coagulation or thrombolysis can lead to either **hypercoagulability** or **bleeding disorders**. A complete discussion of the coagulation and thrombolytic systems is beyond the scope of this chapter. Instead, the focus is on the clinical presentation of the major bleeding disorders and the diagnostic workup of these problems. Hypercoagulability is discussed briefly in Chapter 16.

Bleeding disorders can be classified by the **defect in the clotting cascade**:

- Decrease in clotting factors because of an inherited defect, decreased production, or excess consumption
- Thrombocytopenia
- Abnormal platelet function
- Drugs that activate the thrombolytic pathway (e.g., tissue plasminogen activator) or interfere with the action of activated coagulation factors (e.g., heparin)

ETIOLOGY AND PATHOGENESIS

The most common hemorrhagic disorders in adults are **acquired** rather than hereditary:

- Vitamin K deficiency/anticoagulant therapy
- Coagulopathy associated with liver disease
- Disseminated intravascular coagulation (DIC)

Vitamin K deficiency leads to decrease of the coagulation factors II, VII, IX, and X and the coagulation regulators protein C and protein S. Vitamin K is required for the γ-carboxylation of all these factors. The anticoagulant drug warfarin interferes with the action of vitamin K, leading to a similar defect.

The liver plays an important role in the production and metabolism of coagulation factors. Severe liver failure can therefore result in a bleeding tendency because of factor deficiency. Factor VIII, produced by the endothelium, is preserved in liver disease.

DIC is a condition in which a number of diseases (including sepsis, trauma/tissue injury, neoplasms, and obstetric catastrophes) can trigger **accelerated, unregulated activation of the coagulation cascades**. There is formation of small thrombi and emboli throughout the vascular tree that eventually leads to depletion of coagulation factors and platelets. A severe coagulation defect comprised of thrombocytopenia, decreased fibrinogen, and decreased factor levels is seen.

The **inherited bleeding disorders** include von Willebrand disease (vWD) and hemophilia. The most common inherited bleeding disorder is vWD, the result of a deficiency or qualitative defect in

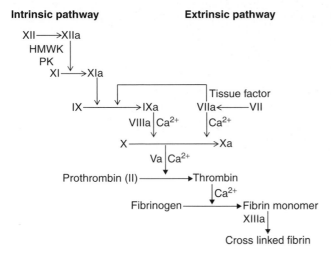

Intrinsic pathway   **Extrinsic pathway**

Figure 66-1 • Coagulation cascade. Two pathways (intrinsic and extrinsic) able to activate the common pathway of factor X. Factor VIIa is also able to activate the intrinsic pathway indirectly through factor IXa. Factors II, VII, IX, and X require vitamin K and calcium for biologic activity. HMWK, high molecular weight kinogen; PK, prekallikrein

von Willebrand factor. This factor is a carrier for factor VIII and a cofactor for platelet adhesion. Hemophilia is an X-linked disease caused by the lack of factor VIII (hemophilia A) or factor IX (hemophilia B).

CLINICAL MANIFESTATIONS

HISTORY

The patient with a bleeding disorder may present with **epistaxis** or **easy bruisability**. The patient often can be totally asymptomatic, and the disorder is suspected by the presence of abnormal laboratory tests of coagulation (see later).

Inherited disorders, such as the classic disorder of hemophilia, tend to present with abnormal bleeding at an early age. Milder inherited coagulopathies are apparent only during times of significant hemostatic stress. Previous surgery or dental extraction without bleeding argues against an inherited disorder. A **family history** of abnormal bleeding is an important clue to an inherited disorder.

A **medication history** may suggest the etiology of the bleeding disorder. Anticoagulants, such as warfarin, are an obvious cause, but patients may unknowingly ingest aspirin in over-the-counter "cold remedies" and "headache remedies." Certain drugs (e.g., sulfa and beta-lactam antibiotics) are associated with **immune-mediated platelet destruction**.

PHYSICAL EXAMINATION

The nature and site of abnormal bleeding can give clues to the nature of the coagulation defect. **Platelet disorders** usually manifest as **superficial bleeding** involving the skin, mucous membranes, and gastrointestinal (GI) and urinary tracts. Typical skin findings include **petechiae** (see Color Plate 23) and small **ecchymoses**. Bleeding occurs immediately after trauma because of the inability to form a platelet plug. Bleeding within the oral mucous membranes (wet purpura) is associated with an increased risk of more serious bleeding.

Disorders involving plasma **coagulation factor defects** generally manifest as **deeper bleeding**, affecting joints and body cavities (e.g., peritoneum). Chronic bleeding into joints, as is seen in hemophilia, can lead to joint deformity. Because platelet function is unaffected, abnormal bleeding does not manifest immediately after trauma but can be delayed hours to days.

The physical examination should also focus on signs of liver disease (see Chapter 42) and the presence of splenomegaly.

DIFFERENTIAL DIAGNOSIS

The differential diagnosis of bleeding disorders can be divided based on the primary abnormality.

Platelet Disorders
• Abnormal function (uremia, vWD, decreased cyclooxygenase activity related to aspirin or nonsteroidal anti-inflammatory drugs [NSAIDs])
• Thrombocytopenia (immune destruction, DIC, splenic sequestration, marrow failure)

Coagulation Factor Disorders
• Defective factors (hemophilia, dysfibrinogenemia)
• Consumption of coagulation factors (DIC)
• Vitamin K deficiency (insufficient dietary intake, intestinal malabsorption, chronic liver disease)
• Interference with vitamin K activity (warfarin administration)
• Interference with activated coagulation factors (heparin administration)

Abnormal Activity of the Fibrinolytic Pathway

- Exogenous plasminogen activator (tPA or streptokinase administration during acute myocardial infarction [MI])
- Abnormal regulation of fibrinolysis (plasmin inhibitor deficiency)

DIAGNOSTIC EVALUATION

The initial workup of a bleeding disorder begins with a complete blood count (CBC), PT, and activated PTT (aPTT) (Table 66-1). The CBC provides analysis of other hematologic lines (white blood cell [WBC] count, red blood cell [RBC] count) as well as the platelet count. With normal platelet function, clinical or spontaneous bleeding usually does not occur until the platelet count is <20,000 per mm^3.

The aPTT assesses the so-called **intrinsic limb** of the coagulation pathway (factors VIII, IX, XI, and XII, high molecular weight kininogen and prekallikrein), whereas the PT assesses the **extrinsic** (factor VII and tissue factor-dependent) **limb**. Both tests assess the adequacy of the final steps of the coagulation cascade, leading to thrombin-mediated cleavage of fibrinogen (factors II, V, and X and fibrinogen). A possible defect in a coagulation factor that leads to an abnormal PT or PTT can be screened for by the addition of normal plasma to the patient's plasma and repeating the test **(1:1 mixing study)**. Normalization by the addition of normal serum indicates a **factor deficiency**, whereas a

continued prolongation indicates the presence of a **coagulation inhibitor**. Specific assays are available for the various coagulation factors that can pinpoint a particular factor deficiency.

Abnormal results of these coagulation tests can narrow the differential diagnosis:

- Prolonged PTT: heparin administration, classic hemophilia (factors VIII or IX deficiency), some cases of vWD
- Prolonged PT: warfarin administration, vitamin K deficiency, factor VII deficiency (factor VII has the shortest half-life and therefore is the first to show deficiency in conditions such as liver disease)
- Prolonged PTT and PT: factor II, V, and X deficiency, severe vitamin K deficiency, higher dose warfarin administration, severe liver disease, DIC, dysfibrinogenemia

When both PT and aPTT are elevated, the level and function of fibrinogen should be tested. Hypofibrinogenemia is seen in DIC, and fibrin degradation products (FDPs) are increased from the accelerated consumption. The cleavage of fibrinogen to fibrin can be specifically tested by the **thrombin time**. Dysfibrinogenemia is a rare cause of a prolonged thrombin time with normal fibrinogen levels.

When the platelet count, PT, and aPTT are normal, the **functional capacity of platelets** needs to be assessed. Uremia or the use of antiplatelet medica-

■ TABLE 66-1 Laboratory Features in Bleeding Disorders

	Platelet Count	PT	aPTT	Thrombin Time	Fibrinogen	Other Features
Thrombocytopenia	Low	Normal	Normal	Normal	Normal	
DIC	Low	Elevated	Elevated	Elevated	Low	Schistocytes on blood smear
Hemophilia A (factor VIII deficiency)	Normal	Normal	Elevated	Normal	Normal	Corrected by mixing study
Von Willebrand disease	Normal	Normal	Normal or slightly elevated	Normal	Normal	Abnormal ristocetin cofactor activity
Vitamin K deficiency (diet or warfarin)	Normal	Elevated	Normal	Normal	Normal	Corrected by mixing study
Dysfibrinogenemia	Normal	Elevated	Elevated	Elevated	Normal	

tions (aspirin, clopidogrel) are potential causes of platelet dysfunction. Von Willebrand disease may be diagnosed with measurement of vWF antigen and ristocetin cofactor activity (a functional measure of the ability of vWF to agglutinate platelets). More unusual causes of platelet dysfunction require more specialized tests of platelet agglutination. The **bleeding time** was previously often used to assess platelet function, but subtle as well as significant abnormalities may be missed. In addition, a preoperative bleeding time does not accurately predict bleeding during surgery.

THROMBOCYTOPENIA

Thrombocytopenia may be caused by increased destruction, decreased production, or sequestration. The first step is to examine the peripheral blood smear. Increased destruction is seen in the microangiopathic hemolytic anemias, such as hemolytic uremic syndrome (HUS), TTP, and DIC (see Chapter 64). **Idiopathic thrombocytopenic purpura** (ITP) is caused by autoimmune destruction of platelets and demonstrates isolated thrombocytopenia, often with platelet counts <20,000 per mm^3. Large (i.e., young) platelets are seen on the blood smears of patients with ITP. A bone marrow biopsy demonstrates increased megakaryocytes in ITP, confirming the accelerated destruction of platelets. Medications, such as heparin or quinidine, are alternative causes of increased platelet destruction. Infiltrative bone marrow disorders, acute leukemias, and myelodysplastic syndromes may also present with thrombocytopenia from decreased production, usually in the context of pancytopenia.

TREATMENT

Once the diagnosis of a coagulation defect is made, attempts must be made to correct the underlying cause if possible. Supportive care with transfusion of blood products can be initiated if indicated. However, in cases of excess consumption (DIC, TTP, HUS, heparin-induced thrombocytopenia), transfusion should be avoided because it adds "fuel to the fire." Plasmapheresis with plasma exchange is the treatment of choice for TTP.

Fresh-frozen plasma contains all the needed coagulation factors and can be used to rapidly replenish factor deficiencies. Its short half-life (4 hours) and risk of viral transmission are disadvantages. **Cryoprecipitate** contains vWF, factor VIII, and fi-

brinogen. It can be used for vWD or hypofibrinogenemia. **Factor VIII concentrate** is specifically used for hemophilia A.

Thrombocytopenia or qualitative platelet defects that cause significant hemorrhage can be managed with platelet transfusions. In general, platelet transfusions are only given for thrombocytopenia when bleeding is present or a procedure is planned. In the case of immune-mediated thrombocytopenia, platelet transfusions are avoided because the platelets are rapidly consumed. **Prednisone**, 1 mg/kg/day, is the treatment of choice for ITP. IV immune globulin can temporarily reduce consumption in patients who do not respond to prednisone. Splenectomy is recommended for patients with ITP when thrombocytopenia recurs after withdrawal of corticosteroids. In patients with refractory ITP, the antiCD20 monoclonal antibody rituximab has been used. In patients with functional platelet dysfunction related to uremia, IV **desmopressin acetate** (dDAVP) at 0.3 µg per kg can improve platelet function for several hours. Patients with a quantitative defect in vWF (type 1 vWD) can often be treated with intranasal dDAVP.

Vitamin K deficiency and excessive anticoagulation with warfarin can be treated by administration of subcutaneous or oral vitamin K. If a more rapid reversal of the defect is required because of clinically significant bleeding or the need for immediate surgery, fresh-frozen plasma can be administered.

KEY POINTS

- DIC causes bleeding by consumption of coagulation factors. PT and aPTT are elevated, and platelets and fibrinogen are decreased.

- A mixing study tests for deficiencies in coagulation factors. Failure to correct an elevated PT or aPTT with normal plasma suggests a factor inhibitor is present.

- Thrombocytopenia usually presents with bleeding when levels are <20,000 per mm^3. Drug effects, microvascular destruction, and autoimmune destruction (ITP) are common causes.

- Standard coagulation tests (PT, aPTT, and platelet count) are usually normal in vWD. A history of bleeding with surgical procedures is often present, and the vWF antigen and function should be measured.

67 Breast Cancer

EPIDEMIOLOGY

Breast cancer is the most common noncutaneous cancer in women and the second most common cause of cancer deaths in women (approximately 41,000 deaths per year). An estimated 12% of women will develop breast cancer and 3.5% will die of it. The incidence of breast cancer increased 1% to 2% per year from 1980 until 2000 (perhaps due to more aggressive screening and estrogen replacement therapy), but more recently it has slightly decreased. The mortality has decreased slightly over the past decade.

RISK FACTORS

The risk of breast cancer increases with increasing age; the median age for breast cancer is 54 years. Family history is also important, with a relative risk of 1.5 to 2 for patients with a first-degree relative with breast cancer. The risk from family history is increased if the relative had an early diagnosis (premenopausal) or bilateral breast cancer. Germline mutations in the *BRCA1* and *BRCA2* genes are responsible for some of the inherited risk of breast cancer. Carriers of these genes were previously informed of a 75% lifetime risk of breast or ovarian cancer, but more recent population-based estimates suggest a 50% lifetime risk. Patients with a previous breast biopsy showing benign proliferative changes appear to be at higher risk, especially those biopsies that show atypical hyperplasia.

Other risk factors are not as strong and appear to have a hormonal basis. These include:

- Early menarche
- Late menopause
- Late age of first pregnancy
- Nulliparity

Combination hormone replacement therapy (estrogen and progestin) increases the relative risk of breast cancer an estimated 25% after approximately 5 years. Unopposed estrogen in women with hysterectomies does not appear to confer a similar risk. Dietary factors, such as fat intake and alcohol consumption, have not been consistently related to increased risk. Despite the emphasis on the preceding factors, approximately half of the patients with breast cancer do not have any identifiable risk factor.

CLINICAL MANIFESTATIONS

HISTORY

An asymptomatic **breast mass** is the most common complaint of the patient with breast cancer. Approximately 20% of the masses prove to be malignant. Important historical points include risk factors (see earlier), duration of mass, change in size, and relation to menses. Patients with intraductal cancer may present with unilateral **nipple discharge**. Bloody discharge increases the concern for malignancy. **Breast pain** without an associated mass is an uncommon presenting sign; less than 5% of these women have cancer.

PHYSICAL EXAMINATION

Physical examination should concentrate on finding an underlying breast mass. Although benign masses are often mobile, soft, or cystic, these features are not specific enough to rule out malignancy. The breasts should be examined for asymmetry or skin changes, such as thickening or dimpling. Lymphadenopathy, particularly axillary, suggests malignancy.

DIFFERENTIAL DIAGNOSIS

In the patient presenting with a **breast mass**, the following diagnoses should be considered in addition to malignancy:

- Cyst
- Fibroadenoma
- Fibrocystic changes

In the patient with **nipple discharge**, the differential includes:

- Ductal papilloma
- Ductal ectasia
- Endocrinopathies, such as prolactinoma (especially if discharge is bilateral)

DIAGNOSTIC EVALUATION

Ultrasonography (US) can be used to differentiate cystic from solid masses. This is helpful for young women who have a high rate of cystic disease relative to cancer. The US may then be used to guide aspiration of the cyst.

Mammography is useful in identifying suspicious lesions or concurrent nonpalpable lesions. An irregular spiculated mass or cluster of microcalcifications suggests carcinoma. However, because of the high false-negative rate (10% to 20%), a normal mammogram does *not* rule out malignancy.

In evaluating a patient with a breast complaint, one must consider the underlying risk of breast cancer. A mammogram is a reasonable start for all women older than 35 years. For younger women or those with findings that suggest cystic disease, a US may identify cysts and guide aspiration. A cyst may be followed closely if the fluid is nonbloody and the cyst resolves completely. **Bloody fluid** or a **nonresolving mass** necessitate further workup.

As mentioned, a normal mammogram does not rule out cancer. Fine-needle aspiration (FNA) or core-needle biopsy may yield a diagnosis, but false-negative samples are possible. If physical examination, mammography, and FNA suggest a benign lesion, the mass can be followed closely. However, if there is suspicious result with any of these tests, **excisional biopsy** remains the definitive diagnostic procedure for a solid breast mass. Positive biopsies should be sent for estrogen and progesterone receptor testing because these tumors respond better to hormonal therapy. Figure 67-1 summarizes the workup of a breast mass.

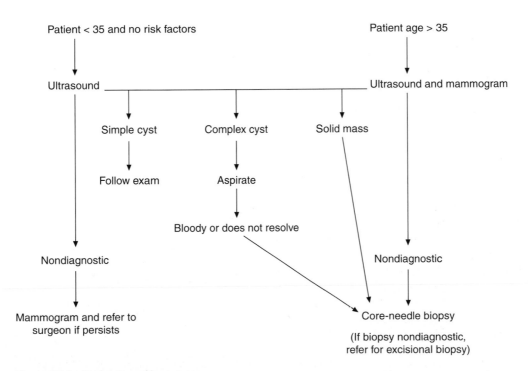

Figure 67-1 • Evaluation of breast mass.

Mammograms have also proven useful to **screen asymptomatic women**. Annual or biannual mammograms decrease breast cancer mortality in women 50 to 74 years of age. Although the use of screening mammography in younger women remains controversial, recent meta-analyses suggest a similar reduction in breast cancer mortality. The American Cancer Society and the United States Preventive Services Task Force recommend annual screening mammography in women older than 40 years. Screening should be started earlier for women with a family history of breast cancer. **Breast magnetic resonance imaging** (MRI) is now recommended to screen women with the BRCA mutations. Although some serum markers (such as CA 15–3) may correlate with breast cancer, there are no accepted blood tests for early detection.

STAGING OF BREAST CANCER

Lymph node involvement, including the number of lymph nodes involved, is strongly correlated with prognosis. Besides absence of lymph node involvement, factors that indicate a **better prognosis** include:

- Small size of tumor (<2 cm)
- Presence of steroid receptors (estrogen receptors [ER] or progesterone receptors [PR]) on tumor
- *Lack* of overexpression of certain oncogenes (e.g., *HER-2/neu*)
- Specific subtypes of ductal carcinoma (e.g., mucinous, tubular)

Staging is completed at the time of surgery (see later) with resection of tumor and lymph node sampling. A chest radiograph, serum calcium, and alkaline phosphatase are often used to screen for advanced disease. Carcinoma in situ is considered stage 0. Tumors <2 cm with negative lymph nodes are classified as stage I. Lymph node involvement and/or larger tumors (2 to 5 cm) are classified as stage II. Tumors >5 cm are considered stage IIB if lymph nodes are negative. Large tumors with positive nodes, any tumor with fixed lymph nodes, and tumor infiltration into the skin or chest wall are classified as stage III. This includes **inflammatory breast cancer**, where tumor infiltration into skin lymphatics causes swelling, erythema, warmth, and peau d'orange appearance. Distant metastases (such as bone, lung, or liver) are classified as stage IV. Five-year survival in stage I is >80% but is reduced to 10% to 15% in stage IV breast cancer.

TREATMENT

Previously, all patients with localized breast cancer underwent a **modified radical mastectomy**. Recent studies indicate that for many patients with localized breast cancer, **lumpectomy** (breast-conserving surgery) **with primary radiation** therapy is equivalent in 10- and 20-year survival to mastectomy. The choice of therapy should be discussed with the patient after the biopsy-proven diagnosis of breast cancer. Important factors in the decision include size of tumor, size of breast, expected cosmetic result, and patient preference. Local recurrence rate is high after lumpectomy if radiation treatment is omitted. Lymph node sampling is necessary for prognosis and treatment, but it can result in substantial morbidity from lymphedema of the affected arm. A technique known as **sentinel lymph node mapping** uses a radioactive substance and/or blue dye injected around the tumor to locate the first lymph node to drain the region of the cancer. This lymph node is excised, and, if it is negative, it indicates a small possibility of additional lymph involvement. This technique can be used to avoid full axillary node dissection in some patients.

ADJUVANT THERAPY FOR EARLY STAGE BREAST CARCINOMA

Adjuvant therapy for early stage breast cancer, which aims to eliminate micrometastatic disease and prevent clinical recurrence, includes chemotherapy and hormonal therapy (tamoxifen, aromatase inhibitors, ovarian ablation). The overall benefit of adjuvant therapy is greatest in women with positive nodes, with a 20% to 30% reduction in the risk of death. In women without lymph node involvement, the decision is more complex because approximately 70% of these women will have no recurrence of their cancer. Adjuvant therapy should be offered to node-negative women with an increased risk of recurrence (e.g., ER/PR negative, tumor >2 cm). In women with small, node-negative tumors, prediction models and genetic profiling (e.g., Oncotype Dx) have been used to identify higher risks of recurrence. Table 67-1 outlines the options for adjuvant therapy.

Tamoxifen, an antiestrogen, is used in women with steroid receptor–positive tumors. Treatment for 5 years appears to be the optimal duration. Side effects include nausea, menopausal symptoms (e.g., hot flashes), thromboembolism, and a small increase in uterine cancer (mandating a workup for any uter-

■ TABLE 67-1 Adjuvant Therapy in Breast Cancer

	Lymph Node Negative	Lymph Node Positive
Endocrine responsive[a]	Hormonal Rx ± chemotherapy[b]	Chemotherapy + hormonal Rx
Endocrine nonresponsive	Chemotherapy	Chemotherapy
HER-2/neu positive tumor	Add trastuzumab	Add trastuzumab

[a]Endocrine responsive tumors express estrogen receptors or progesterone receptors.
[b]Adjuvant chemotherapy is recommended for women with endocrine responsive tumors and negative nodes if high-risk features are present (tumor >2 cm, high-grade histology, HER-2/neu positive, or age <35).
Co-morbid disease should be considered in recommending chemotherapy in women over age 70. Hormonal therapy may be added to any patient's regimen on the basis of prevention of contralateral breast cancer.

ine bleeding). Ovarian ablation is only beneficial as a hormonal treatment in premenopausal women.

The **aromatase inhibitors** (anastrozole, letrozole, and exemestane) are another hormonal treatment available for postmenopausal women with steroid receptor–positive tumors. The drugs block the conversion of androgens to estrogens by the aromatase enzyme. Studies have shown that aromatase inhibitors are more effective than tamoxifen in preventing breast cancer recurrence in postmenopausal women, and they have less adverse effects such as uterine cancer and thromboembolism. Aromatase inhibitors can be used in place of tamoxifen or as sequential therapy (following 2 to 5 years of tamoxifen).

Chemotherapy is the mainstay of treatment for women with high-risk disease (e.g., node positive, ER/PR negative). The benefit is greatest in patients with positive lymph nodes. Standard treatment involves multiple drug regimens for 4 to 6 months. Typical regimens are cyclophosphamide, methotrexate, 5-FU (CMF); cyclophosphamide, Adriamycin (doxorubicin), 5-FU (CAF); and cyclophosphamide and doxorubicin (CA). Regimens with an anthracycline (e.g., doxorubicin) appear to be superior to those regimens without an anthracycline (like CMF). Newer regimens incorporate the taxanes; either cyclophosphamide and doxorubicin (CA), followed by a taxane (paclitaxel or docetaxel), or a combination treatment (cyclophosphamide, doxorubicin, paclitaxel). These taxane-based regimens have shown some benefit in cancer-free survival compared to the standard CAF treatment. Side effects of chemotherapy include nausea, vomiting, and bone marrow suppression. Doxorubicin can cause cardiomyopathy at cumulative doses >400 mg per m^2. Cyclophosphamide (an alkylating agent) can cause hemorrhagic cystitis and carries an increased risk of leukemia many years after treatment. Taxanes can cause peripheral neuropathy.

Trastuzumab (Herceptin) is a monoclonal antibody against HER-2/neu, a growth factor receptor overexpressed in approximately 25% of breast cancers. HER-2/neu expression is associated with an increased risk of recurrence, and trastuzumab may be added to adjuvant therapy for these patients.

METASTATIC BREAST CANCER

In the patient with **metastatic breast cancer**, cure is not possible with standard treatment. Experimental approaches (such as high-dose chemotherapy with rescue by autologous stem cells to replenish the bone marrow) have not been proven superior to standard treatment. In postmenopausal patients with ER-positive breast cancer, aromatase inhibitors are the first-line therapy. Oophorectomy is used in premenopausal women. Patients who become resistant to hormonal treatment or have ER-negative tumors are candidates for salvage chemotherapy, including regimens containing doxorubicin, taxanes (docetaxel, paclitaxel), or both. Additional chemotherapeutic agents with activity in metastatic breast cancer include vinorelbine and capecitabine. Trastuzamab can be added to treat tumors that overexpress HER-2/neu protein. Lapatinib, another agent that targets HER2 as well as the epidermal growth factor receptor, can be used in patients who fail trastuzamab.

CONTINUED CARE

Follow-up involves monitoring the patient for recurrence of breast cancer. Physical examination and mammography should be conducted at regular intervals. These women have five times the baseline risk for cancer in the contralateral breast. For this reason, tamoxifen is also useful for prevention of the second breast cancer (as opposed to the use of tamoxifen as an adjuvant treatment of the primary cancer). Although there is no evidence that early detection of metastatic disease will improve survival, patients should be evaluated for complaints that may indicate metastatic disease. Common sites of spread and clinical scenarios include:

- Bone (back pain, hypercalcemia)
- Brain (seizures, headache)
- Lung (dyspnea, cough)
- Liver (abdominal complaints)

Patients with these symptoms should be worked up with the appropriate tests because systemic treatment or radiation often palliates symptoms. In addition, patients with known bone metastasis benefit from treatment with bisphosphonates (pamidronate, zoledronate) to prevent further morbidity (see Chapter 50).

KEY POINTS

- The asymptomatic breast mass is the most common presentation of breast cancer. A normal mammogram does not rule out malignancy.

- Breast-conserving surgery combined with radiation is equivalent in efficacy to modified radical mastectomy for limited local disease.

- Presence of lymph node involvement significantly increases risk of recurrence and death from breast cancer.

- Adjuvant therapy, such as tamoxifen or chemotherapy, is indicated in node-positive patients; it is used in node-negative patients based on individualized risks and benefits.

- Symptoms such as headaches, seizures, or back pain in the patient with a history of breast cancer may represent metastatic disease.

68 Prostate Cancer

EPIDEMIOLOGY

Prostate cancer is the most common noncutaneous cancer in men and the second most common cause of cancer deaths in men (approximately 27,000 deaths per year). An estimated 15% to 20% of men will develop prostate cancer and 3% will die of it. Many men harbor subclinical prostate cancer, however, and die *with* it, not *of* it. Current diagnostic techniques cannot predict which cancers will cause death and which will remain confined to the gland. Tumor grade by the Gleason score (see later) is one method to evaluate aggressiveness of disease. The incidence of prostate cancer rose sharply from 1989 to 1992 as prevalent cases were diagnosed by routine use of prostate-specific antigen (PSA) testing, but it has recently decreased. Mortality from prostate cancer has gradually declined over the past decade.

RISK FACTORS

The annual risk of prostate cancer increases with increasing age; the median age at diagnosis is 68. Family history is also important, with a twofold risk for patients with a first-degree relative with prostate cancer. African Americans are at higher risk than whites for both developing prostate cancer and dying of it. Dietary factors, especially lack of antioxidants, have been suggested as possible risk factors. Increased dietary fat is one such factor that has been associated with prostate cancer. Increased consumption of tomato products (containing the antioxidant lycopene), vitamin D, and selenium remain possible, but unproven, methods to prevent prostate cancer.

CLINICAL MANIFESTATIONS

HISTORY

Most prostate cancer is detected by screening PSA tests and is asymptomatic at the time of diagnosis. Symptoms of obstruction by locally advanced prostate cancer (urinary frequency, urgency, and nocturia) are indistinguishable from the symptoms of the more common problem of benign prostatic hyperplasia (BPH). Metastatic disease may present as back pain from vertebral body involvement.

PHYSICAL EXAMINATION

Physical examination of the prostate is often entirely normal or reveals a diffusely enlarged prostate consistent with BPH. Prostate cancer sometimes presents as a prostate nodule, but approximately half of the cancers detected in this manner will already be locally advanced.

DIFFERENTIAL DIAGNOSIS

In the patient with an elevated PSA, other prostate diseases may be considered:

- Benign prostatic hyperplasia
- Prostatitis

Acute urinary retention, transurethral resection of prostate (TURP), and prostate biopsy can elevate PSA briefly. Digital rectal examination has no measurable effect on the level of PSA.

DIAGNOSTIC EVALUATION

The **prostate-specific antigen** (PSA) is a serine protease produced by the prostate and can be elevated in a number of conditions (see earlier). The exact characteristics of the test have not been determined, but it is estimated to be 85% to 90% sensitive and 85% to 90% specific for the diagnosis of prostate cancer. Levels <4 μg per mL are often used as a cutoff for "normal" values, and levels >10 μg per mL are highly suspicious for prostate cancer. A PSA between 4 and 10 μg per mL represents a gray zone; only 25% of these patients actually have prostate cancer. Some experts advocate the use of **age-specific PSA** ranges, with 2.5 μg per mL the upper limit of normal in men younger than 50 years, and 6.5 μg per mL the upper limit in men older than 70 years. In addition, PSA in patients with prostate cancer tends to be bound to α_1-antichymotrypsin, and **free PSA** values are usually lower (<25%) in patients with prostate cancer. In men with PSA levels between 4 and 10 μg per mL and a negative initial biopsy, a free PSA fraction >25% indicates a low probability (<3%) of undetected prostate cancer.

Transrectal prostate biopsy is the definitive diagnostic test for prostate cancer. Using transrectal ultrasonography (US) to guide the biopsy, at least six samples (but more commonly 8 to 12) are taken. Prostate cancer is then graded by a Gleason score from 1 (well differentiated) to 5 (poorly differentiated). The two most common patterns are added together to yield a score from 2 to 10.

Prostate cancer screening remains a controversial issue. PSA testing has certainly resulted in an increased detection of early localized cancers. However, no randomized trials of screening have demonstrated that early detection and aggressive treatment can reduce prostate cancer mortality. Patients with well-differentiated tumors may need no treatment (watchful waiting) and patients with poorly differentiated tumors may progress despite early intervention. Men who choose to undergo PSA testing must be aware of the high false-positive rate and potential for unnecessary testing. Also, a normal PSA does not detect all prostate cancers, so false reassurance is also possible. A recent study detected prostate cancer in approximately 15% of men with PSA values <4 μg per mL.

STAGING

The Gleason score is a histologic grade used to predict prostate cancer–related mortality. Prostate cancer is classified as well differentiated (Gleason 2 to 4), moderately differentiated (Gleason 5 to 6), moderately to poorly differentiated (Gleason 7), and poorly differentiated (8 to 10). This grading system correlates with 15-year mortality from prostate cancer (approximately 6%, 9%, 24%, and 75%, respectively, for well to poorly differentiated adenocarcinoma).

Staging (using the tumor-node-metastasis [TNM] system) is also important in prostate cancer prognosis. Disease confined to the prostate is classified as nonpalpable (T1) or palpable (T2). Locally advanced disease is labeled as T3 or T4. Regional lymph node involvement (N0 or N1) is assessed at time of surgery but may also be suggested by radiologic studies. Metastatic disease (M1) often presents in the vertebral bodies. Bone scanning is recommended in some patients with prostate cancer at time of diagnosis but may be avoided in patients with a PSA <10 and Gleason scores <7 (chance of metastatic disease <1%).

TREATMENT

Treatment for prostate cancer consists of surgery, radiation therapy, and/or androgen deprivation therapy. Many treatment options have not been compared directly in randomized trials, so the treatment decision depends on the Gleason score, the likelihood of locally advanced disease, patient co-morbidities, and patient preferences. If the patient has an expected life span of <10 years, it is unlikely that aggressive treatment is warranted. The probability of organ-confined disease (and possible cure with surgery) can be predicted using validated models that incorporate Gleason score, PSA level, and clinical stage.

SURGICAL THERAPY

Radical prostatectomy is an option for patients with disease confined to the prostate gland. The patient should have few co-morbidities and a reasonable 10-year life expectancy. The most common surgery is the nerve-sparing prostatectomy using a retropubic approach through an anterior abdominal incision. However, despite an attempt to preserve the nerve bundles responsible for sexual function, impotence remains the most common side effect of surgery, affecting 50% to 80% of men. Age and prior potency of the patient, as well as skill of the surgeon, are important predictors of postoperative impotence. Urinary incontinence is a significant problem immediately postoperatively and may persist in 8% to 30% of men.

RADIATION THERAPY

Radiation therapy consists of either external radiation beam or interstitial brachytherapy (seed implants). Radiation therapy is acceptable for patients with disease confined to the prostate and appears comparable to prostatectomy for overall survival. Biochemical recurrence (as evidenced by increasing PSA) may be higher in patients treated with radiation (compared to surgery). Radiation treatment can be combined with androgen deprivation for patients with locally advanced (T3 or T4) disease. Side effects of radiation include proctitis, diarrhea, and urinary symptoms. Late effects include impotence (approximately 50%); incontinence is less common.

HORMONAL THERAPY

Testosterone is required for normal development of the prostate, and androgens are believed to promote growth of prostate cancer. Most of the androgens produced in the prostate are derived from testicular sources with a small contribution of adrenal androgens. **Androgen deprivation therapy** is used to treat the patient with locally advanced (T3 or T4), regionally advanced (N1), or metastatic disease (M1). Approximately 80% of patients with metastatic disease initially respond to androgen ablation with a median response of 12 to 18 months. However, hormone-resistant disease eventually develops, and initial chemotherapy regimens were ineffective at improving survival in hormone-resistant disease. Newer treatment regimens with the taxanes (paclitaxel and docetaxel) appear to provide modest increases in survival rates.

Orchiectomy removes the source of testosterone production and remains the gold standard for hormonal treatment of metastatic prostate cancer. The physical morbidity of the procedure is low, but psychological morbidity of surgical castration is high. Therefore, medical castration has gained increasing acceptance.

Luteinizing hormone-releasing hormone (LHRH) agonists (goserelin, leuprolide, triptorelin) act to suppress LH release by providing continued stimulation of the LH receptor (delivered by long-acting injections). Initial treatment may cause a "flare" in LH production and should be combined with additional androgen blockade (see later). The main disadvantage of these medications is their high cost. **Nonsteroidal antiandrogens** (flutamide, bicalutamide, nilutamide) may be added to LHRH agonists or surgical castration to induce "complete androgen blockade" and to prevent a "flare" in disease with LHRH agonists. These drugs also block the small amount of adrenal androgens remaining. Numerous trials have failed to show clearly if "complete androgen blockade" is superior to castration (medical or surgical) alone.

CONTINUED CARE

Follow-up involves monitoring the patient for recurrence of prostate cancer, most commonly using PSA testing. In patients treated for local disease with radiation or surgery, an increase in previously undetectable PSA indicates recurrence. Not all patients with PSA recurrence develop metastatic disease, so the decision for timing of androgen deprivation depends on the individual patient's risks and comorbidities. Furthermore, although several studies suggest that early intervention with androgen blockade may be more beneficial than waiting for clinical recurrence, the risks and potential benefits of androgen deprivation must be weighed for each patient. Any patient with prostate cancer who develops new-onset back pain should be evaluated for bony metastases, which are usually osteoblastic on x-ray and easily detected by bone scan. Palliative radiation or the radioactive isotope strontium-89 can alleviate bone pain in the majority of patients with bony metastases.

KEY POINTS

- The incidence of prostate cancer increases with increasing age. Although it is the second most common cause of cancer deaths in men, most men with prostate cancer die of other competing causes.

- PSA screening for prostate cancer remains controversial. Testing leads to a higher detection of organ-confined disease, but randomized trials showing decreased mortality from prostate cancer have not been completed. Mildly elevated levels (4 to 10 µg per mL) of PSA are usually false positives but must be evaluated further.

- Localized prostate cancer may be treated with radiation therapy, radical prostatectomy, or watchful waiting.

- Androgen deprivation therapy, by medical or surgical castration, is appropriate for locally advanced or metastatic disease. LHRH agonists result in chronic suppression of LH production and are given as long-acting injections.

- The most common site of metastases is the vertebral body. Any patient with known prostate cancer with new-onset back pain should be assessed for bony metastases and possible cord compression.

Leukemia

Leukemias are neoplasms that **arise in the bone marrow** and then spread to the peripheral blood and throughout the body. Leukemias can be broadly classified according to the cell of origin and their clinical course:

- Acute lymphoblastic leukemia (ALL)
- Acute myelogenous leukemia (AML)
- Chronic lymphocytic leukemia (CLL)
- Chronic myelogenous leukemia (CML)

In an older classfication system, AML was divided into eight subtypes: M0, M1, M2 are myeloblastic leukemias of varying differentiation, M3 is acute promyelocytic leukemia (APL) with its unique treatment and clinical features, M4 and M5 are monocytic variants, M6 is erythroleukemia, and M7 is megakaryocytic leukemia. Newer classification systems focus on the presence of preceding myelodysplastic syndrome (MDS) and chromosomal abnormalities.

EPIDEMIOLOGY

Approximately 30,000 new cases of leukemia are diagnosed each year in the United States. CLL is the most common (15,000 cases annually), occurring almost exclusively in patients over the age of 50. The median age of presentation for CML is 45 to 55 years, and for AML is around 65 years.

ETIOLOGY AND PATHOPHYSIOLOGY

In most cases, a specific etiology for a leukemia is not known. Certain environmental exposures have been associated with hematologic neoplasms.

- Radiation exposure: For CML and AML, this appears to be dose related (as seen in the survivors of the atomic bomb in Japan) and has a peak incidence years after exposure.
- Chemotherapy: Use of alkylating agents or topoisomerase II inhibitors has a subsequent risk of AML.
- Chemical toxins: Benzene exposure increases the risk of AML, and Agent Orange (an herbicide used in the Vietnam War) has been associated with CLL.
- Myelodysplastic syndrome (MDS): Many cases of AML are preceded by MDS, which is often associated with chromosomal abnormalities.

The genetic alterations in some hematologic malignancies are well characterized. The **Philadelphia chromosome**, a translocation of chromosomes 9 and 22, is highly associated with CML. This translocation, t(9;22), involves a fusion of the breakpoint cluster (BCR) gene on chromosome 22 with the ABL gene on chromosome 9. The resulting fusion protein is a constitutively activated tyrosine kinase, a finding that has led to therapeutic implications (see later). Acute promyelocytic leukemia (AML type M3) is associated with a translocation, t (15;17), involving the retinoic acid receptor-alpha and the PML genes, resulting in a fusion protein that blocks differentiation. Administration of **all-trans retinoic acid** (ATRA) relieves this block and promotes differentiation.

Chronic lymphocytic leukemia is characterized as a mature B-cell line (CD19+) that also expresses CD5 (which is usually a T-cell antigen). The cells appear to be resistant to apoptosis, resulting in prolonged life and elevated numbers of leukocytes. Certain karyotypes carry a poor prognosis (17p or 11q deletions).

Mutations in the immunoglobulin variable region heavy chain are associated with better outcome.

CLINICAL MANIFESTATIONS

Patients with a **leukemia**, particularly an acute leukemia (ALL, AML), may present with:

- Constitutional symptoms: fever, malaise, dyspnea
- Bleeding: usually related to thrombocytopenia
- Infection: can be as dramatic as overwhelming sepsis
- Bone pain: from the expanding leukemic cell mass within the marrow
- Neurologic symptoms: ranging from headache to seizures and cranial nerve palsies and caused by leukemic cell infiltration of the meninges

The **chronic leukemias** CLL and CML are often clinically silent. Diagnosis may occur when a complete blood count (CBC) is done for another reason and an incidental leukocytosis is found. CML is characterized by a clinically mild phase, followed by a so-called blast crisis when the clinical picture resembles that seen in the acute leukemias. CLL may resemble lymphoma by presenting with painless adenopathy or splenomegaly.

On **physical examination**, a patient with leukemia may exhibit:

- Ecchymoses, petechiae (related to thrombocytopenia)
- Lymphadenopathy, most often with CLL
- Splenomegaly, seen in over 90% of CML, as well as hepatomegaly
- Gingival hypertrophy (because of infiltration) can be seen in the monocytic (M4,M5) types of AML

DIFFERENTIAL DIAGNOSIS

In the patient with an elevated WBC, the differential includes:

- Leukemia
- Leukemoid reaction (may be caused by overwhelming infection or a paraneoplastic syndrome)
- Demargination of neutrophils (physiologic stress, corticosteroids)

DIAGNOSTIC EVALUATION

An **elevated white blood cell (WBC)**, from 15,000 to more than 100,000 per mm^3, is the hallmark of leukemia. Examination of the peripheral smear demonstrates myeloblasts in AML, usually with thrombocytopenia. Blast cells have prominent nucleoli, large nuclear-to-cytoplasm ratio, and lack of granules. An **Auer rod**, a bluish red rod seen in the blast cell, is pathognomonic for AML. In CML, the blood count shows leukocytosis (sometimes with basophilia) and thrombocytosis (see Color Plate 24). The leukocytes in CML lack leukocyte alkaline phosphatase (LAP), in contrast to leukemoid reactions that have a high amount of staining for this enzyme. The blood smear in CLL shows a lymphocyte predominance (>50% lymphocytes, absolute lymphocyte count >5000 per mm^3), and the fragile lymphocytes in CLL are flattened on the blood smear (so-called smear or smudge cells).

Bone marrow biopsy is the definitive study, demonstrating >20% blast cells in AML. Bone marrow biopsy in CML shows a hypercellular marrow with an increase in myeloid cells, and cytogenetic testing reveals the Philadelphia chromosome in over 90% of cases. **Flow cytometry** shows the typical clonal phenotype in CLL (CD5+, CD 23+), and bone marrow biopsy is often not needed.

Additional laboratory abnormalities that may be seen include:

- Hemolytic anemia (CLL)
- Idiopathic thrombocytopenic purpura (CLL)
- Disseminated intravascular coagulation (APL)
- Hyperuricemia (AML)

TREATMENT

Specific therapy for leukemia is constantly undergoing revision secondary to results of clinical trials and is beyond the scope of this discussion. However, the standard approaches are listed here.

LEUKEMIA

Treatment for AML consists of initial **induction therapy** to induce a complete remission, most commonly with an anthracycline (e.g., daunorubicin) and cytarabine (ara-C). Remission can be defined as clinical (<5% blasts in bone marrow) or cytogenetic (absence of associated chromosomal abnormality by polymerase chain reaction). Approximately 70% of patients achieve a complete remission after treatment with cytarabine and an anthracycline. Patients who fail to achieve a complete remission do not usually respond to alternative treatments. Relapse is inevitable in AML, and allogeneic (human lymphocyte antigen–matched relative or unrelated donor) stem cell transplantation (SCT) can be used as consolidation therapy. In other patients, SCT can be performed after the first relapse. Acute promyelocytic leukemia is treated with chemotherapy plus **ATRA**, which results in remission in approximately 75% of patients with much less toxicity than conventional chemotherapy. However, treatment produces newly differentiated WBCs that can lead to the **retinoic acid syndrome** (fever, pulmonary infiltrates, hypoxia), which is treated with corticosteroids. Patients who relapse after treatment for AML have a poor prognosis. A newer treatment for relapsed AML is gemtuzumab ozogamicin, a monoclonal antibody against CD33 linked to a chemotherapeutic agent. This may benefit up to 30% of patients.

Allogeneic SCT is the first-line treatment in young patients (age <40 years) with CML, achieving cure rates of approximately 50%. In patients who are not good candidates for SCT, alpha interferon can lead to cytogenetic remissions in an estimated 25% of cases. The latest treatment for CML is **imatinib mesylate** (Gleevec), a specific inhibitor of the BCR-ABL tyrosine kinase produced in CML. This agent has induced cytogenetic responses in approximately 70% to 90% of patients, including those patients who failed interferon treatment. Two newer tyrosine kinase inhibitors are dasatinib and nilotinib.

CLL, because of its relatively benign course, is generally not treated unless there are complications (e.g., severe cytopenia, bulky adenopathy or organomegaly, severe systemic symptoms). The standard treatment regimen includes **fludarabine**, a purine analogue, which often results in disease regression, but not a cure. Other treatment options (which can be combined with fludarabine) include an alkylating agent (e.g., chlorambucil, cyclophosphamide) and rituximab, a monoclonal antibody against a B-cell marker, CD-20. CLL can transform to a more aggressive disease, at which time the treatment resembles therapy for aggressive lymphoma (Richter transformation). This should be suspected if patient develops B symptoms (fever, night sweats, weight loss) or rapid enlargement of lymph node.

Acute lymphoblastic leukemia is mainly a disease of children, although it can be seen in the blast phase of CML. It is not discussed in this chapter.

KEY POINTS

- CLL, the most common type of leukemia, is often detected during routine blood testing. Blood smear shows lymphocytosis and so-called smudge cells. Treatment is reserved for symptomatic disease.

- CML often presents with an elevated WBC and splenomegaly. CML may now be treated with a drug, imatinib, which inhibits the BCR-ABL tyrosine kinase produced by the 9;22 translocation.

- AML has a number of subtypes. APL (acute promyelocytic leukemia) has the unique feature of presenting with a DIC picture, and responds to treatment with all trans retinoic acid.

Lymphoma

Lymphomas are neoplasms of hematopoietic cells that **arise in peripheral lymphoid tissue** (usually lymph nodes) and may eventually spread to the peripheral blood and bone marrow. Lymphomas can be divided into:

- Hodgkin lymphoma (HL)
- Non-Hodgkin lymphoma (NHL)

NHL is broadly classified into indolent, aggressive, or highly aggressive disease. Classic examples of each type include follicular lymphoma (indolent), diffuse large B-cell lymphoma (aggressive), and Burkitt lymphoma (highly aggressive). There is significant overlap between the clinical features and treatment of indolent NHL and chronic lymphocytic leukemia (CLL) (see Chapter 69). T-cell lymphomas, such as cutaneous T-cell lymphoma, account for less than 10% of the cases of NHL.

EPIDEMIOLOGY

The majority (85%) of lymphomas are NHL, with an estimated 63,000 new cases each year in the United States. The incidence of NHL increases with increasing age, and HL has two peaks of incidence, the first in the second and third decades of life and another in the sixth.

ETIOLOGY AND PATHOPHYSIOLOGY

In most cases, a specific etiology for lymphoma is not known. There is evidence that viral infections play a role in the pathogenesis. Both human immunodeficiency virus infection and immunosuppression for conditions such as organ transplantation are associated with a significantly increased risk of NHL. Human T-cell leukemia virus type-1 has been linked to the development of adult T-cell leukemia/lymphoma. Epstein-Barr virus (EBV) infection has been closely associated with the African form of Burkitt lymphoma and is also associated with HL.

The genetic alterations in some lymphomas are well described. Most follicular lymphomas contain the t(14;18) translocation, which leads to the upregulation of the Bcl-2 proto-oncogene, which is an inhibitor of apoptosis. Mantle cell lymphoma (an aggressive NHL) is characterized by the t(11;14) translocation, which results in production of cyclin D1, a protein involved in cell cycle regulation. Burkitt lymphoma has the t(8;14) translocation, which activates the c-myc proto-oncogene (a transcriptional activator).

CLINICAL MANIFESTATIONS

Patients with **lymphoma** generally present with painless **lymphadenopathy** and/or a mass. Common locations include the axillary, supraclavicular, and cervical nodes. Mediastinal adenopathy can cause cough and respiratory compromise.

The so-called **B symptoms** (named for their use in staging of lymphomas) include fever, night sweats, and weight loss. Other constitutional symptoms, such as malaise, pruritus, and anorexia, may be present. An unusual symptom seen in some patients with HL is increasing pain in lymph nodes with alcohol ingestion.

On physical examination, lymph nodes are usually firm, freely mobile, and nontender. Splenomegaly may be present.

DIFFERENTIAL DIAGNOSIS

The differential diagnosis of lymphoma includes conditions that can lead to lymphadenopathy and is discussed in detail in Chapter 65.

DIAGNOSTIC EVALUATION

The diagnosis of lymphoma is generally made by **biopsy** of suspicious lymph nodes or masses (see Chapter 65). Hodgkin lymphoma is characterized by the presence of the **RS cell**, a large cell with a bilobulated nucleus and "owl's-eye" nucleoli. Excisional biopsy is necessary in the diagnosis of lymphoma to provide architectural information. In addition to determining the histologic appearance, immunophenotyping for cluster differentiation (CD) antigens is used to determine the cell of origin.

Computed tomography (CT) scans and bone marrow biopsy complete the workup of lymphoma to determine the anatomic stage of the disease (Fig. 70-1). Staging laparotomy was often performed to assess splenic involvement in patients with HL. However, more recent evidence suggests laparotomy

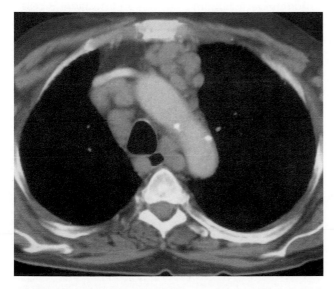

Figure 70-1 • Extensive mediastinal lymphadenopathy caused by lymphoma as demonstrated by CT scan.

is not necessary, and positron emission tomography (PET) scans are reliable indicators of splenic involvement. PET scans may also be used to determine involvement of suspicious lymph nodes. Staging also involves the determination of extranodal disease; common extranodal sites include intestinal tract, skin and bone. The Ann Arbor staging classification for lymphoma is:

- Stage I—single lymph node group or single extranodal site
- Stage II—two or more lymph node groups on same side of the diaphragm
- Stage III—nodal involvement on both sides of the diaphragm, which may include the spleen (IIIS), a contiguous extra-nodal site (IIIE), or both (IIIES)
- Stage IV—disseminated foci of involvement in one or more extralymphatic organs or tissues (such as bone marrow or liver)

Additional tests provide prognostic information for lymphoma. High lactate dehydrogenase (LDH) levels are associated with poorer outctome. All patients with NHL should be tested for the HIV antibody.

TREATMENT

Specific therapy for lymphoma involves consultation with an oncolgist specializing in the disease, and newer chemotherapeutic agents are often added to the standard treatments. General approaches are described below.

The initial treatment of indolent lymphoma resembles CLL. Because these lymphomas are incurable, most patients are followed expectantly until symptoms or cytopenias appear. Fludarabine is the first-line treatment, along with rituximab (see Chapter 69). High grade (grade 3) follicular lymphomas may be curable with systemic chemotherapy.

Limited-stage HL was previously treated with radiotherapy alone, but combination therapy (chemotherapy plus radiotherapy) is used more often now. Standard chemotherapy is ABVD: doxorubicin (Adriamycin), bleomycin, vinblastine, and dacarbazine. Bleomycin can cause long-term pulmonary toxicity, and doxorubicin can cause cardiomyopathy. Patients with no adverse predictors (such as large mediastinal mass, age 50 years or older, elevated erythrocyte sedimentation rate (ESR), and involvement of four or more lymph node regions) may be treated

■ TABLE 70-1 Prognostic Factors for the Lymphomas

Hodgkin Lymphoma	Follicular Lymphoma	Aggressive NHL
Age >45	Age >60	Age >60
Stage IV disease	Stage III or IV	Stage III or IV
Male sex	More than 4 nodal sites	More than 2 extranodal sites
Albumin <4 g/dL	Serum LDH > upper limit	Serum LDH > upper limit
Hemoglobin <10.5 g/dL	of normal	of normal
WBC >15,000/μL	Hemoglobin <12 g/dL	Poor performance status
Lymphocyte count <600/μL		(not fully ambulatory)
5 year survival	5 year survival	5 year survival
0 factors: 90%	0 factors: 90%	0 factors: 75%
4 or more factors: 60%	4 or more factors: 50%	4 or more factors: 25%

with shorter courses of chemotherapy. Advanced HD is treated with ABVD as well. Failure to achieve remission or an early relapse is an indication for autologous stem cell transplantation (SCT).

The standard chemotherapy for aggressive NHL is CHOP (cyclophosphamide, [hydroxydaunomycin], doxorubicin, vincristine [Oncovin], prednisone), which can be improved by the addition of rituximab (R-CHOP), especially in older patients. Patients who do not respond to standard chemotherapy may be considered for additional multidrug regimens or SCT. Prognostic factors are used to help predict outcome and determine aggressiveness of treatment (Table 70-1).

 KEY POINTS

- Lymphoma often presents as painless adenopathy and can be associated with fever, weight loss, or night sweats (B symptoms).

- Important prognostic factors for NHL include age, stage at diagnosis, and LDH level.

- Hodgkin lymphoma is often localized at the time of diagnosis and can be cured with chemotherapy plus radiation therapy.

- Indolent lymphoma, such as follicular lymphoma, is considered incurable and can be managed with watchful waiting for symptoms.

- Aggressive lymphoma, such as diffuse large B-cell lymphoma, is treated with a multidrug chemotherapy called CHOP with the possible addition of the monclonal antibody rituximab.

Part 9

Neurology

Headache

Headache is a very common presenting symptom in outpatient care and emergency rooms. It is vital to distinguish between common benign causes of headache and life-threatening causes. The causes of headache are divided into the primary headache syndromes (migraine, cluster, and tension) and the secondary causes of headache. The main secondary causes are outlined in Table 71-1.

EPIDEMIOLOGY AND RISK FACTORS

The majority of patients presenting for treatment have a primary headache syndrome, most commonly migraine headache. Migraine headaches most often occur in individuals ages 20 to 40, with women affected three times more than men. Cluster headaches are more frequent in men (5:1), and usually present when the patient is 30 to 40 years old. Temporal arteritis occurs in patients over the age of 50.

CLINICAL PRESENTATION

HISTORY

The history is the key to correctly diagnosing the patient with headache. Headache frequency, location, quality, triggers, and associated symptoms are the most important aspects to identify (Table 71-2). Although atypical presentations are possible, the following features are commonly seen in **migraine headaches**:

- Pounding, pulsatile pain
- Unilateral pain
- Worsened with activity
- Associated nausea and/or vomiting
- Phonophobia and/or photophobia

These features have been combined into the mnemonic POUND (Pulsatile quality, 4 to 72 hOurs duration, Unilateral location, Nausea or vomiting, Disabling intensity). Many patients with migraine headaches may have neck or posterior head pain, or complain of "sinus pain." When acute sinusitis causes headaches, there is usually associated nasal discharge and congestion (and fever in about 50% of cases). Patients with recurrent, severe "sinus" headaches likely have undiagnosed migraines. About 20% of migraine sufferers report an "**aura**," which is usually a visual phenomenon (flashing lights, spots, wavy lines) that precedes the headache. Family history is positive for migraines in about 70% of patients with migraine headaches.

Cluster headaches cause unilateral, retroorbital, sharp or knife-like pain and can awaken the patient in the middle of the night. There is associated lacrimation and nasal congestion, and patients often are restless and agitated. **Tension headaches** are dull, often bilateral and radiate from the neck or occiput.

There are several historical features that raise concern for "**worrisome**" headaches:

- Worst headache of life (subarachnoid hemorrhage [SAH])
- Thunderclap (sudden, severe onset) headache (SAH)
- First exertional headache (SAH, carotid dissection)
- New headache after age 50 (brain tumors, temporal arteritis, stroke)
- Associated fever or stiff neck (meningitis, SAH)

■ TABLE 71-1 Secondary Causes of Headache

Vascular causes
Subarachnoid hemorrhage
Subdural hematoma
Cerebrovascular accident
Carotid dissection
Arteriovenous malformations
Temporal arteritis
Intercranial masses
Primary brain tumors
Metastatic disease
Infections
Meningitis
Sinusitis
Severe hypertension
Pseudotumor cerebri

- Behavioral changes (brain tumors)
- Personal history of cancer (metastatic disease)

Medication use should be recorded. Patients taking frequent doses of headache medications (especially butalbital) may develop **medication overuse headaches**. Headaches are side effects of several medications, including beta blockers, nitrates, indomethacin, and phosphodiesterase inhibitors (e.g., sildenafil). Estrogen use (e.g., oral contraceptives) can worsen migraine headaches. Nonsteroidal anti-inflammatory drugs (NSAIDs) and sulfonamides rarely cause an aseptic meningitis. Withdrawal from caffeine may also lead to headache.

Temporal arteritis presents as a general headache in the older patient, sometimes associated with jaw claudication (pain with chewing). The patient may report pain with combing or washing hair, consistent with scalp tenderness. Polymyalgia rheumatica is present in about 50% of patients, with shoulder, hip, and neck stiffness (see Chapter 61).

PHYSICAL EXAMINATION

Since the primary headache syndromes have few physical exam findings, the examination should focus on excluding secondary causes. Blood pressure is measured to rule out a hypertensive emergency. A careful neurologic examination, including fine motor function and cranial nerves, and a funduscopic examination to look for papilledema helps rule out intracranial masses. Papilledema is also seen in hypertensive emergency, and in pseudotumor cerebri, an idiopathic disorder causing intracranial hypertension, most often in obese women. Temporal artery tenderness or absence of pulsation is seen in temporal arteritis.

DIAGNOSTIC EVALUATION

The main diagnostic decision in the evaluation of headache is determining the need for brain imaging. Young patients with typical primary headache syndromes and no worrisome features require no further evaluation. Imaging should be performed in patients

■ TABLE 71-2 Characteristics and Treatment of Primary Headache Syndromes

	Migraine	Tension	Cluster
Quality	Pounding, pulsatile	Pressing, tightness	Sharp, stabbing
Location	Unilateral or bilateral	Bilateral	Unilateral
Associated symptoms	Nausea/vomiting, photophobia, phonophobia	Neck pain	Lacrimation, nasal congestion
Acitivity level	Prefer to rest in dark room	May rest or remain active	Restless, agitated
Acute treatment	Triptans	Acetaminophen, aspirin	Oxygen, triptans
Prevention	Propanolol, amitriptyline	Amitriptyline	Verapamil

with focal neurologic findings, papilledema, or worrisome features on history (see above). Due to the sudden onset of pain, patients with cluster headaches often require imaging as well. Computed tomography (CT) scans can detect subarachnoid hemorrhages, but magnetic resonance imaging (MRI) has a higher yield for aneurysms and neoplasms.

Lab tests are not required in the evaluation of most headaches. The erythrocyte sedimentation rate and C-reactive protein may be elevated in temporal arteritis and should be checked in patients over 50 years old with new onset headache.

A lumbar puncture is required to diagnose meningitis (see Chapter 34). Since the sensitivity of CT scans decreases over time for SAH, lumbar puncture is required to look for xanthochromia (yellow discoloration of cerebrospinal fluid indicative of hemorrhage) or red blood cells.

TREATMENT

MIGRAINE HEADACHES

Over-the-counter (OTC) medications, such as acetaminophen (500 to 1000 mg) or aspirin (650 to 975 mg), are effective treatments for mild to moderate migraine headaches. If nausea is prominent, the addition of prochlorperazine (Compazine) or metoclopramide (Reglan) can be helpful. Headaches that do not respond to OTC medications are treated with triptans, such as sumatriptan, zolmitriptan, or rizatriptan. Triptans are 5-hydroxytryptamine receptor agonists, which result in cerebral vasoconstriction and inhibition of painful nerve stimuli. Side effects include paresthesias and tightness in the throat or chest. Patients should be evaluated for cardiac risk factors and appropriate evaluation completed before use of triptans. Preventive treatment for migraines is indicated for patients with frequent migraines (several per week) or intolerance of medications used for acute treatment. The most studied and effective medications are propanolol 40 to 120 mg bid and amitriptyline 25 to 50 mg at bedtime. Topiramate, an anticonvulsant, is also used for migraine prophylaxis.

TENSION HEADACHES

Tension headaches often respond to acetaminophen, aspirin, or NSAIDs, but caution must be used to avoid medication overuse. Neck stretches and warm compresses are often recommended, and exercise may improve these headaches. In severe cases, muscle relaxants, such as baclofen or tizanidine, can be prescribed, but these medications result in drowsiness.

CLUSTER HEADACHES

Cluster headaches have a unique response to high flow oxygen, which is given by face mask at a rate of 7 to 10 liters per minute. Triptans can also be effective in acute attacks. The drug of choice for preventive treatment is verapamil, 120 to 240 mg daily.

KEY POINTS

- The primary headache syndromes include migraine, cluster, and tension headaches.

- Migraine headaches are often pounding, unilateral, worsened with activity, and associated with nausea, vomiting, photophobia, or phonophobia. Treatment includes aspirin, acetaminophen, or triptans.

- A headache due to subarachnoid hemorrhage is usually maximum at onset (a thunderclap headache), severe ("the worst headache of my life"), and associated with neck pain and low-grade fever. Emergent head CT scan and lumbar puncture are required.

- Imaging is required to rule out intracranial lesions in patients with progressive worsening of headaches, focal neurologic signs, papilledema, and new headaches in patients over 50. Patients with a history of malignancy need imaging to rule out metastasis.

- Pseudotumor cerebri (idiopathic intracranial hypertension) is usually seen in young, obese women. Papilledema and elevated CSF pressure are present, but imaging shows no evidence of intracranial mass or edema.

Delirium

Delirium is a state of impaired consciousness and cognition, developing over hours to days, with clinical fluctuation. The neurologic impairments result from disturbances of medical physiologic condition.

EPIDEMIOLOGY

Delirium is a common finding in the elderly hospitalized population, with up to half of frail elderly experiencing delirium during the course of a hospitalization. In general, the prevalence of delirium increases with increasing medical illness, and a majority of intensive care unit (ICU) patients will experience delirium.

ETIOLOGY, PATHOGENESIS, AND RISK FACTORS

While the exact pathogenic mechanism of delirium is uncertain, diverse causative underlying physiologic abnormalities appear to lead to generalized reduction of cerebral metabolism and global functional derangement. The actual pathogenesis is multifactorial and numerous risk factors have been identified. Risk factors include both those conditions that increase baseline susceptibility to delirium and precipitant factors.

Conditions increasing baseline susceptibility to delirium include:

- Stroke
- Dementia
- Organic brain diseases (Parkinson disease)
- Advanced older age
- Sensory impairment (vision, hearing)

Factors that may precipitate delirium include:

- Medication effects (psychoactive medications, drug-drug interactions, narcotics)
- Medication withdrawal effects (selective serotonin reuptake inhibitors, benzodiazepines, barbiturates)
- Drugs of abuse (both intoxication and withdrawal, including alcohol)
- Sleep deprivation
- Infection (fever)
- Dehydration
- Immobilization (including use of bladder catheters or restraints)
- Metabolic derangements (hyper/hypoglycemia, electrolyte disorders)
- Hypoxemia or hypercarbia
- Cardiac failure, shock
- Hepatic failure
- Renal failure
- Hyper/hypothermia
- Thyrotoxicosis

CLINICAL MANIFESTATIONS

Patients in a state of delirium present with **acute onset** of **confusion and inattention**. They are unable to focus their attention during medical interview, and have difficulty following commands. Other cardinal features include **disorganized thinking** (e.g., incoherence, rambling or tangential speech) and **altered consciousness** (e.g., lethargic or hypervigilant). Patients in delirium may also demonstrate **psychomotor agitation** or retardation, **hallucinations**, and **sleep-wake cycle changes**.

HISTORY

The historical assessment of delirium must explore the patient's medical history and **baseline condition** prior to onset of the acutely confused state. Once the baseline cognitive condition is understood, a **timeline of both acute changes in cognition and possible precipitant exposures** should be identified. Particular attention must be paid to:

- Medication changes (including over-the-counter substances)
- Decompensations of chronic medical illness
- Acute illness
- Medication nonadherence
- Illicit substance use or withdrawal

PHYSICAL EXAM

A careful neurologic and general physical exam should be attempted for all patients with delirium, but patient inability to cooperate can make full examination difficult. The following focused assessments may assist in detection of underlying precipitants:

- Vital signs, including oxygenation
- Hydration status (mucus membranes, skin turgor)
- Cranium (signs of trauma)
- Skin inspection (cyanosis suggesting hypoxia, jaundice suggesting liver failure, needle tracks suggesting IV drug use)
- Neurologic exam (for focal defects suggesting stroke or postictal state)
- Survey for potential sites of infection (meningismus, abscess, infected wound, acute abdomen)
- Mini-Mental Status (if possible, to identify and measure errors of attention and cognition)

DIFFERENTIAL DIAGNOSIS AND DIAGNOSTIC EVALUATION

While dementia also presents with impaired cognition, impaired level of consciousness is not a prominent feature, and the **chronicity of dementia** is distinct from the more acute and fluctuating course of delirium. When baseline dementia is present, careful attention to acute changes in both consciousness and cognition should lead to consideration of superimposed (and treatable) delirium.

In severe cases, **depression** may cause psychomotor impairment and even alterations in consciousness; in such cases, close attention to history with assessment of acuity and fluctuation are helpful for differential decision making. **Psychotic disorders** present with disorganized thinking and hallucinations, but demonstrate less prominent generalized inattention or global cognitive impairment, and tend to present with less acute fluctuation.

Of note, the phenomenon of "**sundowning**," with predictable deterioration of behavioral responses during the night, is not equivalent to delirium. When not an acute change of behavior, sundowning reflects disordered circadian regulation rather than acute metabolic derangement. Acute development of new nocturnal disordered behavior should however be investigated as possible onset of delirium.

Diagnostic evaluation of delirium focuses on detecting the most likely precipitating conditions. Because **medication effects**, drug-drug interactions, and medication withdrawal effects are all common causes of delirium, close attention to prescribed, over-the-counter, and illicit medications is a critical first step in detection of a precipitant. Further testing should be targeted for individual patients. Serum electrolytes, glucose, calcium, complete blood count, and urinalysis are generally indicated to screen for common and treatable conditions. Other **lab testing** should be considered carefully if a precipitant is not readily identified:

- Arterial blood gas
- Thyroid function tests
- Toxicology screen and/or therapeutic drug levels
- Ammonia level, hepatic function testing
- Vitamin B_{12} level
- Bacterial culture surveillance

Lumbar puncture (LP) for assessment of meningitis is indicated when a more likely cause is not clearly evident. In elderly patients with delirium of uncertain etiology, LP should be performed even in the absence of fever, as they may present with delirium without the classic symptoms of fever, headache, or meningismus.

Neuroimaging with **head computed tomography** (CT) or **magnetic resonance imaging** (MRI) may be considered if no apparent diagnostic etiology can be determined, or if treatment of a presumptive etiology does not lead to expected improvement. Neuroimaging is indicated prior to LP if there are examination signs of increased intracranial pressure (papilledema, coma, focal neurologic deficits).

Because nonconvulsive status epilepticus may be confused with delirium, **electroencephalography** (EEG) may be considered for patients defying diagnosis, particularly in patients with a history of prior head trauma, stroke, focal brain lesions, or known seizures.

TREATMENT

The delirious patient requires both acute intervention and supportive care to minimize functional decline and ensure patient safety. **Acute management** starts with **discontinuation of any offending drugs** and **treatment of any noted infections**. Further treatment of underlying detected medical abnormalities is dependent on the results of surveillance studies, as above. **Supportive care** includes maintenance of hydration, reduction of distracting noises, orienting stimuli, and bedside sitters. Immobilizing restraints should be avoided unless mandated by acute patient safety concerns.

When severe agitation interferes with the patient's urgent medical care or compromises patient (or staff) safety, low dose **neuroleptic (haloperidol, respiridone, olanzapine)** may be required. Haloperidol has an onset of action of 30 to 60 minutes; 0.5 to 1 mg (orally or intramuscularly) may be repeated every 30 minutes until sedation is achieved. Doses of haloperidol over 4 mg/day will increase the potential for extrapyramidal side effects, and intravenous administration will increase the risk for QT prolongation. **Benzodiazepines** are generally reserved for acute treatment of delirium in the setting of drug or alcohol withdrawal, as they may themselves lead to confusion and delirium. However, low dose benzodiazepines may be used along with neuroleptics in settings where rapid onset of mild sedation is desired.

PROGNOSIS

While delirium itself is not acutely lethal when supportive care is available, delirium is associated with advanced illness and mortality is generally twice that of similarly ill patients without delirium. Even though the course of delirium is considered to be temporary and treatable, this increase in mortality rate persists even after resolution of the acute event.

KEY POINTS

- Delirium is an acute and fluctuating state of impaired cognition and consciousness.
- The history of the baseline state and the timeline of any potential precipitants are critical to both the diagnosis of delirium and the detection of treatable causes.
- Medication side effects, drug-drug interactions, medication withdrawal, and illicit substance use are common precipitants of delirium.
- Infections may cause delirium in the elderly even in the absence of fever or focal symptoms.
- Supportive care for delirious patients includes maintenance of hydration, reduction of distracting stimuli, and avoidance of immobilization.
- Neuroleptic medications should be used in low doses, only when necessary for patient safety.

Dizziness

Patients with dizziness commonly present to physicians in a variety of inpatient and outpatient settings. Evaluation is complicated by the fact that patients commonly use the term "dizziness" in a nonspecific way for a variety of symptoms including vertigo, presyncope, confusion, weakness, and nonspecific lightheadedness. Therefore, the evaluation of the patient must start with precise delineation of the underlying symptoms that are reported to help narrow the broad differential diagnosis.

ETIOLOGY AND PATHOGENESIS

Since dizziness encompasses a variety of symptoms that have varied etiologies, a number of classification schemes have been developed to allow orderly workup and treatment. One often used scheme divides dizziness into **four subtypes**:

- Vertigo (the false sensation of movement of the body or environment)
- Presyncopal lightheadedness ("impending faint")
- Disequilibrium (a feeling of imbalance generally involving the body, but not the head)
- Other (not fitting into the above categories, many times related to psychological problems, e.g., hyperventilation syndrome)

Although this scheme can be useful it is important to note that patients often have symptoms that do not fit neatly into the subtypes, or may present with multiple subtypes of symptoms. However, using this scheme, we can list **common underlying conditions** that tend to accompany different subtypes of dizziness:

Vertigo: Divided into **peripheral** (due to abnormalities in the vestibular end organs)—benign paroxysmal positional vertigo (BPPV), otitis media, impacted cerumen, labyrinthitis, Meniere disease (endolymphatic hydrops), ototoxic drugs, and **central** (due to abnormalities in the central nervous system)—cerebellar ischemia (hemorrhage/stroke), brainstem ischemia, vertebrobasilar insufficiency.

Presyncope: (also see Chapter 11) dehydration (leading to hypovolemia), vasovagal, medications.

Disequilibrium: medications (especially psychotropic drugs), neuromuscular disease, cerebral ischemia/stroke.

Other: psychological problems (e.g., hyperventilation syndrome), medications, metabolic disturbances (e.g., hypoglycemia).

One important thing to note about the above causes of dizziness is that medications can cause all four subtypes. Medication use is more frequent with increasing age, and many of the underlying cardiovascular causes of dizziness also have increased incidence in older patients. These two facts likely underlie the observation from a number of studies that dizziness has an increasing prevalence in older patients, rising from 10% to 15% patients under 35 years to 30% to 40% of patients older than 75 years.

CLINICAL MANIFESTATIONS

HISTORY

The key component of the history is to try and precisely determine what symptoms the patient is referring to as "dizziness." The patient with vertigo will often describe a sensation of movement or spinning. This can be reported as the environment moving around them (objective vertigo) or that they feel to be spinning relative to their surroundings (subjective vertigo).

Certain characteristics of vertigo can help distinguish between peripheral vertigo (most often BPPV) and central vertigo. Peripheral vertigo generally occurs with sudden onset, significant severity and usually only lasts seconds to minutes. Central vertigo is more gradual in onset with milder intensity but can be chronic, lasting weeks to months. Since peripheral vertigo results from abnormalities in the vestibular system, the patient generally reports that attacks are initiated with movement (see physical exam, below), where this is rare for central vertigo. The involvement of the vestibular system in patients with peripheral vertigo may lead to associated symptoms such as tinnitus, hearing loss, and a full feeling in the ear. Conversely, patients with central vertigo may have associated neurologic symptoms including visual changes, headache, ataxia, and gait disturbances.

Because of the association with medications, a thorough medication history should be taken, including inquiring about over-the-counter and illicit drugs and alcohol. Similarly, a thorough history of cardiovascular disease, diabetes, and other medical problems may reveal predisposing conditions that can aid in diagnosis.

PHYSICAL EXAMINATION

A thorough physical exam is indicated in working up a patient with dizziness, with particular emphasis on the neurologic exam. Cardiovascular examination, is important in detecting predisposing conditions such as carotid bruits, signs of orthostasis, and atrial fibrillation.

The neurologic exam should include tests of sensation, proprioception, coordination (cerebellar function), gait, and motor function. The cranial nerve exam is crucial, particularly in patients with vertigo (see below). Funduscopic exam should be performed, looking for signs of increased intracranial pressure such as papilledema. Otoscopic exam should be performed to exam for cerumen impaction and otitis media. Gross testing of hearing can be accomplished by finger rub, supplemented with Rinne and Weber tuning fork tests as needed.

In patients with vertigo, provocative testing is helpful in diagnosing BPPV. The Dix-Hallpike test (Fig. 73-1) involves provocative stimulation of the vestibular system to make the diagnosis of BPPV. The presumed pathogenesis of BPPV involves the presence of particulate debris within the posterior semicircular canal of the affected side. In the Dix-Hallpike test, the patient is seated on the exam table and the head rotated 45 degrees to align the posterior semicircular canal with the sagittal plane of the body. The patient is then moved from the seated position to the supine and then the neck extended slightly by allowing the examiner-supported head to extend off the exam table. This maneuver is then repeated for the contralateral side. The patient's eyes are to remain open during the test and the examiner looks for the development of nystagmus. In a positive test, the patient will report vertigo and will exhibit a mixed torsional and vertical nystagmus with the upper pole of the eye beating toward the dependent (affected) ear and vertical nystagmus beating toward the forehead.

DIAGNOSTIC EVALUATION

Careful history and physical exam will often help define a cause for dizziness, limiting additional testing to help confirm a diagnosis. When a central lesion (e.g., cerebellar infarction/hemorrhage or cerebral infarct) is suspected, urgent brain imaging is indicated. Magnetic resonance imaging (MRI) angiography can be used to visualize the intracranial vasculature in suspected cases of vertibrobasilar insufficiency. Patients with risk factors for cardiovascular risk factors should have an electrocardiogram (ECG) performed. Routine blood tests aren't necessary in most cases as they rarely lead to diagnosis.

TREATMENT

Treatment of dizziness is dependent on the etiology of the symptom with specific treatment targeted to the underlying cause. For example, presyncope due to hypovolemia is managed by fluid replacement.

For patients with BPPV, a series of maneuvers (first described by Epley) can be performed at the bedside that attempt to relocate debris in the posterior semicircular canal to the vestibule of the labyrinth. This technique (Fig. 73-2) has been

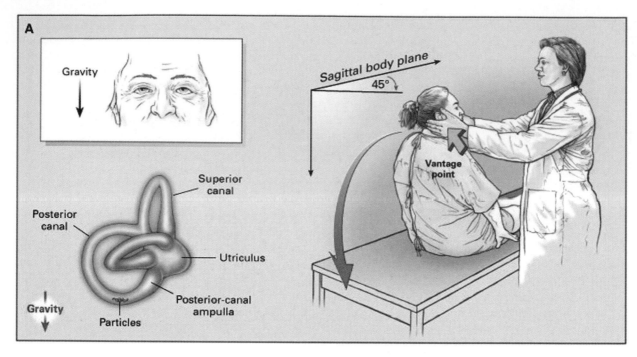

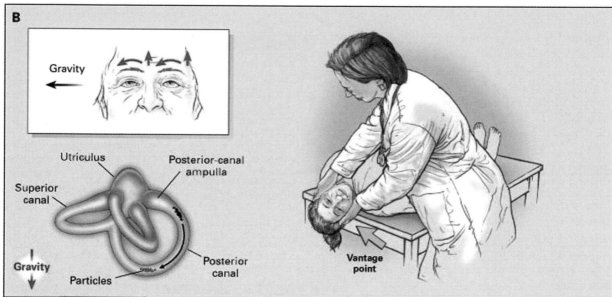

Figure 73-1 • Demonstration of Dix-Hallpike test.

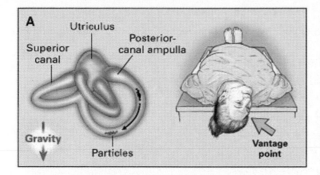

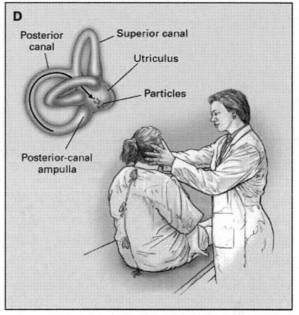

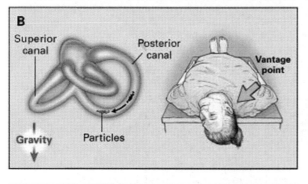

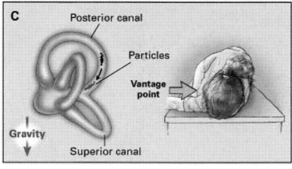

Figure 73-2 • Demonstration of Epley maneuver.
(Image from Furman JM, Cass SP. Benign paroxysmal positional vertigo. N Engl J Med 1999;341:1590. Copyright © 1999 Massachusetts Medical Society. All rights reserved.)

reported to have a high rate of success, although recurrence is relatively frequent. In these patients, repetition of the Epley maneuver can again provide relief.

In rare cases of vertigo without a demonstrable cause, or in cases of patients with severe symptoms and a cause of vertigo expected to resolve shortly (e.g., otitis) short courses of vestibular suppressant drugs (e.g., meclizine) can be given. The use of such drugs is limited by side effects, including sedation and worsening of balance that can put patients with vertigo at greater risk of falls and trauma.

Dementia

Dementia is a disorder of cognitive function. The DSM-IV diagnostic criteria for dementia require both memory loss and at least one other cognitive dysfunction. Other cognitive dysfunction may include aphasia (language disorder), apraxia (disorder of coordination/manipulation despite intact motor function), agnosia (disorder of sensory interpretation despite intact sensory function), or disturbance of executive function (organizing, abstracting, sequencing, planning). In addition, memory loss and other cognitive disturbance must affect social function, represent a decline from prior functional level, and be present not exclusively in the presence of delirium.

EPIDEMIOLOGY AND PATHOGENESIS

Dementia may result from multiple pathologies (Table 74-1). The most common pathology (about 70%) is **Alzheimer** dementia (AD), a disorder characterized by loss of neurons, extracellular **beta-amyloid protein** deposits known as **neuritic plaques** (see Color Plate 26), and intracellular **tau protein** collections known as **neurofibrillary tangles**. While the exact pathogenesis of AD is uncertain, abnormal processing of both tau- and beta-amyloid proteins appears related to neuronal cell death.

Vascular dementia is the next most common pathology (10% to 20%), resulting from ischemic injury. Multiple small-vessel infarcts are the most common vascular defect, but larger vessel occlusion infarcts can result in dementia. Dementias associated with parkinsonism, including both **Lewy body** dementia and **Parkinson disease**, account for approximately 10% of dementia cases. Lewy bodies are intraneuronal inclusions, with aggregations of a synaptic protein (**alpha-synuclein**) the main component.

A variety of other pathologies, including frontotemporal dementia and alcohol-related dementia, are responsible for the remaining small percentage of dementia cases. As suggested by the name, **frontotemporal dementia** (FTD) is characterized by focal atrophy in the frontal and temporal lobes. While FTD comprises a number of pathologies, the presence of **tau** inclusions (**Pick bodies**) or **ubiquitin** inclusions are characteristic. Serotonergic dysfunction is also noted, contributing to cognitive and behavioral abnormalities.

A potentially reversible disease, normal pressure hydrocephalus (NPH) appears to cause dementia in part due to pathology induced in the periventricular white matter.

RISK FACTORS

All dementia syndromes share the common risk factor of advancing age. In addition, the following increase risk for specific conditions:

- Heredity—AD
- Vascular disease including stroke (and atherosclerosis risk factors)—vascular dementia, AD
- Down syndrome—AD
- Female sex—AD
- Renal failure—vascular dementia

Some negative risk factors (factors associated with lowered risk) include:

- Social activity
- Physical activity
- Cognitive activity
- Higher education

■ **TABLE 74-1** Characteristics of Common Dementia Syndromes		
Dementia	**Characteristic Pathology**	**Characteristic Clinical Findings**
Alzheimer	Beta-amyloid (neuritic) plaques, neurofibrillary tangles (tau protein), hippocampal atrophy	Short-term memory loss insidiously progressing to severe deficits
Vascular	Infarcts	Stepwise or insidious progression, possible focal neurologic deficits
Lewy body	Intraneuronal alpha-synuclein aggregations	Fluctuations in cognition, visual hallucinations, parkinsonism
Frontotemporal	Focal frontotemporal atrophy, tau or ubiquitin inclusions	Executive and behavioral or language dysfunction, reduced insight and impaired judgment
Normal pressure hydrocephalus	Enlargement of ventricles	Gait abnormality, incontinence

CLINICAL MANIFESTATIONS

HISTORY

AD usually presents with insidious and progressive memory decline. Short-term memory loss presents early on, progressing to severe memory deficits and total dependence on the care of others for activities of daily living. While classic multi-infarct vascular dementia presents with stepwise decline reflecting successive vascular events, patients may present with insidious decline and without a clear history of stroke. In such cases, it may be difficult to distinguish from AD. Indeed, AD and vascular pathologies may coexist, with overlapping clinical syndromes.

In FTD, memory loss is less prominent early on; patients initially present with executive function impairment and **behavioral or language dysfunction**, possibly with **reduced insight** into deficits. Dementia with Lewy bodies is characterized by **fluctuation of cognition** (drowsiness, staring into space, disorganized speech), visual hallucinations, and parkinsonism. The degree of associated parkinsonism tends to be mild. In dementia associated with Parkinson disease, parkinsonian motor features are more prominent.

For all dementia disorders, neuropsychiatric symptoms may be prominent. These include depression, agitation, hallucinations, and sleep disorders.

PHYSICAL EXAM

While the assessment of dementia is primarily based on history, a Mini Mental Status Examination (MMSE) score of less than 24 out of 30 is confirmatory. MMSE score may also be useful for assessment of degree of decision making capacity, as scores under 19 are predictive of impaired decision making capacity. MMSE is not however sufficiently sensitive for detection of early, mild dementia. Formal neuropsychological examination may be required in cases when routine careful diagnostic history and MMSE are inconclusive.

Some physical findings can be clues to specific dementia diagnoses. Neurologic examination should be performed to detect:

- focal deficits consistent with stroke—vascular dementia
- gait abnormalities—normal pressure hydrocephalus
- parkinsonian rigidity or cogwheeling—Lewy body dementia or PD
- psychomotor retardation—depression

DIFFERENTIAL DIAGNOSIS AND DIAGNOSTIC EVALUATION

Some treatable conditions such as depression, metabolic disorders, and medication effects may result in potentially reversible secondary dementia. Patients should be screened for **vitamin B$_{12}$ deficiency**, **hypothyroidism**, and **depression ("pseudo-dementia")**. When depression cannot be ruled out, formal neuropsychological testing is indicated. Syphilis is an increasingly uncommon cause of dementia, so screening is not indicated unless risk factors are present.

Other potentially reversible causes of dementia include **normal pressure hydrocephalus** (NPH) and chronic subdural hematoma, both of which are detectable on computed tomography (CT). The classic NPH triad includes dementia, gait disturbance, and incontinence. NPH is diagnosed based on the clinical presentation with supporting evidence of pathologically enlarged ventricles on CT and normal opening pressure on LP. Placement of a ventriculoperitoneal shunt may improve the symptoms.

Imaging studies may assist with differential diagnosis of primary dementia, but sensitivity and specificity are imperfect. Brain CT may detect vascular pathology consistent with vascular dementia, but this does not rule out coexistent AD. Magnetic resonance imaging (MRI) can be instructive, revealing bilateral hippocampal atrophy suggestive of AD, or frontotemporal atrophy consistent with FTD. Positron emission tomography (PET) is an emerging modality for the differentiation of FTD and AD, with detection of focal frontotemporal changes suggestive of FTD.

TREATMENT

Cholinesterase inhibitors are the mainstay of medical treatment for AD. Cholinergic augmentation may improve cognition and function for patients with mild to moderate impairment, but it does not affect the overall prognosis. In addition, the NMDA-receptor blocker **memantine** may offer neuroprotective benefit. For patients with advanced disease, high dose **vitamin E** may slow decline; vitamin E is not however used for prevention or for patients with mild disease due to concerns of increased mortality. Vascular dementia may overlap with AD and cholinesterase inhibitors may therefore offer some symptomatic benefit.

FTD may respond to **trazodone**, with alleviation of behavioral changes and depressive symptoms. Because of the prominent decline in judgment and insight early in the course of this disease, patients should be prohibited from driving, and should be relieved of decision making responsibility for employment, financial management, and medical choices.

Dementia with Lewy bodies may also respond to cholinesterase inhibitors; therefore, a trial of cholinergic therapy is indicated prior to neuroleptic agents (which may worsen parkinsonian symptoms) for associated hallucinations.

Avoidance of adverse medication effects is an important component of therapy for all patients; medications with anticholinergic or sedating effects should be discontinued if possible. Secondary dementias may respond with treatment of the underlying disorder. In NPH, selected patients may benefit from placement of a ventriculoperitoneal shunt. While the neuropsychiatric symptoms of dementia disorders may require both behavioral and targeted medical therapy, a full review of psychotherapeutic options is beyond the scope of this chapter.

PROGNOSIS

On average, AD progresses to severe impairment (MMSE of <10 and total dependency for activities of daily living) over the course of 10 years. The prognosis of Lewy body dementia appears similar, with hallucinations and parkinsonian symptoms partly determining the degree of incapacitation and need for institutionalization. Frontotemporal dementia is slightly more rapidly progressive, and vascular dementia is highly variable due to varying degrees of ischemic injury.

KEY POINTS

- Both memory loss and one other cognitive impairment (agnosia, apraxia, aphasia, or loss of executive function) are required for the formal diagnosis of dementia.

- Dementia should be diagnosed in the absence of delirium.

- Alzheimer disease is the most common form of dementia. Its short-term memory loss insidiously progresses to severe dependency for ADLs in about 10 years.

- Dementia with Lewy bodies results in cognition fluctuations, hallucinations, and parkinsonism. Cholinesterase inhibitors should be tried prior to antipsychotics to treat the hallucinations, in order to avoid worsening parkinsonism.

- Frontotemporal dementia impairs decision making capacity early in the disease.

- Reversible causes of dementia, such as normal pressure hydrocephalus, depression, hypothyroidism, and vitamin B_{12} deficiency, should be assessed and treated.

- Anticholinergic medications should be avoided in patients with dementia.

Stroke

Acute stroke, the sudden onset of focal neurologic deficit, is a medical emergency. As with myocardial infarction, passage of time reduces the likelihood that brain tissue at risk can be protected from permanent injury. Therefore, prompt recognition and medical care are paramount.

EPIDEMIOLOGY

Stroke is the third leading cause of death in the United States (after cardiovascular disease and cancer). The annual incidence is approximately 750,000. Because this condition not only leads to hospitalization but often also leads to disability requiring rehabilitation and long-term care, direct costs due to stroke are more than 50 billion dollars annually.

PATHOGENESIS AND RISK FACTORS

Ischemia is the cause of 80% to 85% of strokes. Cerebral ischemia may be caused by intravascular thrombosis, embolism, or generalized hypoperfusion. **Atherosclerotic thrombosis** may occur in the large extracranial or intracranial vessels and leads to progressively restricted distal blood flow. Small penetrating vessels may also thrombose, either due to atherosclerosis at their origin in a large parent vessel or due to hypertension-induced intravascular lipid-hyaline collections. Small vessels can also become occluded when atherothrombosis in a parent artery embolizes distally, also known as **artery-artery embolization**. Because atherosclerotic thrombosis is a major cause of stroke, risk factors for stroke correlate with risk for cardiovascular disease (see Chapter 5). **Embolic** stroke results from

cardiac, aortic, or large arterial sources, and may include thromboembolism or embolism of complex atherothrombotic material. Cerebral **hypoperfusion** may occur in any hypotensive state, such as cardiogenic shock or significant gastrointestinal bleeding. Rare causes of ischemic stroke include hyperviscosity syndromes or arterial dissection.

The remaining 15% to 20% of strokes are caused by **hemorrhage**, including both **intracerebral hemorrhage** (ICH) and **subarachnoid hemorrhage** (SAH). ICH most commonly results from hypertension, but may occur in the setting of amyloid deposits, cocaine/amphetamines, or vascular malformations. SAH usually results from rupture of an arterial aneurysm (Fig. 75-1).

CLINICAL MANIFESTATIONS

Patients presenting with acute focal neurologic deficits must be quickly assessed for potential intervention. Initial triage care must rapidly establish the potential diagnosis of stroke through an abbreviated history and physical, focusing on identifying the presence of new neurologic deficit and differentiating the presentation from seizure or migraine. Hypoglycemia and drug effects may mimic stroke, so a rapid history of prior medical conditions, medications, and substance use should be obtained. Computed tomography (CT) of the brain should then be performed urgently to differentiate ischemic from hemorrhagic stroke, and patients with ischemic stroke should be considered for thrombolytic therapy within 3 hours of onset of neurologic symptoms. Because of this time urgency, some formal elements of the history and physical, such as an extensive history of risk

Common sites of cerebral hemorrhage

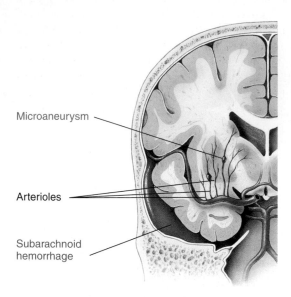

Microaneurysm

Arterioles

Subarachnoid
hemorrhage

Figure 75-1 • Common sites of intracerebral or subarachnoid hemorrhage.
(Asset provided by Anatomical Chart Co.)

factors or complete neurologic exam, may be deferred until urgent therapy is addressed.

HISTORY

After initial triage evaluation is complete, a detailed history may help differentiate between stroke etiologies. (See also Table 75-1.)

- **Sudden severe headache** associated with loss of consciousness or nausea and vomiting suggests

subarachnoid hemorrhage. Focal neurologic motor or sensory deficit is not commonly seen.
- Intracerebral hemorrhage symptoms gradually progress over hours as the hemorrhage spreads.
- Embolic strokes classically present with **sudden severe neurologic deficits** due to a discreet embolic event; symptoms are maximal at stroke onset. Thromboembolic strokes may resolve rapidly due to thrombolysis.
- Intravascular thrombosis classically presents with more of a **stuttering** or **fluctuating** process, due to the active nature of the intravascular clot.

PHYSICAL EXAM

Vital signs on stroke presentation usually reveal **hypertension**. While hypertension may be a causative factor for stroke, it is also a normal physiologic response to stroke, preserving cerebral perfusion pressure. Hypertension therefore is a nonspecific finding. Some exam findings do offer clues to the underlying etiology:

- Hypotension—hypoperfusion
- Poor peripheral or carotid pulse—atherosclerotic disease
- Carotid bruit—atherosclerotic disease
- Atrial fibrillation, displaced point of maximal intensity (PMI) (cardiac enlargement)—cardioembolic disease
- Retinal cholesterol crystals—atheroemboli
- Speckled iris and papillary dilation—ipsilateral carotid artery occlusion
- Meningismus signs or altered level of consciousness—subarachnoid hemorrhage

■ **TABLE 75-1** Characteristics of Common Stroke Syndromes		
Stroke Etiology	**Characteristic History**	**Characteristic Findings**
Ischemic: athero-thrombosis	Stuttering or fluctuating course	Peripheral vascular disease Infarct at penetrating small arteries
Ischemic: embolism	Sudden onset of severe deficits	Atrial fibrillation Retinal cholesterol crystals
Ischemic: hypoperfusion	Shock or other low flow state	Hypotension "Watershed" infarct on CT
Intracerbral hemorrhage	Gradual progression of deficits	Hemorrhage detected on CT
Subarachnoid hemorrhage	Sudden onset of headache Loss of consciousness Nausea and vomiting	Meningismus RBCs noted on LP

Neurologic exam may suggest the location of the neurologic injury. In particular, examination should assess **posterior circulation** territory that would require magnetic resonance imaging (MRI) evaluation over CT. Basilar artery distribution is suggested by **oculomotor** deficits and cerebellar **ataxia**, while ataxia with **dysphagia**, **dysarthria**, or palate/tongue deviation suggest disease in the vertebral artery territory. Also, "**crossed**" presentations, in which one side of the face and the contralateral side of the body are affected, suggest posterior circulation disease.

DIFFERENTIAL DIAGNOSIS AND DIAGNOSTIC EVALUATION

Triage noncontrast head CT should be rapidly performed in all patients suspected of stroke. While imaging of acute ischemic injury on CT may not reveal a discreet infarct, subtle evidence of ischemia includes gray-white matter boundary changes, effacement of cerebral sulci, and even possibly hypodense vessels due to vascular thrombus (Fig. 75-2). CT is highly sensitive for detecting intracerebral hemorrhage (Fig. 75-3), but some small subarachnoid hemorrhages will not be detected. **Lumbar puncture** should therefore be performed to assess for the presence of blood if SAH is suspected and CT is negative. **MRI** is more sensitive than CT, but requires more time and is therefore less desirable for urgent triage; it may be used in follow-up to CT for identifying potentially viable tissue at risk.

If triage head CT is benign, differential diagnosis includes

- Seizure, including Todd paralysis—history of prior seizures, tonic-clonic activity
- Migraine—associated unilateral headache and possible visual prodrome
- Tumor—insidious symptoms noted on more extensive history, history of known primary with potential to metastasize, or examination suggesting melanoma or other primary
- Conversion reaction—psychosocial stressors or prior history of psychiatric disease
- Stroke not detected by CT—posterior infarct, early infarct, or small infarct

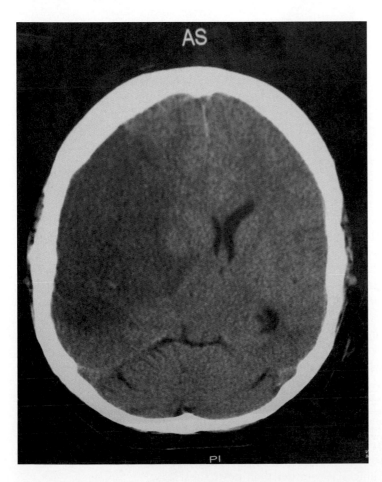

Figure 75-2 • Ischemic stroke—computed tomography (CT) scan of brain showing right-sided infarct and mass effect.
(Image provided by Stedman's.)

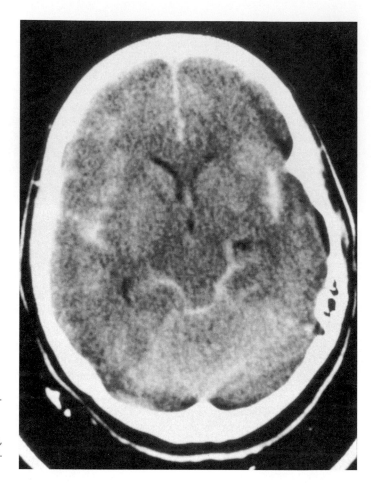

Figure 75-3 • Cranial computed tomographic scan showing diffuse subarachnoid hemorrhage. Note appearance of bright (blood) matter.
(Image from Harwood-Nuss A, MD FACEP, Wolfson AB, MD, FACEP, FACP, et al. *The Clinical Practice of Emergency Medicine*, 3rd ed. Philadelphia: Lippincott Williams & Wilkins, 2001.)

TREATMENT

THROMBOLYSIS

Patients determined to have acute ischemic stroke must be assessed for possible **thrombolysis within three hours** of symptom onset. All patients with significant and not otherwise rapidly improving symptoms should be considered for thrombolysis if the 3-hour window can be met. While direct intra-arterial thrombolysis of occluded cerebral arteries is available in selected centers, systemic intravenous thrombolysis is the primary available therapy. **Intravenous alteplase** (recombinant tissue-type plasminogen activator, a.k.a. **rt-PA**) in selected patients can improve functional outcomes.

Because duration of symptoms is a critical factor in determining thrombolysis eligibility, thrombolysis is contraindicated if the onset of the ischemic event is uncertain, such as when a patient wakes from sleep with symptoms or when no witnesses are available to provide history for noncommunicative patients. Clinical contraindications to thrombolysis primarily relate to **risk of intracerebral** or **life threatening bleeding**:

- Platelet count <100,000, PT >17 on warfarin, or partial thromboplastin time (PTT) elevation on heparin
- Head trauma or stroke within the prior 3 months
- History of intracranial hemorrhage or evidence of hemorrhage on CT
- Major surgery or trauma within the prior 2 weeks
- Gastrointestinal (GI) or genitourinary (GU) bleeding within the prior 3 weeks
- Myocardial infarction (MI) (subacute or acute) or pericarditis
- Pregnancy or lactation
- Lumbar puncture (LP) in the past week
- Arterial puncture in a noncompressible site (e.g., subclavian) in the past week
- Suspicion of subarachnoid hemorrhage (SAH; severe headache at onset of symptoms)
- Seizure at onset of symptoms (unless residual deficits can confidently be ascribed to stroke rather than postictal state)

Thrombolysis in the setting of very large infarct, particularly large territories affected by the middle cerebral artery, is controversial. There is concern that larger ischemic territories are at higher risk for thrombolysis-induced hemorrhage, but larger infarcts are also more likely to cause significant morbidity.

Prior to initiating rt-PA infusion, blood pressure should be below 185/110. As noted above, patients with stroke will often present with hypertension which is physiologically appropriate to maintain cerebral perfusion. Gentle **blood pressure control** with intravenous **labetalol** or low dose nitroglycerin paste may be attempted; if not effective, then thrombolysis is contraindicated.

Secondary stroke prevention following thrombolysis includes **aspirin** 160 mg to 325 mg/d, beginning at least 24 hours after thrombolysis but within 48 hours of symptom onset.

For patients with ischemic stroke who do not undergo thrombolysis, aspirin therapy is also strongly indicated, and should be provided within 48 hours of symptoms. Further antithrombotic therapy with heparin is controversial, given limited evidence of benefit and increased risk for intracerebral bleeding. For patients with evidence of ongoing cardioembolic risk, heparin may be considered for secondary prevention.

Regardless of whether or not a patient undergoes thrombolysis, attention to supportive medical therapy may improve patient outcomes. Standard medical therapy of stroke includes:

- Supine flat position (to maintain cerebral perfusion pressure) for 24 hours
- Glucose control with insulin
- Deep vein thrombosis (DVT) prophylaxis
- Evaluation and treatment of fever to maintain normothermia for several days
- Gentle hypertension control to a goal of under 220/120, otherwise tolerating normal physiologic hypertensive stroke response unless concurrent cardiac ischemia, aortic dissection, or severe heart failure is present.

KEY POINTS

- Stroke is a medical emergency. Initial triage care must rapidly establish the potential diagnosis of stroke through an abbreviated history and physical.

- Triage head CT is performed urgently to assess for intracerebral hemorrhage, and LP should be performed if subarachnoid hemorrhage is suspected.

- Patients determined to have acute ischemic stroke must be assessed for possible thrombolysis within three hours of symptom onset.

- In selected patients, direct intra-arterial thrombolysis of occluded cerebral arteries or systemic intravenous thrombolysis with intravenous alteplase (rt-PA) can improve functional outcomes.

- Secondary prophylaxis following thrombolysis includes aspirin 160 to 325 mg daily, starting 24 hours after thrombolysis. For patients who do not undergo thrombolysis, aspirin is recommended within 48 hours of symptom onset. Frontotemporal dementia impairs decision making capacity early in the disease.

Seizures are sudden, sometimes dramatic, changes in behavior caused by brain dysfunction. **Epileptic seizures** result from abnormal synchronous neuronal firing. Epilepsy is a brain disorder manifesting in two or more unprovoked epileptic seizures. In the medical setting, patients may suffer seizures due to **nonepileptic physiologic** stress, such as severe hypoglycemia or hypoxia. This chapter therefore reviews the general evaluation of medical patients with seizure-type activity, either of epileptic or nonepileptic origin.

EPIDEMIOLOGY

Seizures are common. Approximately 1 in 10 people experience a seizure, and up to 1% develop epilepsy. Men and women are about equally affected. Seizures may present at any age, with about 25% onset in childhood and 25% onset after 60 years of age.

ETIOLOGY, PATHOGENESIS, AND RISK FACTORS

For the majority of patients with epileptic seizures, an etiology cannot be determined. In the minority, a predisposing underlying disorder may be detected:

- head trauma
- brain tumors
- stroke
- intracranial infection
- cerebral degeneration
- drug reactions, including illicit drugs and alcohol
- high fever
- congenital brain malformations (with epilepsy presenting in childhood)

- inborn errors of metabolism (with epilepsy presenting in childhood)

The medical etiologies of nonepileptiform seizures are diverse:

- Hypoglycemia
- Hyperglycemia (e.g., hyperosmolar nonketotic hyperglycemia)
- Rapid changes of sodium level
- Uremia (e.g., renal failure)
- Hypoxia (e.g., cardiac arrest, respiratory arrest, carbon monoxide poisoning)
- Hyperthyroidism
- Acute intermittent porphyria

In addition, nonepileptic seizures may be a manifestation of psychological trauma, resulting in **psychogenic nonepileptic seizures**. Psychogenic seizures have also been called "pseudo-seizures," but it is important to recognize that the vast majority of psychogenic seizures are related to significant psychiatric disease such as dissociative or **conversion disorder**, not malingering or factitious disorder.

CLINICAL MANIFESTATIONS

Seizures may be **partial**, affecting a focal brain region, or **generalized**, affecting nearly the entire brain cortex at once. Partial seizures are further categorized as **simple**, defined by preserved consciousness, or **complex**, defined by impaired consciousness (Table 76-1).

Presentations of **simple partial seizures** vary according to the brain origination site. Symptoms are as diverse as repetitive muscular activity, speech difficulty, déjàvu, or distortions of sound perception.

■ TABLE 76-1 Classification of Seizures

Seizure Subtype	Clinical Presentations	Comments
Partial simple	Preserved consciousness Focal neurologic abnormality Automatisms	May occur as an "aura" prior to partial complex seizure or generalized seizure
Complex partial	Impaired consciousness Focal neurologic abnormality Automatisms	Appears awake but does not respond appropriately
Generalized: absence	Impaired consciousness Staring episodes	Generally limited to pediatric population
Generalized: tonic-clonic	"Yell" at onset Initial tonic back arching Clonic rhythmic motor movement	May develop cyanosis, tongue biting, loss of bowel/bladder control

Simple partial seizures that result in rhythmic motor activity (arm, leg, or face movement) are sometimes called **jacksonian** seizures. Simple partial seizures may progress into partial complex seizures or even generalized seizures. As such, simple partial seizures often represent "aura" symptoms alerting the conscious patient to the imminent onset of a complex or generalized event.

Complex partial seizures are characterized not only by repetitive **automatisms** but also by impaired consciousness. Automatisms may include facial grimacing or facial movements, finger snapping or manual gestures, repetitive speech, or even complex actions such as undressing. A patient with a complex partial seizure will appear to be awake, but will usually stare into space and will not interact normally.

Generalized seizures are further classified as **absence** or **tonic-clonic**. Absence seizures are generalized nonconvulsive seizures that manifest in brief but repeated staring episodes. Primarily a problem in the pediatric population, absence seizures rarely persist into adulthood unless in the setting of developmental brain disorder. Tonic-clonic seizures are also known as **grand mal** seizures. They present quite dramatically, with sudden loss of consciousness and possibly a yell, followed by tonic muscular rigidity that generally arches the back and may impair respiration. After about one minute the tonic phase is followed by rhythmic clonic motor movements

Status epilepticus refers to prolonged (about 10 minutes or more) seizure activity, or seizures reoccurring prior to recovery to an interictal baseline. Due to the physiologic and neurologic stress of continual seizure activity, patients may develop neuronal death (with functional morbidity and/or increased seizure activity), rhabdomyolysis, aspiration pneumonia, lactic acidosis, and respiratory failure.

HISTORY

The historical assessment of a seizure focuses on confirming the occurrence of seizure-like activity, differentiating the likely seizure subtype, and identifying the possible etiology and triggers. As such, the history should fully describe events and behaviors proximal to the seizure, the ictal event, the postictal state, and any predisposing medical history. In addition, family history may reveal an underlying genetic predisposition, particularly for absence or tonic-clonic seizures.

Proximal to an epileptic seizure, patients may note a **seizure aura**, representing a simple partial seizure. Aura "warning signs" vary based on the specific part of the brain involved (see Clinical Manifestations). The presence of simple partial aura symptoms is suggestive of epileptic, rather than nonepileptic, seizures. However, epileptic seizures can occur without aura.

The suspected ictal activity should be described in detail, including level of consciousness and any physical behaviors. A full description of any automatisms, tonic/clonic activity, and degree of consciousness or responsiveness can assist in classifying the suspected seizure type. Differentiation of nonepileptic **psychogenic seizures** by history can be challenging. Underlying significant psychiatric disease is generally present, but not historically diagnostic. Conversion disorder and dissociative disorder are thought to underlie psychogenic seizures, resulting in physical manifestations of psychological stress. Adding to the historical difficulty, psychogenic seizures also occur in patients with a pre-existing diagnosis of epileptic seizures. Such psychogenic seizures may be a stress manifestation response in people with learned behaviors from their epileptic seizures. With this predisposing psychological background, triggers such as family stressors may trigger a nonepileptic seizure event.

The postictal period represents the brain recovery period following seizure activity. Brief (seconds) recovery periods may be noted in young patients with partial seizures. A history of prolonged postictal symptoms (days to weeks) may be noted in older patients with generalized tonic-clonic seizures.

Some historical clues may suggest an underlying seizure etiology. Any known history of conditions increasing seizure risk (see Etiology, Pathogenesis, and Risk Factors) should be assessed. Historical assessment also sometimes identifies a modifiable seizure trigger:

- Flashing lights or video images
- Loud music
- Strong emotions
- Exercise
- Fever
- Menses or perimenstrual period
- Sleep deprivation

PHYSICAL EXAM

Physical examination during the ictal state should focus on assessment of consciousness and ictal behaviors, as well as ensuring physiologic stability and safety from injury. Following triage assessment, attention should rapidly turn to abortive medical interventions (see Therapy.) For evaluation of suspected prior seizure, physical examination does not well differentiate between epileptic and nonepileptic seizures, and examination of psychogenic nonepileptic seizures can be indistinguishable from that of epileptic or physiologic seizures. Neurologic exam may suggest an underlying neurologic injury. Lateralized physical findings in the postictal state suggest a contralateral brain lesion. **Postictal paresis (Todd paralysis)** is a condition of postictal focal neurologic deficit that lasts up to hours or even days.

DIFFERENTIAL DIAGNOSIS AND DIAGNOSTIC EVALUATION

Epileptic seizures must be differentiated from psychogenic seizures, syncope, paroxysmal movement disorders, transient ischemic attacks, and migraine.

The history surrounding the presenting event is often critical to this differential. See the sections on syncope, headache, and stroke for further delineation of characteristic historical features. The history must guide the selection of further laboratory, imaging, and electroencephalogram studies.

Routine laboratory testing for new seizures generally includes:

- Glucose
- Sodium, calcium, magnesium
- Blood urea nitrogen
- Toxicology screen
- Thyroid function tests

Laboratory screening for porphyria is generally reserved for patients lacking a more likely etiology. **Prolactin** levels (elevated within 30 minutes of a seizure and normalized after 6 hours) are sometimes used to confirm the diagnosis of seizure. However, prolactin variation is both insensitive and nonspecific, so must be interpreted with caution. Indeed, in prolonged seizures such as status epilepticus, prolactin levels will normalize and become nondiagnostic.

Urgent **head computed tomography** (CT) is indicated for detection of suspected acute intracranial bleeding, stroke, or mass lesion effect. **Brain magnetic resonance imaging** (MRI) is preferred in nonurgent settings, for assessment of structural brain abnormalities. **Lumbar puncture** should be performed when central nervous system (CNS) infection or metastatic tumor is considered. CNS imaging is generally performed prior to lumbar puncture, both to investigate possible etiologies and to assess for mass effects or possible increased intracranial pressure.

Electroencephalogram (EEG) is the most definitive test for detection of epileptic activity, but even an EEG must be reviewed with caution. While detection of epileptiform activity is highly suggestive of epileptic seizure, nonspecific findings are less diagnostic, and the EEG may in fact be normal between seizure episodes in patients with clinical epilepsy. Provocative measures (sleep deprivation, flashing lights, hyperventilation) may increase EEG diagnostic yield, but even after provocation the resting EEG may be nondiagnostic.

TREATMENT

The first step in seizure therapy is **avoidance of modifiable triggers**. Pharmacologic antiepileptic therapy is not indicated for a first seizure or for a seizure that occurs due to physiologic stressors that are not likely to recur. Antiepileptic medical therapy is generally indicated for those at high risk for recurrent seizures, including:

- Second or frequent seizure
- Structural brain abnormality
- Mental retardation
- History of brain injury with prolonged unconsciousness
- Abnormal EEG

The selection of an antiepileptic drug is dependent on numerous patient and seizure specific factors and is therefore beyond the scope of this chapter. Medications should be selected based on patient preferences for tolerable side effects, efficacy in seizure subtypes, and dosing intervals. While newer medications may have more convenient dosing schedules, less need for monitoring, and in some cases fewer side effects than older medications, clinical superiority is unproven. When cost-effective treatment is desired, older medications titrated slowly to maximal tolerable dose remain a therapeutic option.

Antiepileptic therapy generally requires consistent dosing and avoidance of drug-drug interactions. Medication nonadherance may result in recurrent seizure. Drug levels for medications such as carbamazepine and phenytoin are sensitive to alterations in hepatic metabolism, therefore use of over-the-counter (St. John's wort) or prescription (verapamil, erythromycin) drugs should be accompanied by cautious monitoring of drug levels. Also, many antiepileptic medications themselves induce hepatic enzyme activity (e.g., phenytoin, phenobarbital, carbamazepine, felbamate, topiramate) and therefore the effect on other medications must be closely monitored.

Patients with epilepsy refractory to medical therapy may benefit from surgical procedures, such as focal lesion resection or **temporal lobe resection**. In particular, patients with refractory temporal lobe epilepsy should consider early surgical intervention.

For patients in **status epilepticus, benzodiazepines** are the first-line treatment agent. Diazepam (0.1 mg/kg IV) or lorazepam (0.2 to 0.3 mg/kg IV) is highly effective with rapid onset. Diazepam has a more rapid onset (seconds) compared to lorazepam (up to 2 minutes); however, the duration of diazepam effect is less than 30 minutes. Benzodiazepine loading must be followed by loading of a longer acting antiepileptic drug, such as phenytoin. Alternatives to benzodiazepines and phenytoin include barbiturates (e.g., phenobarbital) or

other neurosuppressive agents (e.g., propofol). In all cases of status epilepticus not rapidly responsive to initial therapy, critical care supports including respiratory and cardiovascular supports are required.

PROGNOSIS

In the adult population, the risk of recurrent seizure following a first seizure is highly variable, depending on the known predisposing factors. Overall, the risk for recurrence is roughly 25% over 5 years, but the risk is likely as low as 10% for those with idiopathic first seizure, and as high as 80% for those with identifiable structural risk factors. For patients in status epilepticus, mortality varies from approximately 20% to considerably higher, approximately 80% for patients with older age and underlying medical co-morbidity.

KEY POINTS

- Both epileptic and nonepileptic (physiologic or psychogenic) seizures are seen in medical patients.
- The majority of psychogenic seizures are related to serious psychiatric disease, such as dissociative or conversion disorder, not malingering or factitious disorder.
- Status epilepticus is a neurologic and medical emergency. Rapid assessment and treatment (preferably with a benzodiazepine) are required. Refractory status epilepticus requires intensive care unit (ICU) support and aggressive pharmacologic intervention.
- For patients with a seizure-like episode, a careful history of the preictal, ictal, and postictal periods informs the assessment of treatable underlying disorders and modifiable triggers.
- While detection of epileptiform activity is highly suggestive of epileptic seizure, nonspecific findings are less diagnostic, and the EEG may in fact be normal in patients with epilepsy. Careful clinical correlation is required.
- Multiple antiepileptic medications are available. Selection should be based not only on the identified seizure subtype, but also on patient preferences, side effect profiles, and potential for consistent dosing schedules.

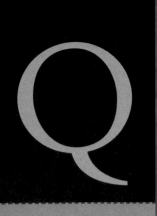

Questions

1. A 69-year-old woman presents to the emergency department with light-headedness and fatigue for the past 3 days while vacationing on Martha's Vineyard, Massachusetts. She denies chest pain, dyspnea, abdominal pain, or fever. Family members have noticed that her skin has looked yellow for the past few days. Her medical problems include hypertension, hyperlipidemia, and a distant history of stage 1 breast cancer, s/p mastectomy. Her medications have been stable for years and include pravastatin, atenolol, and calcium supplements. She denies any other recent travel. Physical examination is significant for pulse 68, blood pressure (BP) 114/70, temperature 98.4°F (36.8°C). There is mild jaundice. Abdominal examination reveals a palpable spleen tip, without hepatomegaly. There is no rash.

    Laboratory values are as follows:

		Normal Values
ALT	53 U/L	(7 to 30)
Alkaline phosphatase	130 U/L	(30 to 100)
Total bilirubin	4.2 mg/dL	(0.0 to 1.0)
Direct bilirubin	1.2 mg/dL	(0.0 to 0.4)
Albumin	3.4 g/dL	(3.1 to 4.3)
LDH	910 U/L	(110 to 210)
Creatinine	1.0 mg/dL	(0.6 to 1.5)
Hematocrit	20.3%	(37 to 48)
WBC count	$8.5 \times 10^3/mm^3$	(4.3 to 10.8)
Platelets	$392 \times 10^3/mm^3$	(150 to 350)
PT	10.6 sec	(8.8 to 11.6)
Reticulocytes	6.8%	
WBC differential		
PMNs	75	
Lymphocytes	12	
Monocytes	7	
Eosinophils	2	

    A peripheral smear is shown in Color Plate 20. What is the most likely diagnosis in this patient?
    a. Hemolytic uremic syndrome
    b. Glucose-6-phosphate deficiency
    c. Babesiosis
    d. Autoimmune hemolytic anemia
    e. Acute mylogenous lukemia (AML)

2. A 35-year-old man comes to your office for follow-up of recent thyroid studies. His laboratory results are as follows:

		Normal Values
TSH	20.2 μU/mL	(0.5 to 5.0)
T_4	5.0 μg/dL	(4.5 to 11.0)
TBG	1.17	(0.77 to 1.23)
FT index	5.9	(4.5 to 11.0)

    He takes no medications. Past medical history is significant for mild intermittent asthma and Hodgkin's disease, treated with mantle radiation therapy for localized disease approximately 10 years ago. He denies recent weight gain, fatigue, change in bowel habits, or changes in skin or hair.

    Which of the following is *true* about this patient?
    a. His thyroid condition will likely improve without treatment.
    b. He has an increased risk of thyroid cancer.
    c. His thyroid examination will likely reveal a goiter.
    d. He is at increased risk for diabetes mellitus (DM).
    e. He should undergo imaging of his pituitary gland to look for an adenoma.

3. A 28-year-old man with a history of type 1 DM for 15 years presents with 2 days of nausea and vomiting following an upper respiratory illness. The patient states he has not been able to take any liquids today and has decreased his insulin dose by 50% because he wanted to avoid hypoglycemia. He denies abdominal pain, fever, cough, headache, or diarrhea. His medications normally include normal pressure hydrocephalus (NPH) insulin 30 U in the morning and 20 U at bedtime, along with 6 to 12 U lispro insulin at breakfast and dinner.

Physical examination shows an ill-appearing young man with BP 104/70, pulse 104, respirations 24 and deep, and temperature 99.4°F (37.4°C). Lungs are clear, heart rate is regular without murmur, and abdomen is soft and nontender.

Laboratory values include:

		Normal Values
Na$^+$	132 mEq/L	(135 to 145)
K$^+$	5.6 mEq/L	(3.5 to 5.0)
Cl$^-$	96 mEq/L	(100 to 110)
HCO$_3$$^-$	10 mEq/L	(22 to 28)
BUN	22 mg/dL	(8 to 25)
Creatinine	1.8 mg/dL	(0.6 to 1.5)
Glucose	328 mg/dL	(70 to 110)
WBC count	8.5 × 10^3/mm^3	(4 to 10)
Hematocrit	44%	(42 to 52)
Amylase	258 U/L	(50 to 120)
Ketones	Positive at 1:4 dilution	

Which of the following is true about this patient?
a. His condition was probably precipitated by pancreatitis.
b. He is likely potassium depleted.
c. Serum ketones should be followed to assess response to treatment.
d. Fluid replacement alone should be sufficient to resolve most of his illness.
e. He is at high risk for cerebral edema.

4. The patient was treated appropriately, and in 4 hours his blood tests reveal the following:

		Normal Values
Na$^+$	134 mEq/L	(135 to 145)
K$^+$	3.7 mEq/L	(3.5 to 5.0)
Cl$^-$	103 mEq/L	(100 to 110)
HCO$_3$$^-$	15 mEq/L	(22 to 28)
BUN	18 mg/dL	(8 to 25)
Creatinine	1.4 mg/dL	(0.6 to 1.5)
Glucose	216 mg/dL	(70 to 110)

Which is the next appropriate step in management?
a. Add bicarbonate to the IV fluid.
b. Discontinue IV insulin and begin subcutaneous treatment.
c. Continue IV insulin at half the current rate.
d. Continue IV insulin and add dextrose to his fluid replacement.
e. Increase insulin drip by 20%.

5. A 72-year-old woman presents to your office for an initial visit. She has a history of type 2 DM, coronary artery disease s/p inferior myocardial infarction (MI) 8 years ago, and

hypothyroidism. She is a lifelong nonsmoker. Medications include atenolol, 50 mg qd; aspirin, 81 mg qd; glyburide, 5 mg qd; and L-thyroxine, 0.1 mg qd. She states she has been feeling well, is compliant with her medications and diabetic diet, and denies chest pain, dyspnea, palpitations, or orthopnea.

Fasting laboratory samples are drawn and the results include:

		Normal Values
HbA1c	7.0%	(3.8 to 6.4)
Glucose	128 mg/dL	(70 to 110)
UA	Albumin negative	
AST	24 U/L	(10 to 40)
Alkaline phosphatase	75 U/L	(45 to 115)
Cholesterol	240 mg/dL	
HDL	46 mg/dL	
LDL	167 mg/dL	
Triglycerides	135 mg/dL	

Which of the following is the next appropriate step for management of this patient's hyperlipidemia?
a. Counsel patient regarding Step 1 Cholesterol Diet and follow up in 3 months.
b. Increase glyburide for better control of glucose.
c. Begin hormone replacement therapy with Premarin, 0.625 mg, and Provera, 2.5 mg daily.
d. Begin niacin, 100 mg three times daily, and increase dose slowly.
e. Begin simvastatin, 10 mg daily.

6. A middle-age homeless man is brought to the emergency department after being found unconscious at the entrance to the subway. He is minimally responsive, withdrawing only to painful stimuli. Temperature is 97°F (36°C) rectally, pulse is 125/min, BP 100/60, respirations 10/minute. On physical examination, the patient's pupils are 6 mm, round, equal, and reactive to light. You note a sweet odor to the patient's breath. Laboratories are as follows:

WBC	7.5
Hematocrit	38%
Glucose	76 mg/dL
Na$^+$	136 mEq/L
K$^+$	3.4 mEq/L
Cl$^-$	104 mEq/L
HCO$_3$$^-$	24 mEq/L
BUN	28 mg/dL
Serum osmolarity	340 mOsm/kg H$_2$O (normal limits 280 to 300)
Serum ethanol	85 mg/dL (legal intoxication ≥80 mg/dL)
UA	2+ ketones, no crystals, no WBC)

Which of the following is the most likely explanation for the patient's condition?
a. Ethanol intoxication
b. Methanol and ethanol intoxication
c. Ethylene glycol and ethanol intoxication
d. Ethanol intoxication and gram-negative sepsis
e. Isopropanol and ethanol intoxication

7. A 43-year-old woman presents to your office with a nine-month history of hand and wrist pain. She complains of stiffness in her hands for 2 hours each morning, improved with activity or warm water. There is no rash, but she has noticed a painless lump on her elbow. She denies dyspnea, cough, chest pain, abdominal pain, back pain, or lower extremity symptoms. She has been taking ibuprofen for 3 months with some relief. There is a family history of arthritis in her mother.

Examination reveals BP 124/70, pulse 84, normal oropharynx, and no adenopathy. Heart, lungs, and abdomen are normal. Joint examination reveals swelling and tenderness of the 3rd and 4th metacarpophalangeal and proximal interphalangeal joints bilaterally. Wrists are tender without obvious swelling. Rest of the joint examination and nailbeds are normal. There is a 2 cm mobile subcutaneous nodule over her right olecranon.

Pertinent laboratories include:

WBC 4.1 (normal 4.3 to 10)
Hematocrit 36 (normal 36 to 48)
Erythrocyte sedimentation rate (ESR) 68 mm/hr (normal for women 1 to 30)
Rheumatoid factor 110 IU (normal <30)
Antinuclear antibody (ANA) positive at 1:80 in a speckled pattern (normal <1:40).

Which of the following extra-articular manifestations is most likely to be present in this patient?
a. Pulmonary nodule
b. Esophageal dysmotility
c. Hypercalcemia
d. Nephrotic syndrome
e. Boutonnière deformity

8. A 56-year-old Vietnamese man comes to your office complaining of fever, cough, and fatigue. He has been your patient for the past 30 years ever since he left his native country. His past medical history is notable for rheumatoid arthritis, which for the past 10 months has been kept under control by the administration of infliximab, which was prescribed to him by his rheumatologist. He takes no other medications. Despite your best efforts, the patient still smokes a pack of cigarettes a day. The patient reports that for the past 3 weeks, he has noted an increasing cough, occasionally productive of yellow sputum, and marked fatigue. He says that he has "felt warm" on occasion but has not taken his temperature.

On physical examination, the patient is a thin Vietnamese man in mild respiratory distress. His vital signs are all within normal limits. Lung examination is notable for diffuse crackles and wheezes bilaterally. The remainder of his physical examination is unremarkable. A chest radiograph is obtained and is shown here.

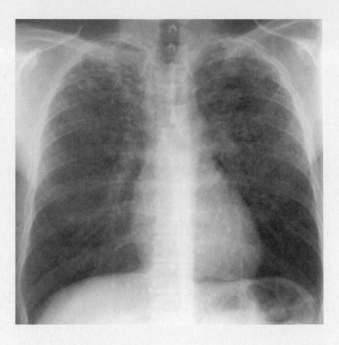

What is the next appropriate step in the management of this patient?
a. Initiate therapy with isoniazid, rifampin, pyrazinamide, and ethambutol.
b. Schedule patient for mediastinoscopy and lymph node biopsy.
c. Initiate therapy with high-dose inhaled steroids.
d. Initiate therapy with azithromycin.
e. Send a serum ACE level.

9. A 54-year-old man presents to your clinic for follow-up of his type 2 DM. You have been adjusting his medications over the past several months, and he has been taking glyburide, 10 mg twice daily, for the past 4 weeks. He feels well without complaints of polyuria or polydipsia, but his fasting blood sugars at home have been 170 to 215 mg/dL. His HbA1c from last month when he was taking 15 mg daily was 9.7% (normal range, 3.8% to 6.4%). He takes no other medications at the present time. On physical examination, his BP is 136/86 and his pulse is 72. Funduscopic examination reveals mild nonproliferative retinopathy. He has mild loss of vibratory sensation in his toes bilaterally without

evidence of ulceration. Pulses are 2 and equal. Other laboratory values from his last visit include the following:

		Normal Values
Na$^+$	138 mEq/L	(135 to 145)
K$^+$	3.8 mEq/L	(3.5 to 5.0)
Cl$^-$	102 mEq/L	(100 to 110)
HCO^3	26 mEq/L	(22 to 28)
BUN	10 mg/dL	(8 to 25)
Creatinine	0.9 mg/dL	(0.6 to 1.5)

You decide to add metformin, 500 mg twice daily, and see the patient again in 1 month. The patient was noted to have 1+ albumin on urine dipstick on his initial visit. Repeat urine studies reveal:

		Normal Values
Urine microalbumin	190 µg/mL	(0 to 40)
Urine creatinine	1.10 mg/mL	(Not determined)

Which is the next appropriate step?
a. Begin treatment with a long-acting calcium channel blocker.
b. Begin treatment with ACE inhibitor.
c. Order 24-hour urine study for protein and creatinine.
d. Order kidney ultrasonography (US).
e. Refer to nephrology for possible kidney biopsy.

10. A 35-year-old previously healthy man presents to the office with back pain for the past 3 days. The pain is located in the lumbar region and radiates down the lateral aspect of his right thigh to his great toe. He works in shipping and delivery and he believes the pain started after a busy day at work. The pain is relieved in the supine position, although it has awakened him at night. He denies change in urination or constipation. He has not taken any medication for the pain.

Examination reveals a healthy-appearing man in moderate discomfort. He is afebrile, with a normal cardiac, pulmonary, and abdominal examination. The pain is reproduced on straight leg raising at 50 degrees. There is paraspinal tenderness at the L4 to L5 level. Neurologic examination shows normal strength, sensation, and reflexes in the lower extremities.

What is the next most appropriate step?
a. Obtain a complete blood count (CBC) and UA.
b. Obtain plain films of the lumbosacral spine.
c. Obtain a magnetic resonance imaging (MRI) scan of the lumbosacral spine.
d. Refer the patient to orthopedic surgery.
e. Conservative treatment with anti-inflammatory drugs and brief period of bed rest.

11. A 58-year-old woman comes into your office complaining of several months of fatigue and dyspnea on exertion. She has an unremarkable past medical history but reports that she has not seen a physician in over 10 years. On examination in the office, you note conjunctival pallor, but the remainder of the physical examination is unremarkable. An electrocardiogram (ECG) is normal, and blood work is obtained with the following results.

Chemistries: Na$^+$ 140; K$^+$ 3.8; BUN 8; creatinine 0.9; ferritin 12 ng/mL (normal 10 to 200 ng/mL); serum iron 450 µg/L (normal 500 to 1,500 µg/L); total iron-binding capacity 4,700 µg/L (normal 2,500 to 3,700 µg/L); total bilirubin 0.7 mg/dL (normal 0.3 to 1.0 mg/dL); LDH 240 U/mL (normal 200 to 450 U/mL)

Hematology: WBC count 6.2 with a normal differential; hematocrit 32%; hemoglobin 10.7 g/dL; platelets 200 K; mean corpuscular volume 76 fl; reticulocyte count 1.2%; red cell distribution width 23% (normal 13% to 15%)

Which of the following would be appropriate initial steps in the evaluation of this patient's anemia?
a. Send a blood sample for hemoglobin electrophoresis.
b. Perform digital rectal examination and schedule patient for colonoscopy.
c. Schedule patient for echocardiography to assess cardiac output and look for valvular abnormalities.
d. Test for the presence of fibrin split products.
e. Schedule patient for a Schilling's test.

12. A 74-year-old woman, recently diagnosed with temporal arteritis by biopsy, presents to your office with leg weakness. The patient states that her headache has resolved since beginning prednisone, 60 mg daily, but she now has difficulty standing up from a chair. She denies back pain, leg numbness, or muscle pain. Physical examination reveals 4/5 strength in the hip flexors bilaterally, with normal muscle tone and preserved reflexes. The rest of the neurologic examination appears normal. Range of motion is normal in all joints, and there is no joint swelling.

What is the next best step?
a. Increase prednisone.
b. Decrease prednisone.
c. Stop prednisone.
d. Perform muscle biopsy.
e. Check creatine phosphokinase (CPK).

13. A 23-year-old woman comes into the emergency department complaining of fever and back pain. The symptoms began the previous day, and the patient noted one episode of nausea and vomiting this morning. She denies any dysuria, urgency, or gross hematuria. She does note a history of urinary tract infections, which she reports were more frequent before she graduated from college. Her only medications are an oral contraceptive.

On physical examination, the patient's temperature is 100.5°F (38°C) orally. She is nontoxic and the only pertinent finding is mild left flank pain.

An abdominal film is ordered and is shown on next page.

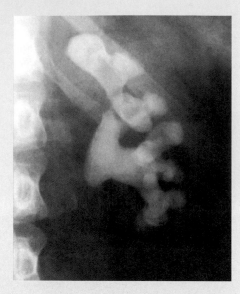

Which of the following has led to the finding seen on the radiograph?

a. A hereditary defect in uric acid metabolism
b. Chronic laxative abuse
c. Preclinical Crohn disease
d. Infection with *Proteus mirabilis*
e. A previous ectopic pregnancy

14. A previously healthy 56-year-old man is admitted to the hospital over the Labor Day weekend for fever and mental status changes. His family noted that he had been complaining of headache, muscle pain, and weakness for approximately 5 days prior to admission. On physical examination, the patient is obtunded, eventually requiring intubation. Neurologic examination is notable for profound proximal muscle weakness. An unenhanced computed tomography (CT) of the head is unremarkable.

A lumbar puncture (LP) is performed, with the following results:

Glucose 70 mg/dL
Protein 56 mg/dL (nl 15 to 45)
Cell count 75 WBC/mm³ 1 RBC/mm³
Differential 95%, lymphocytes 5% polymorphonuclear lymphocytes (PMNs)

Which of the following was the most likely risk factor leading to this patient's presentation?

a. Eating undercooked hamburger
b. Eating poorly prepared red snapper
c. A history of frequent "cold sores"
d. Mosquito exposure
e. Recent travel to New Mexico

15. A 52-year-old woman with a history of recurrent sinusitis presents to the emergency department with three episodes of hemoptysis over the past 24 hours. She has no other significant medical problems, has no history of bleeding disorders, and takes no medicines. She is a nonsmoker. Physical examination reveals a thin woman in moderate distress: BP 162/90, pulse 92, respirations 22, temperature 98.6°F (37°C). Lung examination shows diffuse crackles, and there is a nasal ulceration visualized on speculum examination. Heart, abdomen, and skin examinations are unremarkable.

Laboratory studies sent from the emergency department include:

		Normal Values
Creatinine	2.4 mg/dL	(0.7 to 1.5)
BUN	38 mg/dL	(8 to 25)
Hematocrit	34	(36 to 48)
WBC count	11.3	(4.3 to 10)
ESR	108 mm/hr	(<30)

UA shows marked blood on dipstick. Chest radiograph shows diffuse interstitial infiltrates.

Which of the following tests is the best to confirm the diagnosis?

a. ANA
b. Rheumatoid factor
c. Antineutrophil cytoplasmic antibody
d. Lung biopsy
e. Sputum cytology

16. A 57-year-old woman is brought into the emergency department because of the sudden onset of severe left-sided chest pain and shortness of breath. She had flown back to the United States yesterday following a tour of Southeast Asia. Other than feeling tired after her long trip, she was in her usual state of good health, but this afternoon she had the sudden onset of stabbing left chest pain and noted severe shortness of breath. She denies any previous history of peripheral vascular, cardiac, or respiratory disease. Past medical history is unremarkable, and she is not currently taking any medications.

On examination, the patient is in severe discomfort. Temperature is 100.5°F (38°C) orally, pulse 130, respirations 26, and BP 130/90. Pulse oximetry revealed an O_2 saturation of 88% while the patient was breathing room air. Physical examination is unremarkable other than the patient's tachycardia and tachypnea.

A chest radiograph and ECG are obtained and are as shown on the next page.

What is the most appropriate action at this time?

a. Arrange emergent cardiac catheterization for possible primary percutaneous transluminal coronary angioplasty (PTCA)
b. Ceftriaxone, 1 g IV every 12 hours

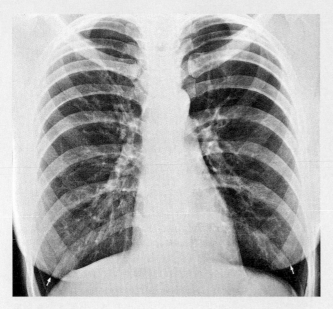

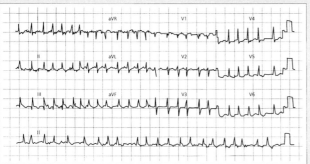

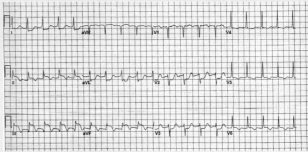

ECG is as shown. Chest radiograph is without evidence of congestive heart failure (CHF).

The patient is given sublingual nitroglycerin, and her BP drops to 80/palp.

17. What is the most likely diagnosis in this patient?

a. Anterior MI
b. Aortic dissection
c. Pericardial tamponade
d. Prinzmetal angina
e. Right ventricular infarction

18. What is the *next* appropriate treatment step in this patient?
a. IV fluid
b. IV nitroglycerin
c. Streptokinase
d. Tissue plasminogen activator
e. Emergent cardiac surgery

19. The patient just described is treated appropriately and stabilized. On hospital day 2, the rhythm is recorded on the cardiac monitor. The patient's BP is 118/70, her pulse is 64, and she is without symptoms of chest pain or dizziness. On hospital day 2, the following rhythm is recorded on the cardiac monitor (see accompanying figure).

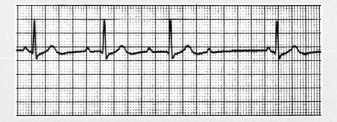

What is the next appropriate step?
a. Atropine, 0.5 mg IV
b. Placement of transcutaneous pacemaker
c. Consult pacemaker service for possible transvenous pacemaker
d. Begin IV isoproterenol at 5 μg/min
e. Continue cardiac monitoring

c. Institute heparin anticoagulation by IV bolus of 6,000 U followed by a maintenance infusion of 1,000 U/hour
d. Emergent pericardiocentesis
e. Emergent upper endoscopy

Questions 17 and 18 relate to the following case. A 63-year-old woman with DM and hypertension presents to the emergency department with nausea and vomiting for the past 4 hours. She has felt waxing and waning symptoms for the past 24 hours, but symptoms have worsened recently. She complains of some dyspnea and diaphoresis, but no chest pressure or back pain. Vomiting is bilious, without coffee-ground material or bright red blood. Her medications include glyburide, captopril, and coated aspirin.

Examination reveals an ill-appearing woman with BP 110/78, pulse 68 and regular, respirations 16. Jugular venous pressure (JVP) is 8 cm, carotid pressures are 2 and equal. Lungs are clear to auscultation; cardiac examination shows S_4 and normal S_1 and S_2, without murmur. Abdominal examination shows no focal tenderness. Pulses are equal bilaterally.

20. A 45-year-old lawyer, who has previously been in his usual state of excellent health, comes in to have abdominal pain evaluated. The patient notes that since joining his new law practice, he has been under increased stress. Because of longer hours in the office, he notes that he has doubled his coffee intake.

For the past 2 months, the patient has experienced what he describes as a "gnawing" pain in his epigastric region. This pain generally occurs approximately 2 hours after meals, in particular after dinner. The patient notes that on occasion, he has awakened in the night with a similar pain. The patient has taken over-the-counter calcium-based antacids and H₂-blockers, which have provided some partial relief. The patient is concerned because his paternal grandfather died at 56 years of age from malignant gastric cancer.

On physical examination the patient's abdomen is nontender with normoactive bowel sounds. Upon rectal examination, brown stool is encountered that is positive for occult blood. Laboratories are as follows:

Routine chemistries within normal limits.
WBC 7.0
Hematocrit 40
Platelets 350 K

The patient is referred for upper endoscopy, and the following is found (see Color Plate 25).
Which of the following is true about the patient?
a. With surgery and chemotherapy, the patient has a 35% chance of surviving 1 year.
b. Genetics plays the most important role in the development of this condition.
c. Coffee consumption resulted in a false-positive fecal Hemoccult test.
d. Antibiotic therapy and administration of a proton pump inhibitor is the preferred treatment for this condition.
e. Intramuscular administration of vitamin B₁₂ is required.

Questions 21 and 22 relate to the following case. A 26-year-old woman presents with a 5-day history of fever and joint pain. Her symptoms began with wrist and hand pain that resolved, and then progressed to right knee swelling and pain. She denies genitourinary (GU) symptoms or diarrhea. There is no history of recent travel, camping, or hiking. She is sexually active and denies alcohol or drug use. On examination, her temperature is 102.0°F (38.8°C), and her oropharynx is without ulcers or exudate. Her right knee is swollen and warm, with pain on flexion. The remaining joints are unremarkable. Skin examination reveals a total of three 5- to 7-mm pustules on the dorsum of her right upper extremity and trunk.

21. The most likely diagnosis is:
a. Disseminated gonococcemia
b. Nongonococcal septic arthritis

c. Lyme disease
d. Reiter syndrome
e. Pseudogout

22. Which of the following is most likely to confirm the diagnosis?
a. MRI of the knee
b. Synovial fluid culture
c. Synovial fluid Gram stain
d. Synovial fluid cell count
e. Synovial fluid crystal analysis

23. A 42-year-old woman with a history of scleroderma for 2 years presents to the emergency department with a chief complaint of headache for 2 days. There is associated fatigue but no fever, neck stiffness, photophobia, chest pain, or abdominal pain. She is on no medications except for acetaminophen recently for her headache. Her scleroderma is characterized by diffuse involvement of the hands, face, and trunk, and she is anti-Scl-70 positive. She has no known visceral involvement from her scleroderma.

Examination in the emergency department shows BP 220/120 in both arms, pulse 96, and regular. Funduscopic examination reveals no papilledema or retinal hemorrhages. Cardiac examination demonstrates normal heart sounds and a 1/6 systolic murmur at the left lower sternal border. Lungs are clear, abdomen benign. There is no edema, and pulses are equal in all extremities. Neurologic examination reveals normal mental status and no focal deficits. Skin thickening and induration consistent with scleroderma are present on the hands, face, and trunk; there are several telangiectasias.

Pertinent laboratory values include:

CBC	Normal
BUN	58 mg/dL (normal, 8 to 25)
Creatinine	2.4 mg/dL (normal, 0.7 to 1.5)
UA	
Specific gravity	1.020
pH	5.5
Protein	1+
	5 to 10 RBC/high-power field (hpf)
	No WBC/hpf

ECG shows normal sinus rhythm, normal axis, and no left ventricular hypertrophy or ischemic changes.

The most appropriate treatment for this patient is to begin therapy with:
a. Captoril
b. Nifedipine
c. Nitroprusside
d. Prednisone
e. D-Penicillamine

24. An 84-year-old nursing home resident is brought to the emergency department after she was found abandoned in her long-term care facility after a severe hurricane 4 days previously. The patient suffers from dementia and is wheelchair bound because of a healing hip fracture but has no other significant medical problems.

On examination the patient is alert but disoriented, weight 60 kg, BP 100/60, heart rate (HR) 100, respiratory rate (RR) 16. You note poor skin turgor but no other acute abnormalities other than related to her hip fracture. Laboratories are as follows:

Na^+ 156 mEq/L
K^+ 3.8 mEq/L
BUN 38 mg/dL
Creatinine 1.3 mg/dL

Which of the following would be the most appropriate orders for the management of this patient's fluid and electrolyte status?
a. 2-L bolus of D5W (5% dextrose solution in water) followed by D5W at 100 mL/hour
b. 3% saline at 100 mL/hour
c. 0.45% saline at 100 mL/hour
d. 2-L bolus of 0.9% saline followed by 0.9% saline at 100 mL/hour
e. D5W at 100 mL/hour with 60 mg furosemide IV × 1.

25. A 67-year-old woman is brought into the emergency department after being found unresponsive at her nursing home. She was intubated in the field by the paramedics. On arrival in the emergency department, stat laboratory samples are drawn and an ECG and portable chest radiograph are obtained. Laboratory results revealed Na 134 mEq/L, K 7.8 mEq/L, glucose 130 mg/dL. The ECG was as shown.

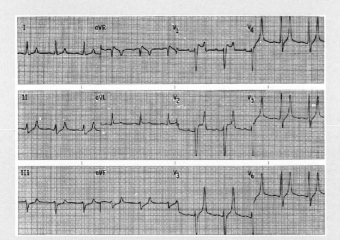

What would be appropriate management of this patient at this time?
a. Prepare for thrombolysis with IV tissue plasminogen activator.

b. Observe patient and redraw laboratory samples because the first sample was probably hemolyzed.
c. Administer calcium gluconate followed by bicarbonate.
d. Administer ceftriaxone, 1 g IV, and perform emergent LP.
e. Attempt DC cardioversion.

26. A 32-year-old man with a history of pheochromocytoma presents to your office for follow-up. He had a successful resection of a unilateral pheochromocytoma 4 years ago and has done well since. He is also s/p thyroidectomy at 5 years of age. His older sister died of medullary thyroid carcinoma, and his father and grandfather had pheochromocytomas.

The family pedigree is as shown in the accompanying figure. Shaded = clinically affected; open = no clinical disease. The arrow indicates your patient.

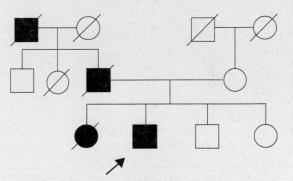

Which of the following is true about this patient's family?
a. The genetic mode of transmission of this disease is X-linked.
b. His unaffected paternal uncle has a 50% chance of passing the disease to his children.
c. Hypercalcemia in this family should be assumed to be from a parathyroid adenoma.
d. Recurrence of hypertension and "spells" in the patient is likely from a malignant recurrence of his pheochromocytoma.
e. This syndrome is most often caused by a mutation in the RET proto-oncogene.

Match the following serology results with the possible clinical history:

	HBsAg	Anti-HBsAg	Anti-HCV	Anti-HAV IgM
A	−	−	+	−
B	−	+	−	−
C	+	+	−	−
D	−	−	−	+
E	+	−	−	−

27. A 19-year-old college student who presents with jaundice, fever, and elevated transaminases after a trip backpacking in Thailand.

28. A 22-year-old nursing student who returns to your office for a routine checkup 2 months after her third dose of hepatitis B virus (HBV) vaccine.

29. A 67-year-old man with cirrhosis, end-stage liver disease, and a history of multiple transfusions in 1983 following an auto accident.

30. A 21-year-old homosexual male who presents with hepatomegaly, jaundice, and elevated transaminases 1 month after acquiring a new sexual partner.

31. Which of the following are *true* about breast cancers?
   a. A patient who presents with bilateral nipple discharge is more likely to have an underlying breast malignancy than one who presents with unilateral nipple discharge.
   b. The use of annual screening mammography has been shown to decrease mortality from breast cancer in women older than 50 years.
   c. When properly performed, mammography-guided fine-needle aspiration has as high a sensitivity as excisional biopsy and is less disfiguring.
   d. Following definitive surgical treatment, estrogen receptor−negative tumors respond more favorably than estrogen receptor−positive tumors to adjuvant therapy with tamoxifen.
   e. A patient who presents with a unilateral breast cancer has minimal increased risk of subsequently developing a tumor in the contralateral breast following appropriate treatment.

32. Which of the following conditions is associated with a non-anion gap acidosis?
   a. Renal tubular acidosis
   b. Salicylate intoxication
   c. Methanol intoxication
   d. Overwhelming gram-negative sepsis
   e. Diabetic ketoacidosis

33. A 34-year-old woman with a history of panhypopituitarism related to postpartum pituitary necrosis (Sheehan syndrome) returns for a routine follow-up. She has no specific complaints but has noticed some increasing fatigue at the end of the day. Her medications include prednisone, 5 mg orally every morning, 2.5 mg orally every evening; L-thyroxine, 0.112 mg orally every day; and ethinyl estradiol/norethindrone daily. Her body mass index (BMI) is 26 kg/m^2, and physical examination appears normal.
   Which of the following is true about this patient?
   a. Adrenocorticotropin hormone (ACTH) stimulation test will probably be normal.
   b. Treatment with a gonadotropin-releasing hormone (GnRH) analog will return her normal gonadal function.

   c. Thyroid medication should be adjusted according to her free T$_4$ level and symptoms.
   d. Replacement with human growth hormone is indicated.
   e. The evening dose of prednisone should be increased.

34. An 18-year-old African American college freshman comes to you for increased asthma symptoms. She has had a diagnosis of asthma since childhood, and prior to coming to the university was well controlled on daily low-dose inhaled beclomethasone with inhaled albuterol as needed. She now notes that she has required once-daily use of her albuterol and has nighttime symptoms approximately twice per week. She thinks that, in part, the increased symptoms are because of the "increased stress of college." She reports that she used to use a peak-flow meter but has not used it for at least a year, and she did not bring it to school with her.
   On examination, the patient is in no apparent distress. Vital signs are normal. Physical examination reveals rare expiratory wheezes. In-office spirometry reveals a forced expiratory volume (FEV$_1$) of 3.56 L (75% of predicted for patient).
   What would be the most appropriate step in the management of this patient?
   a. Maintain current inhaled medications and prescribe low-dose lorazepam to be used as needed for sleep.
   b. Discontinue inhaled steroid and start oral prednisone, 5 mg daily. Reassess the patient in 6 months for possible steroid taper.
   c. Add long-acting inhaled β_2-agonist (salmeterol, 2 puffs every 12 hours).
   d. Discontinue the use of albuterol and prescribe long-acting β_2-agonist (salmeterol) for use on an as-needed basis.
   e. Increase inhaled steroids to high dose and add long-acting inhaled β_2-agonist (salmeterol, 2 puffs every 12 hours).

35. A 23-year-old man presents to the emergency department complaining of "mono." He reports that for the past 5 days he has had a sore throat, fevers (as high as 102°F [39°C]), and "swollen glands" in his neck. Yesterday, he noted a rash consisting of "small red bumps" appeared on his chest, neck, and face. After extensive questioning, you find out that the patient is an injection drug user, mainly heroin. He does admit to sharing needles, "but only with close friends, and never with strangers." Because of his drug use, he has had human immunodeficiency virus (HIV) testing in the past. He notes that his most recent HIV test, performed at a local clinic, was 2 weeks ago and was "negative."
   On examination, the patient is a well-developed white man in mild distress. His temperature is 101.5°F (39°C) orally. His pharynx is hyperemic without exudates. The patient has nontender easily palpable nodes in the anterior and posterior cervical chains. His chest is clear and ab-

dominal examination is unremarkable. A maculopapular rash is present over the patient's torso, neck, face, and proximal upper extremities.

You order a CBC, routine chemistries, and a chest radiograph. What other testing would be appropriate at this time?

a. Repeat HIV enzyme-linked immunosorbent assay (ELISA)
b. West Nile virus titers
c. HIV viral load testing by polymerase chain reaction
d. Bone marrow aspirate
e. Serum immunoelectrophoresis

Questions 36 and 37 relate to the following case. A 70-year-old woman presents to your office with a chief complaint of fatigue and dyspnea on exertion. She denies chest pain, cough, light-headedness, syncope, or orthopnea. She takes no medications. On examination, BP is 128/76, pulse 76, respiratory rate 12. JVP is flat, and lungs are clear. Cardiac examination shows a normal S_1 and S_2 with a 3/6 holosystolic murmur at the left lower sternal border that radiates to the left axilla. There are normal pulses throughout and no edema.

ECG shows left atrial enlargement, no ventricular hypertrophy, and no evidence of ischemia or prior MI.

36. The most likely cause of this patient's heart condition is:
a. Syphilis
b. Rheumatic heart disease
c. Endocarditis
d. Myxomatous degeneration of the valve
e. Rupture of papillary muscle

37. The most appropriate treatment at this time would be to start:
a. Furosemide
b. Captopril
c. Digoxin
d. Antibiotics
e. Warfarin

38. A 42-year-old man with a history of alcohol abuse is brought in by the emergency medical technicians. He was found lying down in his home by his wife. She reports that her husband was binge drinking over the past several days and he was vomiting early today. She reports no bright red blood or coffee-ground material. He takes no medications and has no history of liver disease. His wife is unaware of other drug use.

On examination, he is a lethargic-appearing man who responds to loud voice and who smells of alcohol. Vital signs include BP 76/palp, pulse 170, and respiratory rate 20. Pupils are reactive bilaterally, and tongue is without laceration. JVP is not seen, and carotid pulses are 1 bilat-

erally. Lungs are clear, and cardiac examination shows tachycardia without murmur. Abdomen is soft and nontender, and stool is brown and guaiac negative by rectal examination. Extremities are cool, with intact pulses and no edema. He moves all extremities.

ECG shows normal axis and no ST wave changes. A rhythm strip from lead V_1 is as shown.

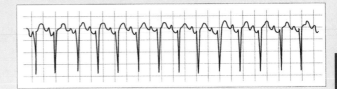

Which is the next appropriate step?
a. Cardioversion
b. Carotid massage
c. IV normal saline
d. Adenosine, 6 mg IV
e. Lidocaine, 75 mg IV bolus

39. A 75-year-old woman presents for routine follow-up. Her medical problems include hypertension, hyperlipidemia, and osteoarthritis. She does not smoke or drink. On further discussion, she describes occasional palpitations without chest pain on exertion. She also notes increasing ankle swelling and fatigue. Her medications include atenolol, amlodipine, pravastatin, and acetaminophen.

Examination reveals BP 142/84, pulse 74, and irregular, respiratory rate 16. JVP is 5 cm, lungs are clear, and cardiac examination shows an irregularly irregular rhythm with no murmur. Extremities show 1+ edema bilaterally without tenderness.

ECG shows normal axis and nonspecific ST wave changes. A rhythm strip is as shown.

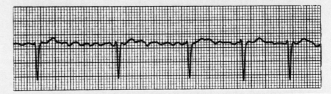

Which of the following medications should be started at this time?
a. Digoxin
b. Diltiazem
c. Procainamide
d. Quinidine
e. Warfarin

40. A 48-year-old man is admitted to the hospital in CHF. After appropriate treatment, the patient is discovered to have a diffusely hypokinetic ventricle with an ejection fraction of 20%. There is moderate mitral regurgitation. Exercise test-

ing is negative for ischemia, and coronary angiogram shows mild epicardial artery disease in all three vessels. Laboratory studies, including iron and thyroid studies, are normal. The patient admits to heavy alcohol use over 20 years but denies tobacco or illicit drug use.

Which of the following medications will improve this patient's survival?

a. Digoxin
b. Enalapril
c. Furosemide
d. Propranolol
e. All of the above

41. A 48-year-old man with a family history of coronary artery disease presents to your office with a complaint of sub-sternal chest tightening with exertion. The pain is associated with dyspnea and is relieved with 5 to 10 minutes of rest. The patient will commonly have symptoms when walking up two flights of stairs or more but not on flat surfaces. Examination is unremarkable, and resting ECG appears normal.

An exercise stress test is ordered. The patient exercises for 10 minutes and his heart rate increases to 150 bpm (with BP of 170/70). He stops because of the occurrence of his pain, which is associated with 1-mm ST depression in the lateral leads that resolves with rest.

The next most appropriate step(s) in the management of this patient is (are):

a. Aspirin, atenolol, sublingual nitroglycerin
b. Aspirin, isosorbide dinitrate, diltiazem
c. Sublingual nitroglycerin as needed
d. Repeat exercise testing with thallium imaging
e. Refer for cardiac catheterization

42. The patient in question 41 returns 2 years later with a complaint of increasing chest pain. Over the past week, he has noticed pain with any exertion, including walking across his office. The pain is relieved with rest or one sublingual nitroglycerin tablet. Most of the time the pain subsides in 5 minutes, although on one occasion the patient did not have his nitroglycerin and the pain lasted approximately 20 minutes. His current medications include aspirin, 81 mg daily; isosorbide mononitrate, 20 mg twice daily; and atenolol, 100 mg daily.

A repeat ECG shows no changes from his previous ECGs. The next most appropriate step in this patient would be:

a. Increase the nitrate dose.
b. Increase the atenolol dose.
c. Add diltiazem.
d. Repeat stress testing.
e. Hospitalize the patient.

43. A 79-year-old woman presents to your office with a 4-month history of weight loss and fatigue. Her weight has

decreased from 142 lb to 120 lb without any specific change in her diet. She denies diarrhea, abdominal pain, cough, dyspnea, fever, or night sweats. Her family members state she appears to have less energy and seems less interested in her usual activities. The patient denies insomnia, inability to concentrate, or feelings of guilt but does admit to lack of energy and some decreased appetite. Past medical history includes hypertension and osteoarthritis. Medications are atenolol, 50 mg daily, and acetaminophen, 500 mg as needed.

On examination, she is a thin, tired-appearing woman. BP is 142/70, pulse 78, and irregular, respirations 12. Cardiac examination reveals an irregular rhythm but no murmurs. Abdominal examination is benign without masses, and rectal examination reveals guaiac-negative stool. Her skin appears within normal limits for her age, and the rest of her examination is normal.

A CBC and chemistry panel were obtained in the office and are significant for:

		Normal Values
WBC count	$8.6 \times 10^3/mm^3$	(4 to 10)
Hematocrit	33%	(42 to 52)
MCV	92 μm^3	(86 to 98)
AST	20 U/L	(9 to 25)
Alkaline phosphatase	135 U/L	(45 to 115)
Albumin	2.8 g/dL	(3.1 to 4.3)
Globulin	4.0 g/dL	(2.6 to 4.1)

Which of the following will likely lead to the diagnosis responsible for this patient's weight loss?

a. Purified protein derivative skin test
b. Thyroid function studies
c. Abdominal CT scan
d. Referral to psychiatrist
e. Discontinuation of atenolol

44. A 38-year-old woman comes to your office complaining of fatigue and pruritus. On review of her history, you note that her only medication is sulfasalazine, which she takes for ulcerative colitis. Her last flare of colitis was 3 years ago. She has not traveled recently, although she does report recently joining a local health club in an attempt to improve her fatigue, which she attributes to "not getting enough exercise."

On physical examination, you note that the patient's weight is unchanged from her last visit 1 year previously. The heart, lung, and abdomen are benign, and you do not find any skin changes. Laboratories are as follows:

WBC: 8.2 normal differential
Hemoglobin: 13.5 g/dL
Electrolytes: within normal limits
Alkaline phosphatase: 383 U/L (normal, 30 to 120)
AST: 45 U/L (normal, <40)
ALT: 38 U/L (normal, <40)
Bilirubin (direct): 0.3 mg/dL (normal, 0.1 to 0.3)

What is the most likely cause of the patient's symptoms and laboratory findings?
a. Surreptitious steroid use
b. Primary biliary cirrhosis
c. Alcoholic cirrhosis
d. Primary sclerosing cholangitis
e. Hot tub folliculitis (cutaneous *Pseudomonas aeruginosa* infection)

45. A 32-year-old man presents with a hematuria and shortness of breath. He was in his usual state of good health until he began to notice progressive dyspnea 4 weeks ago. For the past 10 days, he has noticed intermittent "reddish" urine.

On physical examination, the patient's temperature is 98°F (36.8°C), BP 130/70, RR 16, HR 88. Head and neck examination is normal. Lung examination reveals scattered fine crackles without evidence of consolidation. Cardiac and abdominal exams were normal, and no rash is noted. Laboratories are as follows:

Sodium: 134 mEq/L
Potassium: 4.8 mEq/L
BUN: 54 mg/dL
Creatinine: 6.0 mg/dL
UA: 4+ blood, 2+ protein

A renal biopsy is performed and reveals diffuse crescentic glomerulonephritis and immunofluorescence.
Which of the following tests would *confirm* the diagnosis?
a. C3 complement levels
b. Antiglomerular basement membrane titer
c. ANCA (antineutrophil cytoplasmic antibody) titer
d. Antistreptolysin O titers
e. Stool culture for *Escherichia coli* O157:H7

46. A 56-year-old man with a 40 pack-year smoking history and a history of coronary artery disease requiring cardiac catheterization and stent placement presents to the emergency department with shortness of breath and is found to have a right-sided pleural effusion by chest radiograph. The patient reports that he is not taking any medications. He denies cough, sputum production, chest pain, or fever.

On physical examination, the patient is in moderate respiratory distress.

Temperature: 98°F (36.8°C); oxygen saturation: 90% on room air; BP: 130/86; RR: 18; HR: 94.
Lung examination: scattered fine crackles bilaterally.
Cardiac examination: regular rate and rhythm with 2/6 systolic murmur at left sternal border
Abdominal examination: soft, nontender, bowel sounds present
Extremities: No cyanosis, trace bilateral pretibial edema

ECG: nonspecific ST-segment, T-wave changes.
A diagnostic thoracentesis is performed and analysis of the fluid reveals:
Fluid albumin: 1.3 mg/dL (serum albumin, 3.6 mg/dL)
Fluid LDH: 120 IU (serum LDH: 240 IU)

Which of the following would be a component of the proper management of this patient?
a. Administration of a loop diuretic
b. Emergent cardiac catheterization
c. Large-volume thoracentesis for cytologic examination
d. Administration of IV piperacillin/tazobactam
e. Placement of purified protein derivative testing with controls

For each of the following patients who present with the sudden onset of dyspnea and pleuritic chest pain, decide if:
a. Immediate anticoagulation with heparin is necessary.
b. No anticoagulation is necessary.
c. Pulmonary angiography should be performed.

47. A 19-year-old man who presents after playing in a collegiate hockey game. The patient has a swollen right calf that he attributes to being stuck by a hockey stick early in the game. Chest radiograph is normal; D-dimer test is negative.

48. A 64-year-old woman with a recent diagnosis of ovarian cancer with pelvic metastases is taken to the emergency department following an airplane trip to visit her grandchildren who live across the country. Patient has bilateral leg swelling, right greater than left. V/Q (ventilation-perfusion) scan is high probability, but CT angiography is reported as negative.

49. A 59-year-old businessman who presents with cough and left calf swelling. The D-dimer test is positive; V/Q scan is indeterminant.

50. A 72-year-old man with asymptomatic prostate cancer who has a normal physical examination, indeterminant V/Q scan, negative venous Doppler studies, and negative SimpliRED D-dimer.
Match the cause of the coagulation disorder with the appropriate clinical picture in questions 51 to 55.
a. Disseminated intravascular coagulation (DIC)
b. Type I von Willebrand disease
c. Heparin-induced thrombocytopenia
d. Hemophilia A (factor VIII deficiency)
e. Warfarin administration
f. Antiphospholipid syndrome
g. Drug-induced thrombocytopenia

51. A 65-year-old man with a history of atrial fibrillation and multiple strokes who on results of laboratory specimens

drawn in the office has an international normalized ratio (INR) of 2.5.

52. A 24-year-old woman with an unremarkable medical history who suffers severe bleeding during the birth of her first child.

53. A 72-year-old woman in the intensive care unit for a severe pneumonia who develops widespread ecchymoses and bleeding from IV catheter sites. Laboratory results reveal a platelet count of 15 K and elevated fibrin degradation products.

54. A 57-year-old man who was recently placed on quinidine for cardiac arrhythmias develops easy bruising. A platelet count is found to be 20 K.

55. A 27-year-old woman with a history of three spontaneous first-trimester abortions is noted to have prolonged partial thromboplastin time (PTT). The laboratory notes that the abnormality is not corrected by the addition of normal plasma.

56. Which of the following is true about the prophylaxis of opportunistic infections in HIV-infected individuals?
    a. Opportunistic infections do not occur in HIV-infected individuals started on highly active retroviral therapy.
    b. In a patient on potent antiviral therapy, *Pneumocystis jiroveci* pneumonia (PCP) prophylaxis can be discontinued if the CD4 count increases above 200 cells/μL.
    c. The rise of multidrug resistance has resulted in the loss of effective prophylactic regimens against *Mycobacterium avium* complex (MAC).
    d. Acyclovir is an effective and inexpensive agent for prophylaxis of cytomegalovirus (CMV) retinitis.
    e. Prophylaxis is not required for HIV-infected individuals with baseline IgG titers against *Toxoplasma gondii* because this is correlated with protection against infection.

57. A 64-year-old man with a 100 pack-year history comes in for evaluation. He was hospitalized a month ago with a pneumococcal pneumonia, which was treated with a 10-day course of antibiotics. He now comes into your office for follow-up care. It was noted in the hospital that he had marked hypoxia, which was attributed to his pneumonia. The patient notes that he had not received any medical care for "at least 30 years." Since his hospitalization, he has "cut back" on his cigarette use and notes that he is "only smoking 1 pack a day."

On physical examination, the patient is a thin elderly gentleman, who has moderate difficulty in speaking because of shortness of breath.

Temperature: 98.4°F (37°C); BP: 116/78; HR: 96; RR: 22.
O_2 saturation on room air: 94%; pursed-lip breathing noted
HEENT: within normal limits
Neck: no adenopathy
Respirations: scattered bilateral wheezes, prolonged expiratory phase, no consolidation.
Abdomen: benign
Extremities: no cyanosis

You perform basic spirometry in your office and obtain the following values:

FEV_1: 1.7 L (60% of predicted)
Forced vital capacity (FVC): 2.6 L (84% of predicted)

Which of the following interventions would be most effective in preventing further decline in the patient's FEV_1?
a. Treatment with tiotropium
b. Start nighttime supplemental oxygen
c. Smoking cessation
d. Treatment with inhaled steroids (moderate dose)
e. Treatment with oral steroids (low dose)

58. A 25-year-old woman comes to your clinic after returning from a vacation to Mexico. During this trip, she traveled extensively, taking part in hiking trips, horseback tours, and a white water rafting trip. Just prior to returning home she noted the onset of bloody diarrhea. Which of the following is most likely to be the cause of her illness?
a. *Bacillus cereus*
b. *Staphylococcus aureus*
c. *Vibrio cholerae*
d. *Giardia lamblia*
e. *Shigella dysenteriae*

59. You are asked to evaluate a 78-year-old man who is being screened for admission to a nursing facility. The patient has a history of hypertension and multiple lacunar infarcts. He is referred for admission to the nursing facility because of "multi-infarct dementia" that has made it impossible to live independently. As part of the routine workup, it was noted that the patient had a positive rapid plasma reagin (RPR) test. He is now sent to you for further evaluation.

On physical examination, the patient is a pleasant elderly gentleman, who is oriented to himself only. His temperature is 99°F (37.2°C), BP 176/80, HR 84. HEENT examination is unremarkable, no mucosal lesions are noted, no abnormalities on funduscopic examination. The neck is supple. Lungs are clear to auscultation. Cardiac examination reveals a 1/6 systolic murmur heard along the left sternal border without radiation. Abdominal and GU examination are within normal limits. Neurologic examination is notable for dementia. Coordination appears normal; no focal neurologic findings.

Reviewing his laboratory results that were sent from the nursing home:

WBC: 7.0 with normal differential
Hematocrit: 39%
Platelets: 250,000/mm^3
Electrolytes: within normal limits
BUN: 14
Creatinine: 0.9
RPR: positive at 1:64

You order a FTA-ABS test and it is reported back as positive.

What is the next appropriate step in the management of this patient?

a. Administer 2.4 million U benzathine penicillin G IM in a single dose.
b. Administer 7.2 million U benzathine penicillin G as three doses of 2.4 million U IM each at 1-week intervals.
c. Perform an LP and send cerebrospinal fluid (CSF) for Venereal Disease Research Laboratory (VDRL) testing.
d. Perform an LP and send for immunoglobulin electrophoresis.
e. No additional testing or treatment is necessary.

60. A 38-year-old man comes to your office to evaluate fatigue and nausea. He reports that he was seen at an urgent care clinic 2 weeks previously to evaluate an abrasion on his right arm sustained while working on his car. His arm had become erythematous and painful, and the physician at the urgent care clinic gave him a tetanus shot and a 10-day course of dicloxacillin for cellulitis. The patient reports that the erythema and pain resolved within 5 days, but now the patient reports that for the past 3 days he has noted increasing fatigue. He reports nausea and one episode of emesis. He has not checked his temperature but reports a couple episodes of "feeling feverish" without rigors or sweats. He denies any diarrhea, rash, or cough. He does not take any medications and completed his antibiotics 5 days ago.

On physical examination, the patient is a well-developed man in no apparent distress.

BP: 130/84; HR: 90; RR: 14; temperature: 100.2°F (38°C) orally
HEENT: no oral lesions, funduscopic examination without lesions
Lungs: clear
Heart: regular rate and rhythm (RRR), normal S$_1$ and S$_2$, 2/6 systolic murmur at the left lower sternal border without radiation
Abdomen: soft, nontender; bowel sounds present

Neurologic examination: nonfocal
Extremities: 2+ pitting edema of legs bilaterally
Skin: no rash
Laboratories are as follows:
Na$^+$: 136 mEq/L
K$^+$: 4.2 mEq/L
Cl$^-$: 110 mEq/L
HCO$_3$$^-$: 22 mEq/l
BUN: 34 mg/dL
Creatinine: 2.4 mg/dL
WBC: 8.9 differential 65% PMNs, 20% lymphocytes, 8% eosinophils, 4% monocytes
UA: 2+ blood, 2+ protein, +WBC, negative nitrites by dipstick
Microscopic UA: 50 to 75 RBC/hpf, WBC casts

What is the most likely diagnosis?

a. Acute tubular necrosis from rhabdomyolysis
b. Subacute endocarditis
c. Acute interstitial nephritis
d. ANCA-positive glomerulonephritis
e. Cutaneous larva migrans

61. A 24-year-old man in previous good health is brought in for evaluation of confusion. His roommate said that he awoke this morning complaining of a headache after going out last night to celebrate his admission to business school. During the day he became progressively confused, not remembering receiving his letter of acceptance to business school the previous day and having episodes of nonsensical "babbling."

On physical examination, the patient is uncooperative and only oriented to self. He has a temperature of 101.5°F with a pulse rate of 110 and BP of 118/76. The remainder of the physical examination is normal, including a normal neurologic examination without focal deficits or meningeal signs. Laboratories are as follows:

WBC: 13,000 with 50% PMNs, 40% lymphocytes, 3% monocytes
Electrolytes: within normal limits
Plasma glucose: 97 mg/dL
A LP is performed with the following results:
Glucose: 62 mg/dL
Protein: 64 mg/dL
Cell count: 700 RBC/mm^3, 45 WBC/mm^3 (34% PMNs, 66% mononuclear cells)
CSF: Gram stain, few WBC, no organisms seen.

You start IV *vancomycin and ceftriaxone*. What would be the next appropriate step?

a. Add IV acyclovir
b. Emergent neurosurgical evaluation for drainage of a subdural hematoma

c. Administration of naloxone
d. Forced saline diuresis
e. Institution of an insulin drip

62. Which of the following patients with chronic pulmonary disease would be expected to have **decreased mortality** following the institution of chronic oxygen supplementation?
   a. A 24-year-old African American woman who was recently admitted to the hospital with an asthma flare requiring admission to the intensive care unit. Outpatient management requires high-dose inhaled steroids and a long-acting β₂-agonist inhaler.
   b. A 62-year-old man with emphysema (FEV₁ 70% of predicted). Oxygen saturation is 95% on room air. The patient was recently diagnosed with *Legionella pneumophila* pneumonia and treated with levofloxacin.
   c. A 58-year-old woman with chronic bronchitis. The patient underwent pulmonary function testing as an outpatient. Her baseline Pao₂ on room air was 54 mm Hg.
   d. A 60-year-old woman with emphysema who recently underwent pulmonary function testing as part of evaluation of a possible lung transplant. Baseline Pao₂ on room air was 68 mm Hg. FEV₁ was 1.1 L (50% of predicted), FVC was 2.2 (70% of predicted).
   e. An 18-year-old man who was recently admitted to the hospital with status asthmaticus following accidental aspirin ingestion.

63. A 53-year-old man and his 45-year-old wife come into your office for an initial visit. They are both in good health but have had only irregular routine medical care. They are not currently on any medications, but the man does admit to smoking one pack of cigarettes a day. They bring in a number of articles from magazines and newspapers regarding screening for a number of different cancers.

   Which of the following concerning cancer screening is true?
   a. The woman should have annual screening mammography instituted only if hormone replacement therapy is instituted.
   b. Both the man and the woman should have a screening sigmoidoscopy and annual testing for fecal occult blood, or have a colonoscopy.
   c. The woman requires Papanicolaou smears to screen for cervical cancer.
   d. The man should have an annual chest radiograph and/or sputum cytology to screen for early lung cancer.
   e. You should screen the woman for ovarian cancer by measurement of serum CA-125 and screen the man for prostate cancer with measurement of serum PSA (prostate-specific antigen).

64. A 45-year-old African American man presents to the emergency department with a chief complaint of headache and blurry vision for 2 days. He takes no medications and denies illicit drug use. He has no past medical history but has been told his BP is above normal. He denies dyspnea, chest pain, back pain, or abdominal pain.

   Examination reveals BP 240/126 in both arms, pulse 96 and regular. Funduscopic examination shows arteriovenous nicking without hemorrhages or papilledema. JVP is 6 cm, and carotid pressures are 2+. Lungs are clear, and cardiac examination shows +S₄, with a prominent PMI. Abdominal and extremity examinations are unremarkable. Neurologic examination is nonfocal with clear sensorium.
   Laboratory results include:

		Normal Values
BUN	56 mg/dL	(8 to 25)
Creatinine	2.6 mg/dL	(0.6 to 1.5)
K⁺	4.5 mmol/L	(3.5 to 5.0)
Hematocrit	48%	(42 to 52)
Platelet count	325	(150 to 350)
UA		
Specific gravity	1.010	
pH	6.0	
Protein	2+	
RBC count		5 to 10/hpf
WBC count		0 to 2/hpf

   ECG shows left ventricular hypertrophy with T-wave inversions in leads I, L, V₅, and V₆.
   The most appropriate management for this patient would be:
   a. Captopril
   b. IV propranolol
   c. Morphine sulfate
   d. Sodium nitroprusside
   e. Sublingual nifedipine

65. A 21-year-old man in good health comes to you because his college roommate was admitted to the hospital with meningitis because of *Neisseria meningitidis*. He was told to see his physician about receiving preventative treatment. The patient reports that he has been feeling well but is worried about his roommate. The patient's record indicates that he received the tetravalent meningococcal vaccine his freshman year. A physical examination is completely unremarkable. You call the hospital and they inform you that the patient's roommate did have meningitis with *N. meningitidis* identified as serogroup B by the state laboratory.
   What would be the appropriate next step?
   a. Administer a booster of meningococcal vaccine.
   b. Administer rifampin (600 mg PO every 12 hours for four doses).

c. Admit the patient for ceftriaxone therapy (1 gm IV every 12 hours).

d. Administer *H. influenzae* type b vaccine.

e. Reassure the patient that no treatment is required.

66. A 24-year-old woman presents to you for evaluation of chronic diarrhea. She reports that she had episodic diarrhea during her youth, which was attributed to a "nervous stomach." Over the past 2 years, she has noted an increase in her diarrhea, which she describes as "bulky and foul-smelling." She is somewhat embarrassed to note that her stool tends to float in the toilet bowl, and she often has to flush her toilet repeatedly after a bowel movement to "get it all down." She has also noted increased flatulence and abdominal bloating but denies any abdominal pain or fever. The patient volunteers that she had significantly decreased diarrhea approximately 3 months ago, when she started on a high-protein, low-carbohydrate diet in support of her roommate who was trying to lose weight. However, she "couldn't stand the Atkins diet" and resumed her normal diet, and then had an increase in diarrhea, which prompted her to seek medical attention.

On physical examination, the patient is a thin woman. Her height is 65 inches, weight 97 pounds (BMI 16). The remainder of her physical examination is unremarkable. Laboratories are as follows:

WBC: 6.0 normal differential
Hematocrit: 37%
MCV: 84 fL
Serum iron: 20 µg/dL
Total serum iron-binding capacity: 250 µg/dL

Which of the following laboratory tests is likely to confirm the diagnosis?

a. IgA endomysial antibodies

b. Serum B_{12} levels

c. Stool ova and parasites examination

d. Antimitochondrial antibodies

e. Serum porphyrins

67. A 72-year-old man with a history of chronic obstructive pulmonary disease (COPD) returns to your clinic for follow-up. His only complaint consists of his usual dyspnea on moderate exertion, without chest pain or cough. His medications include ipratropium and albuterol inhalers. On previous visits, his BP has been 170 to 182/76 to 80. Today, his BP is 176/80, pulse 72, and respirations 16. Lung examination shows expiratory wheezes with good air movement. Cardiac examination is normal, pulses are equal bilaterally, and there is no edema. Laboratory studies, including renal function and electrolytes, are normal. ECG shows a normal sinus rhythm without ventricular hypertrophy.

Which of the following is the next appropriate step?

a. Begin dietary treatment with sodium restriction of 2 g sodium daily.

b. Begin treatment with hydrochlorothiazide, 25 mg daily.

c. Begin treatment with captopril, 25 mg twice daily.

d. Order angiogram of the renal arteries.

e. Order morning renin and aldosterone levels.

68. A 55-year-old homeless man with known chronic hepatitis C infection and alcohol dependence presents to the emergency department for evaluation of abdominal distention. He reports that he has noted increasing abdominal girth over the past 2 to 3 weeks. He denies any abdominal pain, fever, chills, or previous history of esophageal varices or ascites.

On physical examination the patient is afebrile and nontoxic but has evidence of chronic liver disease with spider angiomata and obvious ascites. A diagnostic paracentesis is performed, and 60 mL of slightly cloudy, yellow fluid is obtained and sent to the laboratory for analysis.

Ascitic fluid:
Cell count: 400 cells/mL; differential: 75% PMNs, 25% mononuclear cells
Albumin: 0.6 mg/dL
Total protein: 0.8 mg/dL
Gram stain: few WBCs, no organisms seen (centrifuged specimen)

Other laboratories:
Serum albumin: 2.5 mg/dL
WBC: 9.3 differential, 80% PMN, 15% lymphocytes, 3% monocytes
AST: 32 U/liter
ALT: 34 U/liter
BUN: 16 mg/dL
Creatinine: 1.3 mg/dL

What would be the next steps in the management of this patient?

a. Initiation of sodium restriction and administration of spironolactone (100 mg a day) and furosemide (40 mg a day).

b. Contrast CT of the liver to localize probably hepatic neoplasm.

c. Biopsy of the peritoneum to diagnose tuberculous peritonitis.

d. Renal biopsy.

e. Initiate treatment with cefotaxime (2 g every 8 hours).

Match the following patients with the most likely type of renal calculus.

a. Calcium oxalate stone

b. Struvite stone

c. Cystine stone
d. Uric acid stone
e. Ferric chloride stone

69. A 19-year-old male patient with a family history of nephrolithiasis who has hexagonal crystals seen on urinalysis.

70. A 25-year-old woman with a history of chronic urinary tract infection (UTI) who has a urine pH of 8.0 and "coffin lid" shaped crystals on UA.

71. A 56-year-old man who presents with flank pain, knee pain, and is found to have a radiolucent stone by abdominal CT.

72. Which of the following statements regarding small cell lung cancer is correct?
   a. Because of the increased responsiveness of small cell lung cancers to chemotherapy compared to nonsmall cell lung cancers, patients with small cell lung cancers have a higher 5-year survival rate.
   b. TNM (tumor-node-metastasis) staging can predict survival for small lung cancer.
   c. Small cell lung cancer is associated with a relatively high incidence of paraneoplastic conditions (hypercalcemia, syndrome of inappropriate antidiuretic hormone [SIADH]).
   d. Small cell lung cancer is commonly diagnosed during the workup of a solitary pulmonary nodule.
   e. Approximately 25% of small cell lung cancers occur in nonsmokers.

73. A 25-year-old woman presents to your office with severe throat pain for 2 days. She states she had myalgias and a dry cough approximately 10 days ago that have resolved over the past week. Her throat began to hurt 2 days ago and she has some difficulty with swallowing. She feels tremulous and diaphoretic. Examination shows no pharyngeal erythema or exudate but instead a tender nonenlarged thyroid. There is no cervical adenopathy.

The patient has a pulse of 110, temperature 100.8°F (38.2°C), and a slight resting tremor.

The most likely diagnosis is:
   a. Granulomatous thyroiditis
   b. Hashimoto thyroiditis
   c. Lymphocytic thyroiditis
   d. Graves disease
   e. Toxic multinodular goiter

74. A 27-year-old man without past medical history presents to the emergency department with a 1-day history of sharp substernal chest pain. The pain is exacerbated by deep breathing and not associated with dyspnea or diaphoresis. He states that he had a sore throat and myalgias earlier in the week.

Before you can examine the patient, the nurse hands you his ECG, which has just been completed (see accompanying figure).

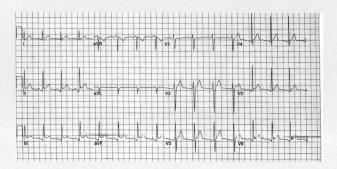

Which of the following would you expect concerning this patient's chest pain?
   a. Pain was maximal at onset.
   b. Pain is reproducible by palpation.
   c. Pain is relieved with sitting forward.
   d. Pain is relieved with lying down.
   e. Pain is associated with feeling of impending doom.

75. A 54-year-old man with a history of type 2 DM and hypertension has been hospitalized for GI bleeding. On hospital day 3, he developed a painful, swollen left toe. There has been no trauma and no previous history of knee or joint problems. His medications include insulin, hydrochlorothiazide, and omeprazole. Examination reveals a temperature of 100.4°F (38°C), no skin rashes, and a swollen, warm, mildly erythematous first metatarsophalangeal joint.

Fluid is obtained by arthrocentesis and reveals the following:

WBC count: 40,000 (84% polymorphonuclear cells)
Gram stain: Abundant polys, no organisms
Fluid analysis: Negatively birefringent needle-shaped crystals

The most appropriate treatment for this patient is:
   a. Prednisone
   b. Colchicine
   c. Indomethacin
   d. Open drainage of joint
   e. Allopurinol

76. A 45-year-old female presents to clinic complaining of epigastric pain that radiates to the right upper quadrant of her abdomen. The pain is dull and crampy. It is worse after eating and will last around 3 hours. The pain has been ongoing for 2 months. She has no weight loss, change in bowel habits, or blood in her stool. On physical examination she is afebrile with normal vital signs; her body mass

index is 40. Her abdomen is obese and nontender. She has no organomegaly.

What is the most likely diagnosis?
a. Acute pancreatitis
b. Biliary colic
c. Nephrolithiasis
d. Colon cancer
e. Viral hepatitis

77. A 40-year-old female presents with abdominal pain, confusion, and yellow skin over the past 36 hours. She has a history of depression and osteoarthritis. Her medications include sertaline 100 mg daily and acetaminophen 1,000 mg six to eight times daily as needed. She denies tobacco use. She drinks 1 to 2 drinks of alcohol daily. On physical examination she is slow to answer questions. She has scleral icterus and ascites.

Laboratory studies are as follows:

AST	8,000
ALT	7,000
Bilirubin, total	10.3
Alkaline phosphatase	40
INR:	4.7
Hepatitis B surface antigen	Negative
Hepatitis B core antibody	Negative
Hepatitis B surface antibody	Positive

What is the most likely diagnosis?
a. Alcoholic hepatitis
b. Acute hepatitis B infection
c. Acetaminophen-induced hepatitis
d. Metastatic breast cancer
e. Autoimmune hepatitis

78. A 25-year-old female who was previously healthy presents to the emergency department with acute onset of substernal chest pain. Pain has been ongoing for 4 hours and is better with sitting up and leaning forward. The patient takes a multivitamin with folic acid daily. She works in a daycare center and reports that the job is stressful. She also notes a recent upper respiratory tract infection that she feels she caught at work.

Physical exam reveals a healthy appearing female in no apparent distress. She is normotensive. Cardiac and pulmonary examination is normal. The patient notes chest discomfort when you lay her flat for the abdominal exam.

Electrocardiogram (EKG) shows diffuse ST segment elevations in all leads with progesterone receptor (PR) depressions in the inferior leads. What is the most likely diagnosis?
a. Acute myocardial infarction
b. Cocaine-induced chest pain
c. Acute pericarditis
d. Generalized anxiety disorder
e. Esophageal reflux

79. A 46-year-old male with a history of type 2 diabetes presents to outpatient clinic for routine follow-up. He takes metformin 1,000 mg twice daily for his diabetes. He checks his blood sugars once daily in the morning and notes values ranging 120 to 220. He is currently without complaints and feels in his usual state of health. On his past several clinic visits over the past 6 months he has been noted to have blood pressure readings greater than 130/80. Today his blood pressure is 136/89. Physical examination is unremarkable. Laboratory studies are as follows:

Glycosylated hemoglobin:	8.0
Glucose:	200
Sodium:	144
Potassium:	4.0
Chloride:	110
Bicarbonate:	24
Creatinine:	1.3
LDL cholesterol:	70
HDL cholesterol:	40
Triglycerides:	120

Urinalysis was notable for 2+ protein.

Which of the following medications should be used to treat the patient's hypertension?
a. Atenolol
b. Lisinopril
c. Clonidine
d. Furosemide
e. Amlodipine

80. A 75-year-old male is admitted to the hospital from primary care clinic with a diagnosis of community-acquired pneumonia. He has a history of diabetes which is well controlled on oral medications. He is a lifelong nonsmoker. He is allergic to penicillin. On physical examination his temperature is 102, pulse 96, respiratory rate 16, oxygen saturation 95% on room air. Lung exam is notable for crackles in the left lower lung field.

Labs are as follows:

WBC:	12,000
Hemoglobin:	13
Hematocrit:	40
Sodium:	142
Potassium:	3.9
Creatinine:	1.0

Which is the most appropriate choice of antibiotic therapy for this patient's community-acquired pneumonia?
a. Oral azithromycin
b. Intravenous ceftriaxone and intravenous azithromycin
c. Intravenous cefepime and intravenous ciprofloxacin
d. Oral ciprofloxacin
e. Intravenous moxifloxacin

81. A 16-year-old female presents to the adolescent health clinic complaining of vaginal discharge. She describes the discharge as clear and foul smelling. There is no pain, pruritus, or vulvar lesions associated with the discharge. She has three lifetime sexual partners and currently is having unprotected intercourse with her boyfriend of 4 months. Pelvic examination is performed and she is noted to have clue cells on wet prep.

Which organism is most likely causing her discharge?
a. *Treponema pallidum*
b. *Chlamydia trachomatis*
c. *Gardnerella vaginalis*
d. *Neisseria gonorrhoeae*
e. *Ureaplasma urealyticum*

82. Which is the best treatment for her discharge?
a. Metronidazole
b. Doxycycline
c. Ciprofloxacin
d. Fluconazole
e. Penicillin

83. A 29-year-old male presents to clinic complaining of low back pain and swelling of his hands. Symptoms have been ongoing for a week. He also notes some blurring of his vision and redness of his eyes. He has no significant past medical history. He has a family history of psoriasis, but not personally. He recently went backpacking through Europe and had sex with numerous prostitutes in Amsterdam. On physical examination he has bilateral conjunctivitis and inflammation and swelling of the joints of his bilateral hands. He has full range of motion of his back.

What is the most likely diagnosis?
a. CMV retinitis
b. Reactive arthritis (Reiter's)
c. Psoriatic arthritis
d. Enteropathic arthritis
e. Ankylosing spondylitis

84. A 35-year-old female presents to clinic noting increasing anxiety for the past several months. Her anxiety is associated with heart palpitations, loose stools, and a 5 kilogram weight loss. On physical examinations she appears anxious with a resting tremor. Her skin is warm and moist. Her patellar reflexes are 3+.

Labs studies are as follows:

Sodium:	140
Potassium:	4.0
Chloride:	100
Bicarbonate:	24
BUN:	12
Creatinine:	1.1
Glucose:	110
TSH:	0.00
Free T4:	4.0
Serum ethanol:	0.00

What is the most likely diagnosis?
a. Alcohol withdrawal
b. Generalized anxiety disorder
c. Cocaine intoxication
d. Grave's disease
e. Hashimoto thyroiditis

85. A 19-year-old female with a history of asthma presents to outpatient clinic for continuing management of her asthma. She reports that she has daily symptoms of her asthma and has nocturnal symptoms once a week. She uses her albuterol rescue inhaler on average twice daily for her symptoms. She does not smoke.

What medication should be added to the patient's regimen next to improve control of her asthma?
a. Inhaled fluticasone
b. Inhaled salmeterol
c. Inhaled tiotropium
d. Oral prednisone
e. Oral montelukast

86. A 61-year-old homeless female with a history of extensive alcohol and tobacco use presents to the emergency department with increasing dyspnea and abdominal distention. She notes that her dyspnea has been gradually escalating over the past several weeks and is associated with a cough. She takes no medications and has not seen a physician in over 20 years. On physical examination she is thin, jaundiced, and has spider angiomata over her upper chest. She has absent breath sounds in her right lower lung field with dullness to percussion. Abdominal exam reveals ascites with an umbilical hernia. Her chest radiograph reveals a right pleural effusion, and she undergoes a thoracentesis. 800 mL of fluid is removed and sent for analysis.

Labs are as follows:

Pleural fluid LDH:	10
Serum LDH:	30
Pleural fluid protein:	2.0
Serum protein:	8.0

What is the most likely etiology of the patient's pleural effusion?
a. Cirrhosis
b. Lung cancer
c. Tuberculosis
d. Bacterial pneumonia
e. Pulmonary embolism

87. A 55-year-old male presents to the emergency department with weakness, dizziness, black stools, and abdominal pain. He describes the pain as a gnawing and burning pain over his epigastrium. He has a history of hypertension, headaches, and anxiety. His medications include lisinopril, paroxetine, and naproxen. He smokes 2 packs of cigarettes a day and drinks 4 beers prior to bed each evening. He works as a stockbroker and describes his job as extremely stressful. On admission to the hospital he is found to be hypotensive with a hematocrit of 19. He is diagnosed with a GI bleed and is admitted to the intensive care unit. EGD is performed which shows a bleeding duodenal ulcer.

In addition to quitting smoking and testing for *H. pylori*, which of the following interventions should be done to prevent future ulcer bleeding?
a. Discontinue the lisinopril
b. Discontinue the paroxetine
c. Discontinue the naproxen
d. Start the patient on diazepam
e. Start the patient on metoclopramide

88. A 65-year-old male presents with generalized fatigue, decreased activity tolerance, and weight loss. He estimates he has lost 15 kilograms in the last 6 months. He has no known past medical history and has not seen a physician in over 25 years. He was adopted and he does not know his family history.

His labs are as follows:

WBC count:	6.0
Hemoglobin:	9.0
Hematocrit:	27
Platelets:	250
MCV:	70
Ferritin:	<5
Iron:	<5
Creatinine:	0.6

What is the most appropriate next step in the patient's management?
a. Oral iron supplementation
b. Erythropoietin injections
c. CT scan of the abdomen
d. Colonoscopy
e. Renal ultrasound

89. An 18-year-old male presents to clinic with abdominal pain and weight loss for the past 9 months. He describes the pain as crampy with intense urges to defecate. On physical examination he is thin. He has small ulcerations of his oral mucosa. His abdomen is thin and scaphoid without masses or organomegaly. He is referred for upper and lower gastrointestinal endoscopy. The report makes note of cobblestone-appearing lesions in the colon separated by areas of normal colonic mucosa. Biopsies of the lesions make note of granuloma formation involving the entire bowel wall.

What is the most likely diagnosis?
a. Ulcerative colitis
b. Crohn disease
c. Irritable bowel syndrome
d. Tuberculosis
e. Sarcoidosis

90. An 80-year-old female with a 100 pack-year history of tobacco use presents to clinic with increasing shortness of breath for 2 months. She especially notes diminished exercise tolerance. On physical examination she is noted to have a thin body habitus, clubbing of her fingernails, and prolonged expiratory phase on her lung exam. Her cardiac exam is normal. Chest radiograph shows increased A-P diameter and flat diaphragms.

Which of the following tests should be ordered to confirm the diagnosis of chronic obstructive pulmonary disease?
a. CT scan of the chest
b. Exercise cardiac stress test
c. Echocardiogram
d. Spirometry
e. Polysomnogram

91. A 65-year-old male presents to an emergency department in a rural hospital with chest pain. Pain is sharp, substernal, and radiates down his left arm and up to his jaw. It started 30 minutes prior to presentation. He notes a history of hypertension and tobacco use. He takes hydrochlorothiazide 25 mg orally a day. On physical examination his blood pressure is 140/90, his pulse is 90, and respiratory rate is 12. Cardiac exam reveals regular rate and rhythm with a normal S1 and S2. Chest radiograph is normal. EKG shows ST segment elevations in leads II, III, and aVF. The patient is diagnosed with an acute myocardial infarction and is given aspirin, nitroglycerin, metoprolol, and morphine. His chest pain improves.

The rural hospital does not have the ability to perform cardiac catheterization. The nearest hospital that does is 3 hours away via ambulance.

What is the most appropriate next step in management?
a. Transfer the patient to the outside hospital for cardiac catheterization
b. Start the patient on a continuous amiodarone infusion
c. Admit the patient to the intensive care unit and continue present medical management
d. Start the patient on warfarin dosed to an INR >2.0
e. Admit the patient to the intensive care unit and start intravenous tenecteplase

92. A 76-year-old female with a prior history of stroke and hypertension presents to outpatient clinic for routine health maintenance. She reports no residual issues with her stroke. She takes metoprolol and hydrochlorothiazide for her hypertension. On physical examination she is found to be in atrial fibrillation. EKG shows a controlled ventricular response with a rate of 65. The patient is without symptoms.

Which of the following medications will provide the greatest risk reduction for recurrent stroke in this patient?
a. Clopidogrel
b. Diltiazem
c. Warfarin
d. Amiodarone
e. Aspirin

93. A 69-year-old male with a prior history of myocardial infarction, hypertension, diabetes, and tobacco use presents to the emergency department with acute onset of shortness of breath. He reports that his shortness of breath worsens with exertion and is worse when sleeping at night. His dyspnea is associated with a cough. Physical examination shows a fatigued appearing male who appears older than his stated age. Blood pressure is 95/60, pulse is 72. Cardiac examination reveals an audible third heart sound and jugular venous distention. Pulmonary exam is notable for inspiratory crackles and wheezing. Hepatomegaly is found on abdominal examination.

Chest radiograph shows cardiomegaly with pulmonary venous congestion.

What is the most likely diagnosis?
a. Sarcoidosis
b. Chronic obstructive pulmonary disease exacerbation
c. Congestive heart failure exacerbation
d. Community-acquired pneumonia
e. Metastatic lung cancer

94. A 56-year-old female with a history of congestive heart failure presents to clinic for management of her heart failure. Currently she has symptoms of dyspnea with minimal activity. Her medications include metoprolol, lisinopril, simvastatin, and aspirin. On physical exam she has a blood pressure of 100/70 with a pulse of 70. On cardiac exam she has an enlarged point of maximal impulse with trace peripheral edema. She has faint basilar crackles on pulmonary exam. Her most recent echocardiogram was notable for an ejection fraction of 25%.

Her labs are as follows:

Creatinine	1.0
Sodium	140
Potassium	3.6
Chloride	101

Which of the following medications would improve the patient's overall mortality?
a. Furosemide
b. Spironolactone
c. Digoxin
d. Amlodipine
e. No further medications are needed

95. After adjusting the above patient's medications at her clinic visit, she returns 1 week later to the emergency department with profound dyspnea. The patient notes that she was recently nonadherent with her low-salt diet while attending a party. Physical examination and diagnostic studies are consistent with congestive heart failure exacerbation. She is admitted to the hospital. In the hospital she is treated for her heart failure and clinically stabilized. During her hospitalization, on telemetry monitoring she is found to have nonsustained runs of ventricular tachycardia. She is asymptomatic during these episodes.

Which of the following interventions would best reduce the patient's mortality?
a. Refer the patient for a Holter monitor with loop recorder
b. Initiate therapy with amiodarone
c. Refer the patient for an automatic implantable cardiac defibrillator
d. Perform an exercise cardiac stress test with nuclear imaging
e. Initiate outpatient dobutamine infusions

96. A 60-year-old female presents to clinic with complaints of low back pain. Pain has been ongoing for 2 weeks. She describes the pain as dull and achy. She has a distant history of peptic ulcer disease. On review of systems she makes note of a 10 kilogram weight loss over the past 3 months; she denies loss of bowel or bladder function. On physical exam she has diminished ankle reflexes.

Which is the most appropriate next step in management?
a. Nonsteroidal anti-inflammatory drugs
b. Warm compress and back exercises
c. Radiograph of the lumbar spine
d. Electromyelogram
e. MRI scan of the brain

97. A 38-year-old male is admitted with acute diffuse abdominal pain after binge drinking. The pain is associated with nausea and vomiting. After his initial evaluation he is diagnosed with pancreatitis.

Which of the following tests should be ordered on admission in order to predict the severity of his pancreatitis?
a. Amylase and lipase
b. White blood cell count, LDH, SGOT/AST, glucose
c. CT scan of the abdomen
d. Complete blood count, abdominal radiographs
e. Lipase, bilirubin

98. A 71-year-old male with chronic obstructive pulmonary disease presents for initial evaluation following his diagnosis. He has quit smoking and is participating in a pulmonary rehabilitation program. He uses inhaled tiotropium daily. Spirometry shows an $FEV_1/FVC = 0.5$ (50%). Arterial blood gas was notable for a $Pao_2 = 45$ mm Hg with a $Paco_2 = 50$ mm Hg.

Which of the following interventions will have a mortality benefit in this patient?
a. Theophylline
b. Continuous oxygen
c. Systemic corticosteroids
d. Inhaled corticosteroids
e. Inhaled beta agonists

99. A 95-year-old male with Alzheimer dementia presents to the emergency department from his nursing home with a productive cough and tachypnea. He is confused and unable to give a history. Based on his nursing home records he has a history of hypertension, renal insufficiency, emphysema, and Alzheimer disease. On admission he has a T = 103°F, pulse 130, blood pressure 80/40. He is combative and you are unable to complete a physical examination. Chest radiograph shows a right lower lobe infiltrate.

What is the most appropriate next step in management?
a. Admit the patient to the intensive care unit for intravenous antibiotics

b. Admit the patient to the general medicine inpatient unit for intravenous antibiotics
c. Admit the patient to the general medicine inpatient unit for oral antibiotics
d. Discharge the patient back to the nursing home on oral antibiotics
e. Discharge the patient back to the nursing home with no treatment due to his dementia

100. A 75-year-old male presents to urgent care clinic complaining of painful urination for 3 days with fevers and chills. He has a history of prostate cancer, which was treated over a year ago with surgery. He had an indwelling urinary catheter for 2 weeks following his surgery. Since the procedure he has been doing well without any urinary problems or the need for further catheterization. His urologist has told him that he has negative surgical margins. His last PSA a week ago was undetectable. On physical examination he has normal vital signs. His prostate is surgically absent, and he has no rectal tenderness. Urinalysis is notable for white blood cells, leukocyte esterase, and nitrites. There is no blood. Cultures are ordered.

What is the most appropriate next step in management?
a. 7 days of fluconazole
b. 7 days of metronidazole
c. 3 days of trimethoprim-sulfamethoxazole
d. 3 days of ciprofloxacin
e. 10 days of ciprofloxacin

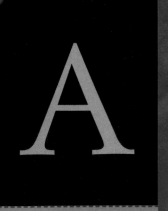

Answers

1. d (Part 8)

Diagnose autoimmune hemolytic anemia. The elevated reticulocyte count, lactate dehydrogenase (LDH), and indirect bilirubin all suggest hemolysis as the etiology of this patient's anemia. The corrected reticulocyte count is 3.4%, which is still high. All of the answers are etiologies of hemolytic anemia except acute myelogenous leukemia (AML). There are no blasts in the peripheral smear to suggest AML. The peripheral smear shows spherocytes, formed by partial phagocytosis of the red cell membrane in the spleen. There are no intracellular pathogens (as seen in babesiosis) or schistocytes (as seen in hemolytic uremic syndrome). Platelet count is often decreased in acute leukemia and hemolytic uremic syndrome. Glucose-6-phosphate deficiency can present as a similar hemolytic anemia with spherocytes on the smear, often after ingestion of an oxidizing drug (such as sulfa drugs). However, it is an X-linked trait and is seen in men only. Autoimmune hemolytic anemia is most often idiopathic but may be secondary to drugs (such as penicillins, quinine, or methyldopa); infections (mononucleosis, *Mycoplasma*); or hematologic malignancies. The diagnosis can be confirmed by a Coombs' antiglobulin test. Treatment is prednisone, 1 mg/kg daily. Although babesiosis is common on Martha's Vineyard, severe disease is usually limited to splenectomized and immunosuppressed patients.

2. b (Part 6)

Recognize the patient with postirradiation hypothyroidism. This patient has iatrogenic hypothyroidism (related to previous radiation treatment) that is unlikely to resolve on its own. Primary hypothyroidism is diagnosed by a high thyroid-stimulating hormone (TSH) with a low-normal free T_4 level. Examination in this case should reveal a small thyroid, if it is palpable at all. The risk for diabetes mellitus (DM) is seen in autoimmune thyroiditis and usually precedes the thyroid disease (type 1 DM). The risk of thyroid cancer is increased in patients with radiation injury of the thyroid. The thyroid should be closely followed for the development of nodules.

3. b (Part 6)

Know the diagnosis and treatment of diabetic ketoacidosis (DKA). This patient has a clinical picture of DKA along with laboratory findings of an increased anion gap of 26 and positive ketones. Although potassium is 5.6, total potassium stores are almost always low in patients with DKA because of loss through osmotic diuresis and dehydration. Serum levels are high initially because of a lack of insulin and acidosis. There is no abdominal pain to suggest pancreatitis, and amylase is often falsely elevated in DKA. Serum ketones are not useful to assess response because they measure only acetoacetate and not hydroxybutyrate. Treatment leads to a shift toward acetoacetate, and therefore serum levels may rise despite adequate therapy. The anion gap should be followed instead. Insulin is an absolute requirement to treat DKA. Although cerebral edema is a common cause of death in children with DKA, it is rare in adults.

4. d (Part 6)

The patient's laboratory results show a decreasing, but not normal, anion gap. Therefore, treatment with IV insulin should be continued. However, because glucose is decreasing to the low 200s, dextrose should be added to the fluids to prevent hypoglycemia. If the IV insulin is discontinued at the same time subcutaneous insulin is given, DKA will likely recur because of the lag time in peak action of subcutaneous insulin. There should be several hours of overlap. Bicarbonate is not necessary in the treatment of DKA.

5. e (Part 6)

Know the treatment goals for cholesterol in patients with coronary artery disease (CAD). The low-density lipoprotein (LDL) goal for patients with coronary artery disease is less than 100 mg/dL. Secondary prevention with cholesterol reduction clearly reduces cardiac events and deaths from CAD. The evidence for this treatment is most convincing for the HMG-CoA reductase inhibitors, such as simvastatin. Further reduction in the patient's glucose is not appropriate and will likely have little effect on her cholesterol. Likewise, the patient already follows a low-fat diet, making it very unlikely that diet alone could achieve the 35% reduction she needs (average reduction through diet is approximately 5% to 10%). The effect of hormone replacement on cardiovascular disease remains controversial, but given the early termination of a part of the Women's Health Initiative because of increased incidence of breast cancer, stroke, and pulmonary embolism, hormone replacement cannot be generally recommended. Niacin can lower LDL and raise high-density lipoprotein (HDL) but would increase this patient's glucose level and is difficult to take because of side effects.

6. e (Part 3)

Know how to evaluate possible toxic ingestions. Ethanol intoxication is common, but the clinician needs to be aware of possible multiple ingestions along with ethanol. The patient in this question presents with a depressed level of consciousness out of proportion to the measured serum ethanol, raising the likelihood of a second toxic agent. Methanol, isopropanol, and ethylene glycol can all cause a possible fatal intoxication. All three will raise the plasma osmolar gap (normally <10 mOsm/kg H_2O), which is calculated as:

$$\text{Osmolar gap} = \text{Measured plasma osmolarity} - \text{Calculated plasma osmolarity}$$

Where the calculated plasma osmolarity is calculated from the formula:

$$2 \times \text{Na glucose (mg/dL)}/18 + \text{BUN (mg/dL)}/2.8 + \text{ethanol (mg/dL)}/4.6$$

In this case, the osmolar gap is markedly elevated at approximately 35 mOsm/kg H_2O. Methanol and ethylene glycol are associated with an elevated anion gap acidosis. Isopropanol intoxication, in comparison, does not usually cause acid–base abnormalities because isopropanol is neutral and does not raise the anion gap. Ketonuria and a fruity odor can result because of metabolism of the isopropanol to acetone. Sepsis is also associated with an acidosis with increased anion gap caused by lactate accumulation.

7. a (Part 7)

Know the extra-articular manifestations of rheumatoid arthritis (RA). This patient has RA with a symmetric arthritis involving hands and wrists, more than three joints affected, morning stiffness, and a positive rheumatoid factor (RF). The positive ANA is present in up to 30% of patients with RA and should not be overinterpreted. The pulmonary manifestations of RA include pulmonary nodules, pleural effusions, and interstitial lung disease. Esophageal dysmotility is most commonly associated with scleroderma. Hypercalcemia may be seen in sar-

coidosis, and nephrotic syndrome can be present in a number of rheumatologic diseases, including systemic lupus erythematosus (SLE). Boutonnière deformity describes the deformity of the hand seen in RA: flexion of the proximal interphalangeal joint and extension of the distal interphalangeal joint. It is an articular (not extra-articular) manifestation.

8. a (Part 3)

Know the complications of treatment with antitumor necrosis factor alpha (TNF-α) agents. Treatment of chronic inflammatory conditions including rheumatoid arthritis and Crohn disease with agents that antagonize the activity of the key inflammatory cytokine, TNF-α represents a major advance in management of these conditions. The use of these agents (etanercept, infliximab, and adalimumab), however, has been associated with the development of serious infections because of global suppression of the cellular immune response. Clinically significant infections normally kept in check by the cellular arm of the acquired immune system (e.g., tuberculosis, histoplasmosis, cytomegalovirus, and *Pneumocystis* species) have been reported in patients on anti-TNF-α therapy. The patient in this question presents with evidence of miliary tuberculosis, which most likely represents reactivation that occurred related to the initiation of infliximab therapy.

9. b (Part 6)

Know the treatment of diabetic nephropathy. The patient described has approximately 180 mg albumin in the urine daily. This is estimated by the albumin-to-creatinine ratio: Multiply both measurements by a factor of 1,000, leading to milligrams of albumin per gram of creatinine (approximate amount excreted in a day). This falls within the range of microalbuminuria (30 to 300 mg/day) and may be missed by routine dipstick. Treatment with angiotensin-converting enzyme (ACE) inhibitors has been shown to decrease the rate of progression to overt nephropathy (>300 mg/day) even in patients with normal blood pressures (BPs). Calcium channel blockers have not been conclusively shown to have similar efficacy. Proteinuria could be confirmed in this patient but is probably not necessary (because he had a positive dipstick earlier). Borderline values should be confirmed with repeat microalbumin. Because the patient has known retinopathy and normal urine sediment except for protein, the diagnosis is fairly certain and further testing is not indicated.

10. e (Part 7)

Know the appropriate evaluation and treatment for sciatica. This patient likely has a disk herniation of the L4 to L5 disk as evidenced by radiation of his pain in the L5 distribution (to the great toe) and positive straight leg raise. Most patients will recover with time (over weeks), and aggressive di-

ANSWERS

agnostic workup or treatment is not usually indicated. Laboratory studies are often not necessary unless referred pain is suspected. Plain films may be useful in older individuals, patients with trauma, or patients on corticosteroids to rule out compression fractures. Magnetic resonance imaging (MRI) is the test of choice to look for disk herniation. The patient has no warning signs for cauda equina, such as urinary retention or saddle anesthesia, to prompt urgent MRI. In addition, indiscriminate use of MRI is discouraged because many *asymptomatic* patients have abnormal disks and bulges that may be misinterpreted in the acute setting. A surgical referral would be appropriate if the patient's condition is worsening, diagnosis is uncertain, or surgery is being considered after failure of conservative treatment.

11. b (Part 8)

Know the evaluation and treatment of microcytic anemia. When evaluating a patient who presents with anemia, the underlying cause can be suggested by the results of several routine hematologic laboratory tests. The complete blood count (CBC), in particular the red blood cell (RBC) parameters, can indicate what type of anemia is present. It is often useful to divide anemias into microcytic (manifested by a low mean corpuscular volume [MCV]), normocytic, and macrocytic. In this patient, the presence of a low MCV, as well as a low ferritin and a low iron saturation (serum iron ÷ total iron binding capacity; normally 20% to 40%) all indicate that this patient has an iron deficiency anemia. In men and postmenopausal women, an iron deficiency anemia should be worked up by screening for occult gastrointestinal (GI) malignancy, in particular colon cancer. Hemoglobin electrophoresis is useful for screening for a thalassemia; however, this is associated with normal serum ferritin and iron studies. Hemolytic anemia can appear secondary to valvular abnormalities, but hemolytic anemias are suggested by elevated serum LDH and a reticulocytosis, which are not seen in this patient. Signs of disseminated intravascular coagulation (DIC) are not present, and therefore testing for fibrin split products is not appropriate. If the patient had a macrocytic anemia, testing for B_{12} and folate levels and scheduling a Schilling's test if the B_{12} level was low would be appropriate.

12. b (Part 7)

Recognize common side effects of glucocorticoid treatment. Prednisone is often used to treat rheumatic diseases effectively, but it has numerous side effects, including hyperglycemia, insomnia, psychosis, and osteoporosis. This patient demonstrates the side effect of proximal weakness. Treatment is to decrease the dose slowly over weeks. Abruptly stopping the prednisone could result in a flare of her temporal arteritis. Polymyositis can also result in proximal muscle weakness and would be diagnosed by biopsy. However, it is unlikely she has developed a second new med-

ical problem. Creatine phosphokinase is usually normal in prednisone-induced myopathy.

13. d (Part 3)

Know the pathogenesis of urinary infection with *Proteus mirabilis*. The patient presented with a large struvite stone—commonly referred to as a "staghorn" calculus. *P. mirabilis* produces an enzyme called urease, which catalyzes the breakdown of urea into carbon dioxide and ammonia. The ammonia reacts with water and this alkalinizes the urine. This increase in pH results in decreased solubility of phosphate, which initiates formation of magnesium ammonium phosphate stones (struvite). These stones can grow rapidly over a period of weeks to months and can lead to permanent damage to the affected kidney. The stones themselves are colonized with bacteria, which contributes to the rapid growth of the stones. Medical therapy alone (i.e., antibiotic therapy) is generally not recommended. Open surgical removal of the stone has been largely replaced by percutaneous nephrolithotomy and/or extracorporeal shock wave lithotripsy. Open procedures are generally reserved for the removal of a unilateral, chronically infected, and poorly functioning kidney because of the presence of a large struvite stone.

14. d (Part 4)

Recognize the presentation of encephalitis caused by West Nile virus (WNV). Since the first recognized outbreak of WNV in 1999, the virus has become endemic in the United States, rapidly spreading across the country in a few short years. Although the majority of infected patients are asymptomatic, approximately 20% of infected individuals exhibit symptoms. The most common presentation is that of a self-limited febrile illness often with notable fatigue, headache, and myalgias. Less than 1% of patients develop neuroinvasive disease, which can be fatal. Treatment of all forms of the disease is supportive. As with all arboviruses, transmission is via a mosquito vector.

15. c (Part 7)

Recognize and be able to diagnose Wegener granulomatosis. The patient described has several features consistent with the diagnosis of Wegener granulomatosis: pulmonary hemorrhage, sinusitis, nasal involvement (ulceration), and renal involvement (elevated creatinine and blood on dipstick suggest rapidly progressive glomerulonephritis). The erythrocyte sedimentation rate (ESR) is nonspecific but is often seen in vasculitis. The diagnosis is confirmed by a serum test for antineutrophil cytoplasmic antibody (ANCA). In Wegener granulomatosis, the ANCA is often in the cytoplasmic pattern (C-ANCA). Antinuclear antibody and rheumatoid factor are nonspecific and are seen in many rheumatic diseases. They are unable to confirm a diagnosis by themselves. Lung cytology may show hemosiderin-laden macrophages and red cells but has no value in diagnosing Wegener granulomatosis. Finally, lung biopsy could be diagnostic, showing vasculitis with necrotizing granuloma. However, this invasive test is not necessary if the scenario is very typical, considering the high sensitivity and specificity of ANCA.

16. c (Part 2)

Recognize acute pulmonary embolism as a cause of chest pain. When evaluating a patient with chest pain, a number of must-not-miss diagnoses should be considered, including coronary artery disease (angina or myocardial infarction [MI]), pulmonary embolus, and aortic dissection. These diseases should be considered because of their potentially fatal nature. Once appropriate consideration has been given to these conditions, other, less potentially fatal diagnoses can be considered. In this patient, a number of clues on initial presentation pointed to pulmonary embolus as a possible cause of this patient's chest pain. The acute onset of severe pleuritic chest pain coupled with the patient's tachycardia, tachypnea, and hypoxia are all suggestive of pulmonary embolism. A historical clue is that the patient just had a long plane ride, which could predispose to the development of a lower extremity deep vein thrombosis (DVT). However, myocardial ischemia and aortic dissection could also present with this clinical picture. The chest radiograph is normal. The majority of patients with pulmonary embolism present with a normal chest radiograph or with atelectasis. A normal chest radiograph is also common in the setting of myocardial ischemia, unless it results in acute pulmonary edema. In the setting of aortic dissection, it is sometimes possible to see an abnormal aortic contour on chest radiograph, as well as possible predisposing vascular abnormalities such as calcifications. The electrocardiogram (ECG) is notable for atrial fibrillation as well as the presence of a deep S wave in lead I, a Q wave in lead III, and an inverted T wave in lead III. This "S1Q3T3" pattern, caused by right heart strain, is highly suggestive of pulmonary embolism. The atrial fibrillation is suggestive of right atrial overload, also compatible with pulmonary embolism. A new right bundle branch block (not seen here) is another typical ECG sign of right heart strain. However, in a large number of cases of pulmonary embolism, the only finding on ECG is sinus tachycardia. To confirm the diagnosis of pulmonary embolism, a Doppler US of the lower extremities could detect a proximal DVT. A V/Q (ventilation-perfusion) scan can identify a mismatch between areas that are ventilated but not perfused. Helical computed tomography (CT) is being evaluated as an alternative to V/Q scanning. If these tests are negative, pulmonary angiogram is the gold standard for the diagnosis of pulmonary embolism. Because the clinical picture is highly suggestive of pulmonary embolism, treatment with heparin anticoagulation should be started as definitive diagnostic evaluation is initiated. No contraindications for anticoagulation are apparent in this patient. Primary percutaneous transluminal coronary angioplasty (PTCA) is not indicated because

the ECG is not suggestive of acute MI. This clinical picture is not suggestive of a pericardial effusion or a gastric problem.

17. e (Part 1)

Recognize a patient with a right ventricular infarction. This patient presents with atypical symptoms for angina but is clearly having an inferior MI. Patients with inferior infarctions often have a predominance of vagal symptoms, such as nausea, vomiting, and bradycardia. The ECG shows ST elevations in the inferior leads (II, III, aVF) and reciprocal ST depressions in the anterior leads (V_1, V_2). The anterior changes represent a more extensive infarct, showing either true posterior ischemia or concurrent disease in the left anterior descending artery. The clues to the diagnosis of right ventricular infarction are the elevated jugular venous pressure (JVP) without pulmonary congestion on examination or chest radiograph and the drop in BP with nitroglycerin. Patients with right ventricular infarctions are very dependent on preload, and nitroglycerin can decrease this preload and cause hypotension. This diagnosis may be confirmed by placing the normal precordial leads on the right side of the chest instead of on the left ("right-sided leads"). ST elevation of 1 mm in right lead V_4 is sensitive and specific for right ventricular infarction. An anterior MI would present with ST elevation in leads V_1 to V_4. Prinzmetal angina, caused by vasospasm, can mimic a MI. However, it is much less common than atherosclerotic coronary disease (especially in an elderly diabetic patient), and it would be expected to resolve with nitroglycerin. An ascending aortic dissection can involve the right coronary artery and result in an inferior MI. This patient does not have any features of a dissection, such as pain radiating to the back, unequal BPs, or severe hypertension. Pericardial tamponade is another condition that would present with dyspnea and elevated neck veins and may result in hypotension from a drop in preload. This cannot explain the ECG findings, however.

18. a (Part 1)

Know the treatment for right ventricular infarction when the patient becomes hypotensive. This patient needs aggressive fluid replacement to restore the preload that she needs. The patient is likely volume depleted from the vomiting, and nitroglycerin has further reduced the preload to the right ventricle, which is not functioning normally. Further nitroglycerin will worsen the hypotension. Thrombolysis, with either tissue plasminogen activator or streptokinase, should not be given in a hypotensive patient with an MI. If BP cannot be restored to normal, then emergent cardiac catheterization, not cardiac surgery, is indicated for possible angioplasty. If BP is restored to normal, then thrombolysis may be appropriate. Although the initial symptoms have been present longer than 12 hours (the usual window for thrombolysis), further history should be obtained to pinpoint the time of worsening of symptoms (likely representing complete occlusion).

ANSWERS

19. e (Part 1)

Recognize and know the appropriate treatment for type 1 (Wenckebach) second-degree atrioventricular (AV) block. The rhythm strip shown demonstrates type 1 second-degree AV block, in which the PR interval gradually increases until a P wave fails to conduct to the ventricles. This type of block represents poor conduction at the AV node. It is commonly seen in situations with high vagal tone, such as an inferior MI. It does not represent worsening ischemia and rarely progresses to complete heart block. Because it is self-limited and the patient is stable during the rhythm, no pacing is needed. Atropine is indicated for unstable bradycardia, such as in hypotensive patients. Isoproterenol is a β-agonist and can worsen myocardial ischemia. It is no longer recommended for treatment of bradycardia.

20. d (Part 5)

Know the presentation of peptic ulcer disease (PUD). The patient presents with a classic history for PUD. The epigastric pain that occurs within 2 to 3 hours following a meal is highly suggestive of a duodenal ulcer, which is confirmed by endoscopy. The vast majority of duodenal ulcers are associated with *Helicobacter pylori* infection. The patient's grandfather had gastric cancer, which is also associated with *H. pylori* infection, but the current theory is that early childhood infection is a risk factor for the development of gastric cancer, but adult infection with *H. pylori* leads to ulcer disease. In patients with a proven peptic ulcer that is found to be infected with *H. pylori* (most commonly by serology or by urease test on an endoscopic biopsy), eradication of the organism by antibiotic administration coupled with antacid therapy is the standard of care.

21. a (Part 7)

Recognize and diagnose gonococcal arthritis. Although definitive diagnosis requires arthrocentesis and fluid examination, the most common cause of septic arthritis in young adults remains gonococcal arthritis. This woman has the typical migratory polyarthralgias, which eventually settle into one joint as a monoarthritis. The characteristic skin rash is also present, although it sometimes resolves before the patient seeks attention. She has no risk factors for Lyme disease (tick exposure) or nongonococcal septic arthritis (e.g., IV drug use). Lyme disease also tends to have the typical erythema chronicum migrans rash, which is 5 to 15 cm in diameter. Pseudogout tends to affect older individuals and has no rash. Reiter syndrome is characterized by conjunctivitis, urethritis, and arthritis.

22. b (Part 7)

The diagnosis of gonococcal arthritis is confirmed by culturing the organism in a normally sterile site, such as the synovial fluid or blood. However, the synovial fluid is only positive in 50% of cases of purulent arthritis. A higher yield of the organism (although indirect evidence) comes from a cervical culture in women, which is positive in approximately 90% of cases. Synovial fluid crystal analysis will be negative, and fluid cell count will show a nonspecific elevation of the white blood cell (WBC) count (usually 50,000 to 100,000), also seen in nongonococcal septic arthritis and crystalline arthritis. Gram stain is rarely positive in gonococcal arthritis. MRI is of no value in diagnosing infectious arthritis; it is most useful for soft-tissue damage, such as a meniscal tear.

23. a (Part 7)

Know the treatment for scleroderma renal crisis. This patient with known scleroderma presents with new renal failure and accelerated hypertension, consistent with the clinical diagnosis of scleroderma renal crisis. It is more common early in the course of scleroderma (first few years) and in the diffuse variant of scleroderma. The typical features of nonspecific headache, malaise, and nausea are accompanied by oliguric renal failure and accelerated hypertension. Urine analysis results are usually benign but may show small amounts of protein and red cells. Blood count may show a microangiopathic hemolytic anemia (not seen here). No further workup is needed, and prompt treatment is indicated. ACE inhibitors have dramatically reduced the mortality from this condition, and they are the treatment of choice, even in the acute setting. Nitroprusside is used in the treatment of hypertensive urgency, but it does not address the underlying physiology of a scleroderma renal crisis. Nifedipine is not used in this setting and may precipitously drop the BP in the acutely hypertensive patient. Immunosuppression with prednisone or D-penicillamine is not indicated.

24. c (Part 3)

Know the evaluation and management of hypernatremia. Hypernatremia results from a deficit in water relative to solute (generally sodium). To correct this condition, it is useful to calculate the free water deficit, which in this patient is approximately 4 L. If the patient is clinically stable, as in this case, replenishment of water can be accomplished gradually, replacing half of the free water deficit over the first 24 hours and the remainder over the next 24 to 48 hours. For this patient, a bolus is not required, and in any case, a 2-L bolus would be excessive. The choice between isotonic saline, hypotonic saline (e.g., 0.45% sodium) or "pure" free water (e.g., D5W) is generally not important (provided the patient does not have significant renal failure); rather the rate of the free water replacement should be the major consideration. Even though the serum sodium concentration is elevated, in most cases this is not because of a net overload of sodium, especially in a case where it is clear that access to water was restricted; therefore diuretic treatment would not be appropriate.

25. c (Part 6)

Know how to diagnose and treat severe hyperkalemia. The ECG reveals widening of the QRS complex and peaked

T waves. This can progress to loss of P waves and an eventual sine wave pattern. This ECG is not representative of an arrhythmia that requires cardioversion, nor does it represent an acute MI. Although hemolysis can often be a cause of a spurious elevated potassium measurement, the ECG changes and clinical picture indicate this is true hyperkalemia. Although bacterial meningitis can result in altered mental status, it would not be associated with the elevated potassium level and the ECG changes.

The emergent therapy of life-threatening hyperkalemia includes administration of calcium, insulin, glucose, and sodium bicarbonate to drive potassium intracellularly, and administration of calcium gluconate to stabilize membranes from the effects of hyperkalemia. None of these measures serves to eliminate potassium from the body. Administration of a cation-exchange resin into the GI tract will bind potassium and reduce serum potassium levels. In certain cases, particularly patients with renal failure, dialysis may be necessary to prevent recurrent hyperkalemia.

26. e (Part 6)

Recognize the clinical features of the MEN type 2 syndrome. This patient has the MEN syndrome type 2, which consists of pheochromocytoma and medullary carcinoma of the thyroid, either in association with hyperparathyroidism (type 2A) or mucosal neuromas (type 2B). When hyperparathyroidism occurs, it is because of hyperplasia, not an adenoma. The pheochromocytomas are bilateral in approximately 50% of MEN patients, and this is a more likely cause of recurrence than a malignant pheochromocytoma. MEN type 2 is an autosomal dominant disease, as seen in the pedigree shown (approximately 50% affected, both genders). If his paternal uncle has not manifested the syndrome, it is unlikely that he will pass on the disease to his children. Penetrance is not 100%, however, so genetic testing is required to diagnose the disease definitively. Mutations in the RET proto-oncogene are the most common cause of MEN type 2, seen in approximately 95% of families. Once the specific mutation in a family is known, genetic testing can rule out disease in other family members definitively.

27. d (Part 5)

28. b (Part 5)

29. a (Part 5)

30. e (Part 5)

Know the use of serology in the diagnosis of acute and chronic hepatitis. The pattern of tests in (A) represents a patient who has had exposure to hepatitis C virus (HCV) sometime in the past. HCV was generally transfusion related in the era before testing of donated blood for HCV became routine and often leads to a chronic hepatitis that can result in cirrhosis and end-stage liver disease. (B) represents a patient

who has had hepatitis B virus (HBV) in the past and had controlled the infection or, more commonly now, represents a patient who has been immunized against HBV using a recombinant vaccine that consists of HBsAg. The pattern in (C) is unusual but may be seen in a subset of patients with chronic HBV infection that generate a weak, nonprotective antibody response against HBsAg. The pattern in (D) is diagnostic for acute HAV infection. The pattern in (E) can be seen either in acute HBV infection or in patients with chronic HBV infection. Distinction between the two can be made by measurement of antiHbcAg IgM, which is generally present in acute HBV infection but not in chronic HBV.

31. b (Part 8)

Understand the epidemiology and presentation of breast cancer. Breast cancer is the second most common cause of cancer mortality in women in the United States. Screening of women older than 50 years with an annual or biannual mammogram has been shown to decrease the mortality from breast cancer. The data for women younger than 40 years who do not have a family history of early breast cancer are less convincing, but these women also probably benefit. Patients who present with unilateral nipple discharge are more likely to have an underlying breast cancer (generally an intraductal tumor) compared with those who present with bilateral nipple discharge (who may have an endocrinopathy such as a prolactinoma). Excisional biopsy remains the gold standard for diagnosis because of the unacceptably high false-negative rates for fine-needle aspiration. Patients with estrogen receptor–positive tumors are more likely to respond to hormonal adjuvant therapy with tamoxifen. In a patient who presents with a tumor in one breast, the risk of developing a tumor in the opposite breast is elevated fivefold.

32. a (Part 3)

Know the causes of elevated anion gap metabolic acidosis. In a patient with acidosis, the calculation of the anion gap can provide a clue as to the etiology. An elevated anion gap is caused by the presence of a nonvolatile acid. This can be because of metabolic abnormalities (e.g., ketoacidosis, lactic acidosis) or intoxications (e.g., methanol, ethylene glycol, salicylates). In contrast, the loss of alkali (e.g., related to diarrhea) or decreased acid excretion by the kidney (as in renal tubular acidosis) does not increase the anion gap.

33. c (Part 6)

Know the appropriate treatment of panhypopituitarism. TSH production is suboptimal in panhypopituitarism, and it cannot be used to monitor treatment as in primary hypothyroidism. Free T_4 levels and symptoms, which are less exact, are used to guide treatment. Although the adrenals are not primarily affected, atrophy occurs and adrenocorticotropin hormone (ACTH) stimulation will be suboptimal. The lower dose of prednisone in the evening is used to mimic the normal amount of cortisol production at that time. There is no indication to increase the dose, and overdosage of prednisone leads to osteoporosis, cataracts, and hyperglycemia. Treatment with a GnRH analog will not improve gonadal function because the pituitary is required to produce luteinizing hormone and follicle-stimulating hormone from GnRH treatment. Treatment of panhypopituitarism with human growth hormone (hGH) is controversial in adults. There does seem to be some measured benefits in terms of body mass and lipids with hGH, but treatment is very expensive and long-term effects are unclear.

34. c (Part 2)

Know the management of asthma and how to step up therapy for inadequate control. The patient presents having previously been adequately controlled on therapy for mild persistent asthma, as per National Heart, Lung, and Blood Institute guidelines. She is currently reporting poor control and thus needs an increase in therapy. Regimens involving the use of oral steroids or high-dose inhaled steroids are generally reserved for patients with severe persistent asthma. The addition of a long-acting β_2-agonist is an appropriate step up in therapy and may be particularly useful in the setting of nighttime symptoms. An alternative would also be an increase of the inhaled steroid to medium dose. Long-acting β_2-agonists are only used as "control" therapy and never on an as-needed basis.

35. c (Part 2)

Recognize the presentation of acute human immunodeficiency virus (HIV) infection. Acute HIV infection presents as a mononucleosis type of illness with generally nonspecific symptoms. Unless the clinician has a high index of suspicion, this diagnosis can be missed. It is important to question patients with such a nonspecific illness about sexual activity and injection drug use. During acute HIV infection, the HIV screening enzyme-linked immunoabsorbent assay (ELISA) is usually negative because the patient has not yet developed antibody responses. The diagnosis thus needs to be made by detecting the virus directly, generally via viral load testing.

36. d (Part 1)

Recognize mitral regurgitation and know its possible etiologies. This patient's clinical scenario is consistent with mitral regurgitation. The murmur is holosystolic and radiates to the axilla. The left atrial enlargement supports this as well. In this patient's age group (>65 years of age), the most likely cause is myxomatous degeneration of the mitral valve. Rheumatic heart disease often involves the mitral valve but usually presents earlier in life. Mitral stenosis and atrial fibrillation (not seen here) are additional features that might be seen in such patients. Endocarditis can affect any valve and has a predilection for damaged valves. However, the patient has no other findings suggestive of endocarditis, either acute or subacute. Rupture of a papillary muscle is an acute event that usually results in marked pulmonary edema. It is often seen in the setting of an MI. Syphilis does not affect the mitral valve. In its late stages (tertiary syphilis), it can affect the aortic root, leading to aortic regurgitation.

37. b (Part 1)

Know the treatment options for mitral regurgitation. The most important aspect of this patient's management will be afterload reduction. ACE inhibitors, such as captopril, can reduce afterload and therefore slow progression of mitral regurgitation. They may also improve symptoms and exercise tolerance. If the patient is in congestive heart failure, diuretics would also be helpful. However, this patient demonstrates no pulmonary findings (crackles or rales) or elevated neck veins to support the need for diuresis. Digoxin is an inotropic agent useful in patients with low ejection fraction. There does not appear to be a need for this agent in this case. Warfarin is not used routinely for patients with valvular disease. It is useful in patients with atrial fibrillation or in patients with a previous history of embolic stroke. Antibiotics would be appropriate for any patient with valvular disease who is undergoing dental work or any invasive procedure to prevent endocarditis. However, without evidence for current endocarditis, they are not needed here. This patient should also have an echocardiogram to evaluate left ventricular dimensions and ejection fraction. If she is interested in valve replacement, the timing of the surgery would depend on these factors.

38. c (Part 1)

Recognize sinus tachycardia. The rhythm strip shows a tachycardia with a rate of 170 beats per minute. It is narrow complex, and P waves are clearly seen before each QRS. This patient's rhythm is sinus tachycardia, and treatment should be focused at treating the underlying cause, not the rhythm. In this case, alcohol abuse and vomiting have led to profound dehydration and hypotension. IV fluids, such as normal saline, should be rapidly administered. Carotid massage and adenosine both act to increase AV node refractories and therefore are useful in diagnosing or treating narrow-complex tachycardias. In AV reentrant tachycardias or AV nodal reentrant tachycardias, these agents often abruptly terminate the tachycardia, with a return to normal sinus rhythm. However, they are ineffective in sinus tachycardia, which is mediated through adrenergic drive and not nodal reentry. Lidocaine is a class 1B antiarrhythmic that is used to treat ventricular arrhythmias, which are wide-complex tachycardias. Tachycardia and hypotension are often said to be an indication for emergent cardioversion (for "unstable tachycardias"). This refers to tachycardias that cause the hypotension and will respond to cardioversion. In this case, it is the hypotension that is leading to the tachycardia, not vice versa.

39. e (Part 1)

Know the appropriate treatment of atrial fibrillation. The rhythm strip shows no atrial activity and an irregular rate consistent with atrial fibrillation. In many patients with atrial fibrillation, the ventricular rate is 130 to 150 beats per minute at first presentation. However, the combination of a β-blocker already prescribed for hypertension and likely underlying AV nodal disease has resulted in a controlled rate in this patient. Therefore, further rate control with either digoxin or diltiazem is not indicated in this patient. Once rate control is established, treatment focuses on restoration of sinus rhythm if possible. Procainamide and quinidine are both class IA antiarrhythmics that are effective in converting atrial fibrillation to sinus rhythm. However, patients who have been in atrial fibrillation for >48 hours (or an uncertain amount of time) should be anticoagulated first. Thrombus can form during atrial fibrillation and be released into the arterial circulation after the restoration of sinus rhythm. Others advocate a transesophageal echocardiogram to rule out thrombus before cardioversion without anticoagulation. If sinus rhythm cannot be restored, long-term anticoagulation would be indicated for stroke prevention. This patient has risk factors for stroke that include age and hypertension.

40. b (Part 1)

Know the indications for medical treatment of dilated cardiomyopathy. This patient has a dilated cardiomyopathy, presumably secondary to alcohol abuse. Randomized controlled trials have convincingly shown that ACE inhibitors reduce long-term mortality in patients with congestive heart failure (CHF) and low ejection fractions. This also appears to be the case in patients with ischemic cardiomyopathy and in patients with asymptomatic cardiomyopathy (i.e., no previous CHF). Furosemide, a loop diuretic, is certainly a necessary drug in many of these patients and has never been formally evaluated for survival benefit. Digoxin has been studied in patients already taking ACE inhibitors and diuretics and was shown to decrease hospitalizations but not deaths. β-Blockers have recently gained popularity because of several studies showing improved survival in dilated cardiomyopathy. However, these studies have used longer-acting agents, and therefore they cannot be extrapolated to the short-acting, nonselective agent propranolol.

41. a (Part 1)

Know the appropriate treatment for the patient with stable angina. This patient presents with typical symptoms of angina, and a stress test confirms the diagnosis. The angina would be classified as class II (moderate exertion) and should be initially treated with medication. This treatment would consist of aspirin and a β-blocker, such as atenolol. If symptoms persist, long-acting nitrates such as isosorbide dinitrate could be added. Diltiazem is also an effective antianginal

agent, but it is considered a second-line agent to β-blockers. Repeat exercise testing with imaging is not needed because the pretest probability of disease was high (typical story in a patient with risk factors), and initial testing was in agreement with this. Cardiac catheterization would be indicated if the patient failed medical management and angioplasty was considered. Initial catheterization is also advocated for patients with a high probability of three-vessel disease who may benefit from bypass surgery. The patient's excellent exercise tolerance and ischemia only in lateral leads argue against the presence of severe three-vessel disease.

42. e (Part 1)

Know the appropriate treatment for the patient with unstable angina. This patient now returns on an appropriate chronic medical regimen with unstable angina, as indicated by increasing severity and intensity of anginal pain. Because of the known coronary disease and escalating nature of the symptoms, the patient should be hospitalized for further evaluation and IV heparin. Possible precipitants, such as anemia or tachycardia, should be looked for. Cardiac catheterization often reveals severe stenosis of one or more coronary arteries in these patients. Repeat stress testing may eventually be ordered but should never be obtained in the unstable patient because it may precipitate a MI. Adding diltiazem or increasing current antianginals are possible interventions that may be undertaken in the hospital.

43. b (Part 6)

Recognize apathetic hyperthyroidism in the elderly as a cause of weight loss. Hyperthyroidism should be ruled out in all elderly patients with a nonspecific syndrome of weight loss and fatigue. It often presents without the classic symptoms of tachycardia, tremor, frequent bowel movements, and diaphoresis. This patient also appears to have atrial fibrillation (as suggested by the irregular pulse), which may be the only sign of hyperthyroidism. The increased alkaline phosphatase (from high bone turnover) and normocytic anemia are also consistent with this diagnosis. There is no suggestion of tuberculosis, although a chest radiograph could be performed if initial evaluation was unrevealing. An abdominal CT scan would be a secondary test if symptoms led in this direction. Depression should always be considered in the elderly but would not explain the laboratory or physical examination findings. Atenolol is a selective β_1-blocker with less central nervous system (CNS) penetration and is less likely to cause depression.

44. d (Part 5)

Know the extraintestinal manifestations of inflammatory bowel disease. Both Crohn disease and ulcerative colitis are associated with the development of many extraintestinal manifestations. Many of these are felt to arise from the underlying immune dysregulation that is central to the

ANSWERS

pathogenesis of IBD. Thus conditions such as inflammatory arthritis, uveitis, and erythema nodosum all can be encountered in patients with IBD. Primary sclerosing cholangitis (PSC) occurs in approximately 5% of patients with ulcerative colitis and less often in patients with Crohn disease. Although often diagnosed in patients who are asymptomatic by an unexplained cholestatic laboratory picture, pruritus and fatigue are among the most common symptoms. Antimitochondrial antibodies, which are common in primary biliary cirrhosis, are not generally seen in patients with PSC. Diagnosis of PSC is generally confirmed by a "beaded" appearance of the bile ducts on cholangiography because of multifocal structures and dilations. PSC is a progressive disease, eventually leading to cholestatic complications and, ultimately, liver failure.

45. b (Part 3)

Know the differential diagnosis of rapidly progressive glomerular nephritis (RPGN). RPGN is the clinical endpoint of a number of pathogenic conditions that all lead to subacute glomerular inflammation and renal failure. Clinically, patients present with subacute renal failure, an active urinary sediment, and subnephrotic proteinuria. On renal biopsy, the presence of crescent formation involving the majority of glomeruli is common. Immunofluorescence (IF) and various serologic tests can confirm the diagnosis. The most common cause of RPGN is immune-complex disease, which is associated with granular deposition of immunoglobulin by IF, low serum C3 and negative ANCA, and antiglomerular basement membrane (anti-GBM) titers. If postinfectious, antistreptolysin O titers would be positive, but many other diseases can result in immune-complex deposition as well (e.g., SLE, endocarditis, cryoglobulinemia). So-called pauci-immune glomerulonephritis is characterized by a positive ANCA, negative antiGBM, normal C3, and minimal or absent glomerular staining by IF. In antiGBM disease, serology would show a positive antiGBM titer, negative ANCA, normal C3, and linear deposits of immunoglobulin are seen by IF. Hemolytic uremic syndrome can cause RPGN, but all serologies would be negative and no staining would be seen by IF.

46. a (Part 2)

Know the distinction between exudative and transudative pleural effusions. Analysis of the pleural fluid reveals a transudate (fluid-to-serum albumin ratio <0.5, fluid-to-serum LDH ratio <0.6, and LDH <200). The differential diagnosis of a transudative pleural effusion includes CHF (most likely given the patient's presentation), cirrhosis, and nephrotic syndrome. Exudative pleural effusions can be caused by pneumonia, tuberculosis, malignancy, or pulmonary embolism.

47. b (Part 2)

48. a (Part 2)

49. c (Part 2)

50. b (Part 2)

Know methods of diagnostic testing for the confirmation or exclusion of acute pulmonary embolus (PE). Pulmonary angiography is the gold standard for the diagnosis of acute PE. A variety of noninvasive tests have been developed, but all lack appropriate sensitivity and specificity. The inclusion of clinical pretest probabilities has been used to increase the sensitivity and specificity of given tests. Additionally, the use of multimodal testing, whether or not supplemented with clinical probability, has been studied to develop accurate diagnostic algorithms for PE. In the first patient, the clinical probability is low. With a negative D-dimer test, PE is effectively ruled out. In the second patient, a high clinical probability (malignancy, immobility, signs of DVT) and a high probability V/Q scan rule in the diagnosis. CT angiography is generally of high sensitivity, but there can be variation in reader expertise, and, overall, the technique has not been as well studied as V/Q scan. In the third case, the clinical probability is moderate. Coupled with an indeterminant V/Q scan, PE cannot be ruled in or excluded. A positive D-dimer is insufficient to rule in PE as well, and thus pulmonary angiography is indicated. In the final case, studies have indicated that anticoagulation is not necessary in patients with a low clinical probability (a score of 1.0 by modified Wells' criteria) with a non–high-probability V/Q and negative D-dimer and/or venous Doppler.

51. e (Part 8)

52. b (Part 8)

53. a (Part 8)

54. g (Part 8)

55. f (Part 8)

Know the evaluation of coagulopathies. The evaluation of a coagulation disorder generally requires a combination of history and selected laboratory tests. A medication history is particularly important. Therapeutic administration of warfarin for indications such as prevention of cardiogenic thrombi because of prosthetic valves or atrial fibrillation is a common cause of an elevated PT, international normalized ratio (INR), or both. Certain drugs such as quinidine, methyldopa, and sulfathiazole are associated with an immune-mediated thrombocytopenia.

Severe thrombocytopenia and spontaneous bleeding are seen in the setting of DIC, a potentially life-threatening consumptive coagulopathy that can be associated with bacterial sepsis, severe trauma, and cancer. The widespread intravascular coagulation leads to an increase in serum levels of fibrin degradation products as the fibrinolytic system attempts to handle the inappropriate fibrin deposition.

Patients with classic hemophilia A (factor VIII deficiency) generally manifest with spontaneous bleeding episodes early in life. However, patients with type I von Willebrand disease (which represents a relative rather than an absolute coagulopathy) often have evidence of overt coagulopathy only at times of severe hemostatic stress, such as surgery or childbirth.

56. b (Part 3)

Know indications for prophylaxis to prevent opportunistic infections in HIV-infected patients. Although the advent of highly active antiretroviral treatment (HAART) has decreased the incidence of opportunistic infections (OIs), OIs remain a significant cause of morbidity and mortality in HIV-infected patients. HAART has resulted in changes in the recommendations for prophylaxis. In patients who experience immune reconstitution on HAART (defined by sustained increases in CD4 count), prophylaxis for *Pneumocystis jiroveci* pneumonia (PCP), toxoplasmosis, *Mycobacterium avium* complex (MAC), and cytomegalovirus (CMV) can be safely discontinued. Although there is an increase in multidrug resistance in *Myobacterium tuberculosis,* the macrolides remain as effective prophylactic drugs against disseminated MAC. In the preHAART era, CMV prophylaxis required the use of ganciclovir or foscarnet, which can be highly toxic agents when used chronically. Immune reconstitution via HAART is the most effective prevention strategy for CMV. Toxoplasmosis in HIV-infected patients is almost universally secondary to relapses of latent infection. Therefore, patients with serologic evidence of latent disease (manifested by positive anti*Toxoplasma gondii* IgG titers) are at greatest risk for toxoplasmosis and require prophylaxis if their CD4 counts fall below 100 cells/μL.

57. c (Part 2)

Understand the pathogenesis of chronic obstructive pulmonary disease (COPD), which encompasses two clinical conditions: chronic bronchitis and emphysema. The patient in this question presents with likely emphysema. Although the pathophysiology of the two conditions differs, the common link between chronic bronchitis and emphysema is the causal role of cigarette smoking in both conditions. In COPD, the only intervention that slows the rate of decline in pulmonary function (as measured by forced expiratory volume [FEV_1]) is the discontinuation of cigarettes. Unfortunately, quitting generally does not reverse the functional limitation, but by slowing the progression of pulmonary decline, patients may not decline to the levels that are associated with high short-term mortality. Therefore, smoking cessation is a key component of the management of any patient who presents with COPD.

58. e (Part 5)

Know the clinical manifestations of infection with various agents of acute gastroenteritis. Along with an exposure history, the clinical presentation of gastroenteritis can give clues about the underlying etiologic agent. In this patient, the key manifestation is bloody diarrhea. *Bacillus cereus* and *Staphylococcus aureus* can be responsible for acute "food poisoning" manifested as vomiting after ingestion of preformed toxin in poorly prepared/stored food. *Vibrio cholerae* is generally responsible for a profuse, watery diarrhea, whereas diarrhea associated with *Giardia lamblia* is characterized by a bulky nonbloody diarrhea caused by malabsorption. Bloody diarrhea is generally caused by invasive organisms or organisms that trigger a strong mucosal inflammatory response. In addition to *S. dysenteriae,* bloody diarrhea can also be a manifestation of infection with *Entamoeba histolytica, Campylobacter jejuni,* or enterohemorrhagic *Escherichia. coli.*

59. c (Part 3)

Know how to differentiate latent syphilis from neurosyphilis. Patients who have positive serologic tests for *Treponema pallidum* but without signs or symptoms are said to have latent disease. Latent syphilis can be divided into early latent, which refers to latent syphilis discovered <1 year after primary infection, or late latent, which is seropositivity discovered >1 year after primary infection (or disease of unknown duration). CNS disease can occur at any stage of syphilis, from primary, to secondary, to tertiary. A common scenario is to find a patient who has a positive syphilis serology of unknown duration (latent syphilis). This can be complicated by findings that suggest possible neurologic involvement, as in the current case. Although the patient has an explanation for his dementia (a history of lacunar infarcts), CNS syphilis needs to be ruled out. If the patient is found to have a positive cerebrospinal fluid (CSF) Venereal Disease Research Laboratory (VDRL) test, treatment with IV penicillin G (18 to 24 million U a day in divided doses or via continuous infusion) needs to be initiated. If the CSF VDRL is negative, then the patient could simply be treated as for late latent syphilis with 2.4 million U of IM benzathine penicillin weekly for three doses total.

60. c (Part 3)

Know the presentation and diagnosis of drug-induced acute interstitial nephritis (AIN). The majority of cases of interstitial nephritis are caused by drugs, most commonly penicillins (in particular the antistaphylococcal penicillin, methicillin) and nonsteroidal anti-inflammatory drugs (NSAIDs), although a large number of different drugs have been implicated. The development of drug-associated AIN is not dose dependent and can occur within 3 to 5 days after a second exposure to the offending agent, or as long as several weeks after an initial exposure to a drug (presumably related to the length of time required to develop an immune response to the agent). Although much less common, several infectious agents have been associated with the development of AIN, including *Legionella* infection and CMV infection.

The clinical presentation of drug-induced AIN is often subtle with nonspecific symptoms and signs caused by an allergic-type reaction and varying degrees of renal impairment.

Despite the immune-mediated renal injury because of the allergic-type reaction, rash is actually relatively rare, as is fever or eosinophilia. The urinalysis is usually notable for the presence of white cell casts and subnephrotic-range proteinuria. If special stains are obtained, it can be demonstrated that the white cells present in the urine are eosinophils.

Treatment of drug-induced AIN involves immediate withdrawal of the suspected offending agent. Steroid treatment has been tried with variable success, and most experts recommend following patients with AIN and only moderate renal impairment for improvement in renal function. For patients with severe renal impairment or those who do not begin to improve within 3 to 5 days, steroid treatment may be beneficial (often following a renal biopsy to confirm the diagnosis).

61. a (Part 4)

Recognize the presentation of herpes simplex virus type 1 encephalitis, the most common fatal sporadic encephalitis in the United States. Recognition is important because the majority of patients die without appropriate treatment. Even with acyclovir administration, mortality is approximately 25%, and a large number of survivors have residual neurologic deficits. HSV encephalitis generally presents with the rapid onset of fever, headache, altered mental status, and focal neurologic findings. The tropism of the virus for the temporal lobes (which can be seen by MRI) can lead to symptoms related to involvement of this area of the brain, including amnesia and the Klüver-Bucy syndrome. CSF examination generally shows a lymphocytic pleocytosis with increased RBCs and an elevated protein. Definitive diagnosis was formally made by brain biopsy, but this has generally been supplanted by the development of HSV-specific PCR assays.

62. c (Part 2)

Know the indication for oxygen therapy in the setting of chronic pulmonary disease. Although it can be a component of the acute care of flares of disease, oxygen therapy is rarely indicated in patients with asthma. In patients with COPD (either emphysema or chronic bronchitis) a mortality benefit for supplemental oxygen therapy has been demonstrated from a number of clinical trials in patients with baseline hypoxia (a Pao_2 <60 mm Hg at rest while breathing room air).

63. c (Part 8)

Understand the usefulness and limitations of cancer screening. Screening can be defined as a means of detecting a disease in asymptomatic individuals, with the goal of early detection to decrease morbidity and mortality. A great deal of attention has been paid to screening for a variety of cancers. These screening methods have been tested in a number of clinical trials, not all of which have ideal trial design. The best data from studies concern screening for breast, cervical, and colon cancer. For breast cancer, a number of studies have shown that routine mammography for women older than 50 years decreases mortality.

Similarly, routine Papanicolaou smears have been shown to decrease mortality from cervical cancer. Although it is not known if there is an upper age limit after which Papanicolaou screening is no longer effective, many experts suggest that screening should be continued until at least 65 years of age. Both fecal occult blood testing and sigmoidoscopy have been shown to decrease mortality in people older than 50 years. Both routine chest radiographs and the use of sputum cytology have been tested as methods for lung cancer screening. Unfortunately, none of the studies to date has shown that either of these methods is associated with reduced mortality, even in smokers. More recent data suggest that high-resolution, low-dose helical CT may be a more sensitive screening test. However, the results are preliminary, and no recommendations can be made yet as to the usefulness and cost effectiveness of this approach as a mass screening method. The use of serum cancer markers such as CA-125 and prostate-specific antigen (PSA) has been promoted as a screening method. Although these markers are elevated in patients with these tumors, the use of these markers for screening has been associated with a significant false-positive rate that has experts divided over whether their use is truly efficacious and cost effective.

64. d (Part 1)

Know the treatment of a hypertensive emergency. This patient presents with markedly elevated BP and evidence of end-organ damage (as indicated by renal failure). This constitutes a hypertensive emergency, and it requires immediate treatment with IV medication. Patients with a hypertensive emergency often have previous histories of hypertension, either treated or untreated. The headache and visual changes are likely manifestations of CNS dysfunction, although no papilledema is seen. Treatment of choice is IV nitroprusside (a vasodilator), which can be closely titrated. Continued use of nitroprusside must be done with caution because of the risk of thiocyanate toxicity (a metabolite of nitroprusside), especially in patients with renal failure. Propranolol is not an effective treatment for hypertensive crisis, but β-blockers may be useful in conjunction with nitroprusside. Captopril, an ACE inhibitor, can be used for urgent situations in which BP control is desired over several hours. The onset of action is approximately 60 minutes. Treatment is more emergent in this case, and the renal failure also argues against use of ACE inhibitors. Sublingual nifedipine can result in rapid and dangerous drops in BP and should not be used in this situation. Morphine would only be useful if pain or CHF were contributing to the patient's presentation.

65. b (Part 4)

Understand the principles for the prevention of bacterial meningitis. The currently available vaccine against *Neisseria meningitidis* is a tetravalent vaccine containing polysaccharides representing serotypes A, C, Y, and W-135. Unfortunately, the capsular polysaccharide of serogroup B (which represents approximately a third of *N. meningitidis* in the United States) is poorly immunogenic and not included in the current vaccine. In certain areas, the tetravalent vaccine is recommended for all first-year college students. Postexposure prophylaxis for close contacts of cases of invasive meningococcal meningitis is accepted as a means to prevent development of disease in contacts and to eradicate possible pharyngeal carriage and transmission. Besides rifampin, single doses of ciprofloxacin or ceftriaxone can be administered. There is no cross protection offered by the *Haemophilus influenzae* vaccine (Hib). The routine use of Hib has resulted in a remarkable decrease in the incidence of meningitis caused by *H. influenzae* type b in the pediatric population.

66. a (Part 5)

Know the manifestations and diagnosis of celiac disease. In a patient who presents with probable malabsorption as in the case presented here, celiac disease (also known as gluten-sensitive enteropathy) figures prominently in the differential diagnosis. In patients with celiac disease, the pathogenesis depends on ingestion of gluten, the alcohol-soluble fraction of wheat protein. Exclusion of gluten from the diet, which is often difficult to do without the advice of a dietician, results in resolution of symptoms and the histopathologic lesions associated with celiac disease. The diagnosis of celiac disease is usually based on the presence of serology sometime combined with small bowel biopsy, via endoscopy. For many years, the presence of antigliadin antibodies was used as a marker for celiac disease. Because of higher sensitivity and specificity, IgA endomysial antibodies have largely replaced the antigliadin antibodies as routine serology in the diagnosis of celiac disease. Definitive diagnosis is generally made by histologic examination of a small bowel biopsy that reveals villous atrophy and variable degrees of inflammation. In patients with highly suggestive symptoms and clinical picture and positive IgG endomysial antibodies, some practitioners forgo obtaining a biopsy and use the institution of a gluten-free diet (with resolution of symptoms) as confirmation of the diagnosis.

67. b (Part 1)

Know how to treat the patient with isolated systolic hypertension. This patient has demonstrated elevated systolic BP on several occasions. Nonpharmacologic treatments, such as diet and exercise, are unlikely to reduce this patient's systolic BP significantly to the goal of less than 150 mm Hg. These measures may result in improvements of 6 to 8 mm Hg on average and in association with drug treatment may help achieve BP goals. The most appropriate treatment, however, is to begin treatment with a thiazide diuretic, which is considered first-line treatment for systolic hypertension. These drugs, along with β-blockers, reduce the risk of stroke in elderly patients with isolated systolic hypertension. β-Blockers are not preferred in this case because of the patient's co-morbid condition of COPD. Captopril, an ACE inhibitor,

could be used but not as much evidence supports its use in these patients. ACE inhibitors may be most useful in patients with diabetes to prevent progression of renal failure or in patients with CHF. There is no suggestion that the patient has a secondary cause for hypertension that would require further workup before treatment is started. A renal angiogram for renal artery stenosis might be indicated if the patient had a dramatic increase in BP, known vascular disease, or difficulty in controlling BP. Renin and aldosterone levels, to look for hyperaldosteronism, should be sent when a patient has spontaneous hypokalemia.

68. e (Part 5)

Know how to evaluate ascites in a patient with cirrhosis. In the United States, approximately 80% of cases of ascites are related to cirrhosis (i.e., portal hypertension). Other causes include malignancy, CHF, pancreatitis, and the nephrotic syndrome. The serum ascites-albumin gradient (SAAG) is useful in helping determine the cause for ascites. In cirrhosis and CDF, the serum ascites-albumin gradient (SAAG) is ≥1.1. If the SAAG is <1.0, this is suggestive of malignancy, tuberculosis, or the nephritic syndrome. In this case, the SAAG of 1.9 supports a diagnosis of ascites caused by cirrhosis. Additionally, however, the polymorphonuclear lymphocytes (PMN) count of >250 is consistent with spontaneous bacterial peritonitis, and the patient needs to be treated empirically, even in the absence of signs and symptoms of infection. In patients who present with ascites and evidence of infection (e.g., fever, abdominal pain, altered mental status), therapy should be initiated even before the results of ascites fluid count are obtained.

69. c (Part 3)

70. b (Part 3)

71. d (Part 3)

Know the presentation of specific forms of nephrolithiasis. Although calcium oxalate crystals are the most common, other causes of nephrolithiasis have specific historical features and may present with distinguishing laboratory findings. Cystinuria is a rare genetic defect but results in familial nephrolithiasis with hexagonal crystalluria. Urinary tract infections with urease-producing organisms such as *Proteus* can lead to a persistently alkaline urine with magnesium ammonium phosphate crystals in the urine that look like a coffin lid. Uric acid stones often present in patients with known gout and are notable in that they are radiolucent.

72. c (Part 2)

Know the pathophysiology and clinical characteristics of small cell lung cancer. Whereas a small percentage of non-small cell lung cancers can occur in nonsmokers, virtually all small cell lung cancers are associated with cigarette smoking. Small cell cancers are notable for their rapid growth rate and earlmetastasis. Therefore, the tumor-mode-metastasis (TNM) staging system that is used for nonsmall cell cancers is not a clinically useful method for staging small cell lung cancers. This feature of small cell cancers also explains why they are much less frequently found during the workup of a solitary pulmonary nodule compared to nonsmall cell lung cancers, where the identification of a T1N0M0 tumor is associated with an up to 40% long-term survival rate. One biologic feature of small cancers is that they are associated with the development of paraneoplastic syndromes, making it not infrequent that the primary diagnosis of small cell cancer is made in a patient who presents with symptoms related to the paraneoplastic syndrome.

73. a (Part 6)

Know how to diagnose granulomatous thyroiditis. The development of hyperthyroid symptoms (tremor, diaphoresis, tachycardia) and a tender thyroid after a viral illness are most consistent with granulomatous (de Quervain) thyroiditis. Lymphocytic thyroiditis shows no tenderness on examination and often occurs in the postpartum period. Hashimoto thyroiditis uncommonly leads to hyperthyroidism (it is the most common cause of hypothyroidism, however). Graves disease is common in young women but is usually less acute in its presentation and shows an enlarged nontender gland. Toxic multinodular goiter is seen more often in the elderly with a nodular, nontender gland.

74. c (Part 1)

Recognize the clinical picture of pericarditis. This patient's ECG shows the typical features of pericarditis. Diffuse ST elevations are present in multiple leads, and PR depression can be seen in II and aVF. The clinical picture is consistent with pericarditis, considering the preceding flulike illness and pleuritic substernal chest pain. Therefore, it would be expected that the pain would be relieved with sitting forward, which is typical for pericarditis. Chest pain that is maximal at onset is more typical of aortic dissection, and musculoskeletal pain can be reproduced with palpation. Panic disorder sometimes manifests as chest pain, palpitations, or both. A common feature of this diagnosis is a feeling of impending doom. The patient may also have associated agoraphobia, or fear of open spaces.

75. b (Part 7)

Know the appropriate treatment for acute gout. This man presents with the typical symptoms of gout: a painful, swollen first metatarsophalangeal joint. Attacks may be precipitated by increased alcohol or protein intake, diuretics (such as thiazides), or acute illness. The diagnosis is confirmed by finding urate crystals (needle-shaped negative birefringence) on examination of the synovial fluid. The treatment options normally include NSAIDs or colchicine. In this case, the recent GI bleeding makes NSAIDs less desirable, especially if the bleeding was from an upper intestinal source. Colchicine is well tolerated in patients without renal or liver disease. Prednisone would certainly treat gout in this case but has more side effects and often results in a flare when removed. The addition of prednisone is unnecessary and could worsen the patient's diabetes. Open drainage of a joint is the treatment for a nongonococcal septic joint, not gout. Allopurinol is used to reduce uric acid level in patients with gout to prevent attacks. It is not effective in acute treatment.

76. b (Chapter 37)

Know the differential diagnosis of abdominal pain. Biliary colic is characterized by steady epigastric abdominal pain that is worse after eating and at night. Obese, premenopausal females are at higher risk for gallstone disease. Acute pancreatitis can be precipitated by gallstones, but would not last for 2 months and have a normal abdominal exam. Kidney stones typically manifest as escalating flank pain and would not relate to food. Colon cancer is usually not associated with abdominal pain, and would feature weight loss and possibly a change in stool caliber or rectal bleeding. Viral hepatitis pain also would not relate to food and would be associated with jaundice or chronic liver disease.

77. c (Chapter 41)

Recognize the toxic dose of acetaminophen. When taken in doses of greater than 4 grams a day, acetaminophen can be hepatotoxic. The drug-induced hepatitis associated with acetaminophen typically features liver transaminases over 1,000. Alcoholic hepatitis causes an AST:ALT ratio of 2:1 and is not generally seen in people who consume 2 or less glasses of alcohol daily. The patient's hepatitis B labs are indicative of prior immunization to hepatitis B. Autoimmune hepatitis and metastatic liver disease typically do not present abruptly or with such profound elevations of the liver transaminases.

78. c (Chapter 1)

Know the differential diagnosis of chest pain and how to diagnose pericarditis. Acute pericarditis is often clinically manifested as chest pain relieved by sitting forward with ST segment elevations in all leads on EKG. Pericarditis is often preceded by a viral illness. Myocardial infarctions are seen in patients with cardiac risk factors such as diabetes, hypertension, and tobacco use; the ST elevations reflect the coronary anatomy affected ischemia. Cocaine-induced chest pain is usually associated with hypertension and a history of cocaine use. While the patient does report job stress, anxiety is not associated with EKG changes. Esophageal reflux also is not associated with EKG changes; the chest pain is associated with eating.

79. b (Chapter 8)

Understand the indications for ACE inhibitors. According to the JNC-7 guidelines, in patients with diabetes and hypertension ACE inhibitors are first line therapy for the treatment of hypertension. This also applies to patients with chronic kidney disease. Beta-blockers, alpha-blockers, loop diuretics, and calcium channel blockers are all second-line agents in this case.

80. e (Chapter 28)

Know the appropriate therapy for community-acquired pneumonia (CAP). Given this patient's age, fever, and white count he warrants inpatient admission for pneumonia with IV antibiotics. Standard therapy for CAP is a third generation cephalosporin plus a macrolide, or a respiratory quinolone. Since this patient has a penicillin allergy the quinolone should be chosen. Azithromycin is for use in outpatients with pneumonia. Cefepime and cipro are used for healthcare-associated pneumonia.

81. c (Chapter 29)

Know the clinical syndromes seen in sexually transmitted infections. *Gardnerella vaginalis* causes bacterial vaginosis which commonly features a malodorous, clear, thin discharge with clue cells on wet prep. *Treponema pallidum* causes syphilis, which features painless genital ulcers. *Chlamydia trachomatis, Ureaplasma urealyticum,* and *Neisseria gonorrhoeae* typically cause urethritis.

82. a (Chapter 29)

Know the treatment for bacterial vaginosis. Either oral or intravaginal metronidazole is the treatment of choice for bacterial vaginosis. Doxycycline and ciprofloxacin are treatments for urethritis. Fluconazole is an antifungal used for vulvovaginitis.

83. b (Chapter 59)

Differentiate the seronegative spondyloarthropathies. The clinical features of reactive arthritis are urethritis, conjunctivitis, and arthritis; the syndrome typically occurs after an infection, in this case a likely STI. Enteropathic arthritis is associated with inflammatory bowel disease which the patient is not having symptoms of. Ankylosing spondylitis is more chronic in nature and presents as back pain with limited flexion and extension of the back. Psoriatic arthritis is characterized by scaly lesions on extensor surfaces typical of psoriasis. CMV retinitis is associated with advanced HIV infections and is not typically associated with back pain and arthritis.

84. d (Chapter 47)

Know the clinical features and lab abnormalities of hyperthyroidism. The symptoms of hyperthyroidism include palpitations, anxiety, loose stools, weight loss, tremor, hair loss, heat intolerance, and menstrual irregularity. Clinical signs include hyperreflexia, tremor, and warm skin. Graves disease causes an autoimmune hyperthyroidism and will feature a suppressed TSH and an elevated T4. Alcohol withdrawal, cocaine intoxication, and anxiety will feature palpitations and tremor, but they will not feature hyperreflexia and a suppressed TSH. Hashimoto thyroiditis causes hypothyroidism.

85. a (Chapter 15)

Understand the stepwise treatment of asthma. Patients with moderate persistent asthma (as in this case) need to be on a daily medication for control of their symptoms. Inhaled steroids such as fluticasone are first-line therapy for the chronic airway inflammation from asthma. Beta-agonists such as salmeterol and leukotriene modifiers such as montelukast should be assessed after inhaled steroids. Oral prednisone should not be used chronically in asthma; it is only indicated for acute exacerbations. Tiotropium is an anticholinergic used in COPD.

86. a (Chapter 18)

Apply the Light criteria for pleural effusions. Exudative pleural effusions will have a pleural fluid LDH >200, a fluid to serum protein ratio >0.5, or a fluid to serum LDH ration >0.6. The fluid in this case is transudative. Cirrhosis is the only transudative cause of pleural effusions listed. The other 4 choices would cause exudates. Additionally the patient has several features of chronic liver disease such as ascites and spider angiomata.

87. c (Chapter 39)

Know the causes of peptic ulcer disease. Nonsteroidal anti-inflammatory medications are common precipitants for bleeding ulcers. Naproxen is likely contributing to the patient's GI bleed in this case and should be stopped. Lisinopril and paroxetine are not known to be major causes for GI bleeding; both are needed to treat the patient's chronic health conditions. Metoclopramide is an anti-emetic and is not used in ulcer treatment. Benzodiazepines such as diazepam should be avoided for the long-term treatment of anxiety.

88. d (Chapter 45)

Know the alarm symptoms of colorectal cancer. In patients over 50 with weight loss and anemia, malignancy evaluation is warranted. This patient has the features of iron deficiency anemia, which is due to chronic blood loss from colon cancer. While iron supplementation can treat iron deficiency, the underlying cause of the iron deficiency needs to be evaluated in this case. Erythropoietin is used to treat the anemia of chronic kidney disease. Renal ultrasound is not indicated as there is no sign or symptom of renal dysfunction. Colonoscopy

ANSWERS

is the procedure of choice for colon cancer screening, not CT scan.

89. b (Chapter 40)

Know the typical organ involvement and pathologic features of Crohn disease. The diagnosis of inflammatory bowel disease is made by endoscopic visualization of the GI tract as well as pathology. Crohn disease can involve any segment of the GI tract; in this case it involves the mouth (ulcers) and the colon. Ulcerative colitis involves only the colon. Crohn disease features "skip lesions" on endoscopy while ulcerative colitis features continuous lesions. On pathology, Crohn lesions are granulomatous and involve the entire bowel wall. Tuberculosis and sarcoidosis rarely involve only the intestines. Irritable bowel syndrome is a clinical spectrum as defined by the ROME criteria and would not have abnormal endoscopic changes.

90. d (Chapter 14)

Understand how to make a definitive diagnosis of COPD. According to the Global Initiative for Chronic Obstructive Lung Disease, spirometry is required to establish a diagnosis of COPD. Spirometry provides lung volume and flow rates to quantify the extent of lung obstruction. Stress testing and echocardiogram is used to evaluate cardiac function and exercise capacity. Polysomnogram is used to diagnose sleep apnea. CT scan of the chest may show changes consistent with emphysema, but it does not establish the diagnosis like spirometry does.

91. e (Chapter 2)

Recognize that expected time for reperfusion in a myocardial infarction is 90 minutes or less. Options for reperfusion include thrombolytics or primary percutaneous intervention (PCI). In this case thrombolysis is the treatment of choice to open the artery since it would take the patient more than 90 minutes to get to a facility that offers PCI. There is no indication for amiodarone or warfarin in the setting of an acute MI.

92. c (Chapter 7)

Understand that patients with atrial fibrillation are at an elevated risk for embolic stroke. Risk factors for embolic stroke in atrial fibrillation include: congestive heart failure, hypertension, age greater than 75, diabetes, and prior stroke. Warfarin is indicated in any patient with atrial fibrillation with more than one of these risk factors. In this case the patient has hypertension, advanced age, and prior stroke. Aspirin can also be used to prevent stroke in atrial fibrillation, but it does not provide as significant a risk reduction. Amiodarone is used as an antiarrhythmic in atrial fibrillation, not to prevent stroke. Diltiazem is used for heart rate control in atrial fibrillation, not to prevent stroke. Clopidogrel has not been proven to prevent stroke in atrial fibrillation.

93. c (Chapter 5)

Know the clinical and radiographic features of congestive heart failure. Congestive heart failure signs and symptoms are typically due to pulmonary vascular congestion. One of the most common causes of heart failure is prior ischemic heart disease. Radiography usually shows alveolar infiltrates with a "bat wing" pattern, cephalization of pulmonary venous fluid, cardiomegaly, and peribronchial cuffing. Chest films in sarcoidosis typically do not show cardiomegaly, and more commonly feature perihilar lymphadenopathy. COPD will feature flattened diaphragms and increased anterior, posterior diameter. Pneumonia will feature lobar consolidations in a patient with sudden onset dyspnea and fevers. Metastatic lung cancer will feature lung masses and lymphadenopathy.

94. b (Chapter 5)

Know the medications that provide a mortality benefit in heart failure versus medications for symptom control. The RALES trial established that aldosterone antagonists provide a mortality benefit to patients with New York Heart Association (NYHA) Class III and Class IV heart failure. ACE inhibitors and beta-blockers provide a mortality benefit as well. Furosemide and digoxin provide symptom relief and decreased hospitalization, but no mortality benefit. Amlodipine is a calcium channel blocker used to treat hypertension.

95. c (Chapter 5)

Understand that defibrillators reduce mortality for patients with ventricular tachycardia and advanced CHF. Automatic implantable cardiac defibrillators (AICDs) reduce mortality for patients with heart failure who have an ejection fraction <35% (MADIT II trial) as well as patients with CHF who experience ventricular arrhythmias. In this case the patient meets both criteria and should be considered for an implantable defibrillator. Holter monitors are used in patients who have symptomatic arrhythmias. There is no evidence that suppressing arrhythmia with amiodardone would improve mortality. Stress testing can provide information on the patient's cardiac function, but would not improve mortality. Dobutamine is used in heart failure to improve hemodynamics, but does not prolong life.

96. c (Chapter 56)

Know the indications to image in back pain. Patients over the age of 50 and with weight loss should have a lumbar spine film when they present with low back pain. NSAIDs and a warm compress are treatments for low back pain only if the case is nonworrisome. MRI of the brain would be indicated if this patient had stroke symptoms, while electromyogram (EMG) would be indicated for isolated neurologic symptoms.

97. b (Chapter 44)

Apply Ranson's criteria. Ranson's criteria are WBC, LDH, SGOT/AST, and glucose. These parameters are used to predict mortality in cases of pancreatitis. Amylase, lipase, and liver function tests are useful in the diagnosis of pancreatitis, but they do not predict mortality. CT scan of the abdomen is indicated in acute pancreatitis to rule out pancreatic pseudocyst, but does not predict mortality directly.

98. b (Chapter 14)

Know the role of oxygen therapy in COPD. In patients with hypoxemia (Pao_2 <60 mm Hg), supplemental oxygen therapy has been shown to prolong survival. Theophylline, steroids, and beta agonists are used in the treatment of COPD symptoms, however they do not provide a mortality benefit.

99. a (Chapter 28)

Understand triage criteria for patients with pneumonia. Patients with advanced age, numerous co-morbidities, altered mental status, fever, hypotension, and tachycardia can have mortality rates of up to 30% from pneumonia. This warrants intensive care unit (ICU) admission for IV antibiotics. Since the patient resides in a nursing home he needs to be treated for healthcare-associated pneumonia with IV antibiotics. Sending the patient home would not be advised given his high mortality. Dementia is not an indication not to treat the pneumonia unless the patient has a documented treatment limitation. There is no evidence of that in this case.

100. e (Chapter 30)

Recognize a complicated urinary tract infection. The major risks for development of a urinary tract infection in a male are urinary tract abnormalities or prior procedures on the urinary tract. Any urinary tract infection (UTI) in a male is defined as complicated and warrants a longer course of antibiotics; in men 10 to 14 days is indicated. Quinolones and trimethoprim-sulfamethoxazole are the therapies of choice for urinary tract infections as most are caused by aerobic gram-negative bacteria.

ANSWERS

Index

Page numbers followed by *f* refer to illustrations; page numbers followed by *t* refer to tables.